Diagnostic Atlas of
Common Eyelid Diseases

Diagnostic Atlas of
Common Eyelid Diseases

Jonathan J. Dutton
University of North Carolina–Chapel Hill
Chapel Hill, North Carolina, USA

Gregg S. Gayre
Kaiser Permanente Medical Group
San Rafael, California, USA

Alan D. Proia
Duke University Medical Center
Durham, North Carolina, USA

informa
healthcare

New York   London

Informa Healthcare USA, Inc.
52 Vanderbilt Avenue
New York, NY 10017

© 2007 by Informa Healthcare USA, Inc.
Informa Healthcare is an Informa business

No claim to original U.S. Government works
Printed in the United States of America on acid-free paper
10 9 8 7 6 5 4 3 2 1

International Standard Book Number-10: 0-8247-2839-4 (Hardcover)
International Standard Book Number-13: 978-0-8247-2839-7 (Hardcover)

Library of Congress Cataloging-in-Publication Data

Dutton, Jonathan J.
   Diagnostic atlas of common eyelid diseases/Jonathan J. Dutton,
Gregg S. Gayre, Alan D. Proia.
      p. ; cm.
   Includes bibliographical references and index.
   ISBN-13: 978-0-8247-2839-7 (hardcover : alk. paper)
   ISBN-10: 0-8247-2839-4 (hardcover : alk. paper)
   1. Eyelids--Diseases--Atlases. I. Gayre, Gregg S. II. Proia, Alan D.
III. Title.
   [DNLM: 1. Eyelid Neoplasms--diagnosis--Atlases. 2. Eyelid
Neoplasms--diagnosis--Handbooks. 3. Eyelid Diseases--diagnosis--
Atlases. 4. Eyelid Diseases--diagnosis--Handbooks. 5. Eyelid Diseases--
therapy--Atlases. 6. Eyelid Diseases--therapy--Handbooks. 7. Eyelid
Neoplasms--therapy--Atlases. 8. Eyelid Neoplasms--therapy--Handbooks.
WW 17 D981da 2007]
   RE121.D88 2007
   617.7'71--dc22   2007005810

Visit the Informa Web site at
www.informa.com

and the Informa Healthcare Web site at
www.informahealthcare.com

Preface

For any clinician dealing with ophthalmic diseases, individual lesions of the eyelid and conjunctiva can be extremely confusing. From a practical perspective such lesions are either benign or malignant, and can be cystic or solid, melanotic or amelanotic. Certainly the most important diagnostic question is whether the lesion represents a malignant tumor that requires biopsy and more definitive treatment. Often, following biopsy, the histopathologic diagnosis is difficult to interpret since most are histologically based on specific tissue cells of origin. The question arises, of course, as to the clinical relevance of the diagnosis. For the majority of benign lesions the treatment will be the same; that is, observation or, if of cosmetic or functional significance, surgical excision. Some lesions may be amenable to ancillary therapy such as steroid injection, cryotherapy, laser ablation, or radiotherapy.

Malignant tumors of the eyelid present a special category of concern. Some, like the basal cell carcinoma, rarely metastasize, but can be locally aggressive; when small they are less of an immediate threat. Others, such as sebaceous cell carcinoma and malignant melanoma, have a metastatic potential that requires more immediate and aggressive intervention. A high index of suspicion and a low threshold for biopsy will lead to a correct diagnosis much of the time.

In the pages that follow we present the current state of our knowledge on a number of eyelid diseases with which all ophthalmic clinicians should be familiar. Several introductory chapters discuss eyelid anatomy, examination, evaluation and decision making, and biopsy and reconstructive techniques. The main body of the atlas is divided into two sections, eyelid malpositions and eyelid lesions. In Chapter 7: Eyelid Malpositions, we discuss congenital and acquired dystopias of the eyelids, such as ptosis, ectropion, epicanthus, and lagophthalmos. In Chapter 8: Eyelid Lesions, we present conditions such as seborrheic keratosis, basal cell carcinoma, and hemangioma.

The concept of this book grew out of the need for a quick and easy-to-use reference to specific clinical and histopathologic information on common eyelid malpositions and diseases. For each condition we give an introduction, clinical presentation, and treatment, with appropriate illustrations. For eyelid lesions, we also include histopathology and differential diagnosis. Available information has been condensed into minimal text without cited references. Within each section, diseases are arranged alphabetically to make it easier to find specific entries. The reader will find the same information, such as clinical presentation or histopathology, in the same sequence for every disease. At the end of each disease entry we include selected references with no attempt at presenting a comprehensive literature review.

Jonathan J. Dutton
Gregg S. Gayre
Alan D. Proia

Acknowledgments

The authors are grateful to the following colleagues for kindly allowing us to use clinical photographs for this volume.

Richard L. Anderson, M.D.	Melanocytic nevus; Microblepharon; Plexiform neurofibroma; Squamous cell carcinoma
Seymour Brownstein, M.D.	Mucoepidermoid carcinoma
Arthur Chandler, M.D.	Metastatic tumor
Kenneth Cohen, M.D.	Herpes simplex
Robert Dryden, M.D. and Brett Koltus, M.D.	Rosacea; Trichoepithelioma
Tamara Fountain, M.D.	Intravascular papillary endothelial hyperplasia
Grant Gilliland, M.D.	Necrotizing fasciitis
Robert A. Goldberg, M.D.	Actinic keratosis; Angiosarcoma; Blue nevus; Dermtofibroma; Ectopic dermatitis; Epidermoid cyst; Erythema multiforme; Hemangiopericytoma; Herpes simplex; Lupus erythematosus; Merkel cell carcinoma; Pyogenic granuloma; Syringoma; Xanthogranuloma
Morris Hartstein, M.D.	Juvenile xanthogranuloma; Rosacea; Trichoepithelioma
John Holds, M.D.	Necrotizing fasciitis
Gordon K. Klintworth, M.D., Ph.D.	Nodular fasciitis; Pemphigus vulgaris
David Lyon, M.D.	Juvenile xanthogranuloma
Bettina Meekins, M.D.	Eccrine nodular hidradenoma
Richard B. O'Grady, M.D.	Primary mucinous carcinoma
Jay J. Older, M.D.	Chondroid syringoma
Henry D. Perry, M.D.	Plasmacytoma
Peter Rubin, M.D.	Pilomatrixoma
Stefan Seregard, M.D.	Phakomatous choristoma
Richard S. Smith, M.D., D. Med. Sc.	Kaposi's sarcoma
Charles S. Soparkar, M.D.	Cicatricial pemphigoid; Epidermoid cyst; Erythema multiforme; Insect bite; Leukemia cutis; Lupus erythematosis; Mucoepidermoid carcinoma; Papilloma

Contents

Chapter 1

Anatomy of the Eyelids

INTRODUCTION

The eyelids serve several valuable functions. Most importantly they provide mechanical protection to the globe. They also provide vital chemical elements to the precorneal tear film, and help distribute these layers evenly over the surface of the eye. During the blink phase the eyelids propel tears to the medial canthus where they enter the puncta of the lacrimal drainage system. The eyelashes along the lid margins sweep air-borne particles from in front of the eye, and the constant voluntary and reflex movements of the eyelids protect the cornea from injury and glare.

In the young adult the interpalpebral fissure measures 10 to 11 mm in vertical height. In middle age this is reduced to only about 8 to 10 mm (1) and in old age the fissure may be only 6–8 mm or less. The horizontal length of the fissure is 30 to 31 mm. The upper and lower eyelids meet at an angle of approximately 60 degrees medially and laterally. In primary position of gaze the upper eyelid margin lies at the superior corneal limbus in children and 1.5 to 2.0 mm below it in the adult. The lower eyelid margin usually rests at the inferior corneal limbus or just slightly above it.

The margin of each eyelid is about 2 mm thick. Posteriorly the marginal tarsal surface is covered with conjunctival epithelium, interrupted by the meibomian gland orifices (Fig. 1). Anteriorly the margin is covered with cutaneous epidermis from which emerge the eyelashes. The gray line is a faint linear zone separating these two regions. Between the skin and conjunctiva at a level 5 mm above the tarsus are, layered from front to back, the orbicularis muscle, the orbital septum, the preaponeurotic fat pockets, the levator aponeurosis, and Müller's supratarsal muscle.

EYELID SKIN

The skin covers the external surface of the body and provides significant protection against trauma, solar radiation, temperature extremes, and desiccation. It also allows for major interaction with the environment. The skin of the eyelid is the thinnest in the body owing to only a scant development of the dermis and subcutaneous fat.

The epidermis is the outer layer of the skin averaging about 0.05 mm in thickness on the eyelids, compared to the palms and soles where it can attain a thickness of 1.5 mm. It contains no blood vessels and is dependent upon the underlying dermis for its nutrients (Fig. 2). There are four layers to the epidermis consisting of keratinocytes layered from deepest to most superficial in progressive stages of differentiation. These keratinocyte cells proliferate and push more formed cells upward into successively higher layers. As they move upward the keratinocytes produce a fibrous protein, called keratin. Bundles of tonofilaments help distribute stress enabling the epidermis to withstand a fair amount of surface abuse. The layers of the epidermis are from top to bottom:

- Stratum corneum
- Stratum granulosum
- Stratum spinosum
- Stratum basale

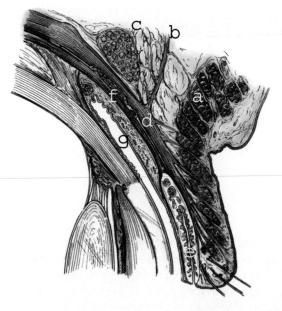

Figure 1 Sagittal cross-section of the upper eyelid. **a.** Orbicularis muscle; **b.** orbital septum; **c.** preaponeurotic fat pad; **d.** levator aponeurosis; **e.** tarsal plate; **f.** Muller's supratarsal muscle; **g.** conjunctiva.

At the base of the sequence is the stratum basale (= basalis) containing cuboidal or columnar cells arranged in a single row and containing large nuclei (Fig. 3). The basal layer of columnar cells with mitotic figures serves for keratinocytic proliferation and was formerly referred to as the stratum germinativum. Together, the strata basale and germinativum are called the basal cells. The stratum spinosum is the next higher layer and is composed of polygonal cells which form spines when they shrink during histologic preparation because of the presence of desmosomes between adjacent cells. The cytoplasm is filled with tonofilaments and phospholipids. The stratum granulosum is 3 to 5 cells thick; these cells contain keratohyalin granules rich in histidine and precursors of the protein filaggrin that promotes keratin filament aggregation. Toward the top of this layer the cells lose their nucleus and become more flattened. Changes in enzyme function cause cell death as the cells enter the upper-most layer, the stratum corneum. This layer is made of dead, flattened keratinocytes that shed about every few weeks in a process known as desquamation. This layer provides a waterproof covering that also resists minor abrasions. In thicker skin such as the palms and soles a layer called the stratum lucidum is found between the granular and cornified strata; this appears as a clear homogeneous amorphous zone.

The epidermis also contains several specialized types of cells. Melanocytes of neural crest origin are scattered among the keratinocytes in the stratum basale and the deeper layers of the stratum spinosum. They are pale cells which produce long processes that extend between the keratinocytes, and produce melanin which is stored in granules called melanosomes. These

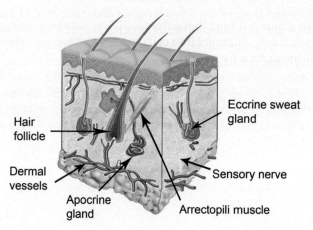

Hair follicle

Dermal vessels

Apocrine gland

Arrectopili muscle

Eccrine sweat gland

Sensory nerve

Figure 2 Anatomic section of eyelid skin showing major dermal adnexal structures.

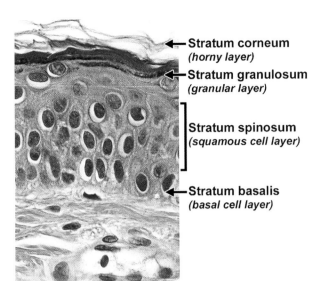

Figure 3 Histologic section of eyelid skin showing the four layers of the epidermis, and the dermis.

are ultimately transferred to the keratinocytes where they accumulate on the sun-exposed side of the nucleus to protect it from UV radiation. Langerhans cells, or epidermal dendritic cells, are macrophages that originate in the bone marrow and migrate to the epidermis. They are present in all epidermal layers, but are concentrated in the stratum spinosum. They serve as antigen-presenting cells that ingest and process foreign antigens and present them to lymphocytes for activation of the immune system. The function of the Merkel cell is not completely understood. They are derived from neural crest cells and are attached to keratinocytes by desmosomes. They are found throughout the epidermis but are particularly abundant in the basal layer. Merkel cells are associated with nonmyelinated nerve endings with which they form the Merkel disc which may act as a mechanosensory receptor for light touch.

Beneath the epidermis is the basement membrane and below that the dermis. The stratum basale is connected to the basement membrane by protein fibers. On the dermal side anchoring fibers of collagen tether the dermis to the basement membrane. The basal membrane is irregular and epidermal extensions project into the dermis to form a system of rete ridges. These are more prominent in areas where the skin undergoes shearing stress.

The dermis lies beneath the basement membrane and on the eyelids is about 0.3 mm in thickness compared to other parts of the body where it may be up to 3 mm thick. It contains three types of tissues that are not layered: collagen, elastic tissue, and reticular fibers. The upper papillary dermal layer contains a thin arrangement of collagen fibers. The lower reticular dermal layer is thicker and contains thick collagen fibers arranged parallel to the surface. The reticular layer also contains fibroblasts, mast cells, nerve endings, lymphatics, and epidermal appendages surrounded by a ground substance of mucopolysaccharides, chondroitin sulfates, and glycoproteins.

The fibroblast is the major cell type in the dermis. These secrete elastin and a procollagen that is then cleaved by proteolytic enzymes into collagen which becomes cross-linked. Collagen makes up nearly 70% of the dermis by weight.

A number of epidermal appendages lined with epithelium lie within the dermis. These include hair follicles associated with an arrectopili muscle attached to the dermal-epidermal junction. Apocrine sweat glands of Moll are coiled glands in the deep dermis that empty via a long ductule into the uppermost portion of the hair follicle. Apocrine glands secrete by cellular decapitation with the apical portion of the secretory cell mixed with sialomucin producing a more viscous secretion with cellular debris. They are concentrated along the eyelid margins.

Sebaceous glands contain epithelium that is an outgrowth of the external root sheath of the hair follicle. These are holocrine glands that shed the entire epithelial cell along with secretory products of complex oils, fatty acids, wax, and cholesterol esters called sebum. A large sebaceous gland is associated with each hair follicle and empties its secretions directly into

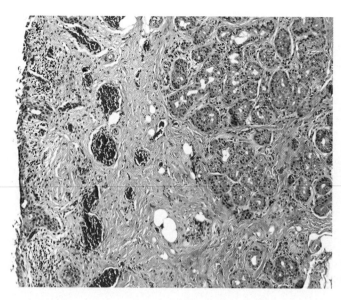

Figure 4 Histologic section of the conjunctiva with numerous glands of Wolfring.

the follicle. The hair follicle along with the sebaceous and Moll glands form the pilosebaceous unit. Additional small sebaceous glands called glands of Zeis are present between follicles and discharge their contents directly onto the skin surface. Eccrine sweat glands are also present in the dermis but they are not associated with the hair follicle. They open directly onto the epidermal surface via a long straight ductule. Eccrine glands secrete a clear fluid composed of water, salts, glycogen, and sialomucin.

Blood vessels and nerve endings course throughout the dermis where they derive from similar structures in the sub-dermis and deep fascia. Specialized sensory structures called Meissner's and Vater-Pacini corpuscles within the dermis transmit sensations for touch and pressure.

Beneath the dermis is a subcutaneous layer of fat and connective tissue. Subcutaneous fat is very sparse beneath the preseptal portion of the eyelid skin, and absent from the more distal pretarsal portions. Beneath the skin within the eyelid are also found other structures that can be the focus for disease processes. On the subconjunctival side of the eyelid these accessory structures include the accessory lacrimal glands of Krause and Wolfring beneath the conjunctiva and are concentrated on the lateral side (Fig. 4), and the meibomian glands which are modified sebaceous glands within the tarsal plates (Fig. 1).

THE ORBICULARIS MUSCLE

The orbicularis oculi is a complex striated muscle that lies just below the skin. It is divided anatomically into three contiguous parts—the orbital, preseptal, and pretarsal portions (Fig. 5). The orbital portion overlies the bony orbital rims. It arises from insertions on the frontal process of the maxillary bone, the orbital process of the frontal bone, and from the common medial canthal tendon. Its fibers pass around the orbital rim to form a continuous ellipse without interruption at the lateral palpebral commissure, and insert just below their points of origin.

The palpebral portion of the orbicularis muscle overlies the mobile eyelid from the orbital rims to the eyelid margins. The muscle fibers sweep circumferentially around each lid as a half ellipse, fixed medially and laterally at the canthal tendons. Although this portion forms a single anatomic unit in each eyelid, it is customarily further divided topographically into two parts, the preseptal and pretarsal orbicularis.

The preseptal portion of the muscle is positioned over the orbital septum in both upper and lower eyelids, and its fibers originate perpendicularly along the upper and lower borders of the medial canthal tendon. Fibers arc around the eyelids and insert along the lateral horizontal raphé. The pretarsal portion of the muscle overlies the tarsal plates. Its fibers originate from the medial canthal tendon via separate superficial and deep heads, arch around the lids and

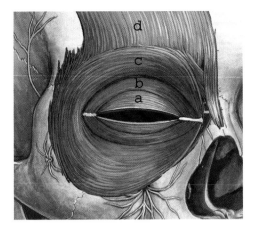
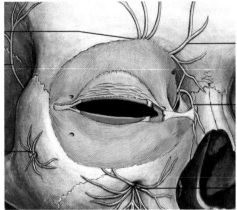

Figure 5 Orbicularis and frontalis muscles.
a. Pretarsal portion; **b.** preseptal portion;
c. orbital portion; **d.** frontalis muscle.

Figure 6 The orbital septum originating
from the arcus marginalis of the orbital rim.

insert onto the lateral canthal tendon and raphé. Contraction of these fibers aids in the lacrimal pump mechanism (2). Medially the deep heads of the pretarsal fibers fuse to form a prominent bundle of fibers, Horner's muscle, that runs just behind the posterior limb of the canthal tendon. It inserts onto the posterior lacrimal crest. Horner's muscle helps maintain the posterior position of the canthal angle, tightens the eyelids against the globe during eyelid closure, and may aid in the lacrimal pump mechanism (3).

THE ORBITAL SEPTUM

The orbital septum is a thin fibrous multilayered membrane anatomically beginning at the arcus marginalis along the orbital rim and represents a continuation of the orbital fascial system. Distal fibers of the orbital septum merge into the anterior surface of the levator aponeurosis (Fig. 6) (4,5). The point of insertion is usually about 3 to 5 mm above the tarsal plate, but may be as much as 10 to 15 mm (6). In the lower eyelid the septum fuses with the capsulopalpebral fascia several millimeters below the tarsus, and the common fascial sheet inserts onto the inferior tarsal edge (7,8).

The septum can always be identified at surgery by pulling it distally and noting firm resistance against its bony attachments. Immediately behind the septum are yellow fat pockets that lie immediately anterior to the levator aponeurosis in the upper lid and the capsulopalpebral fascia in the lower lid. This anatomic relationship is important to note since identification of the levator aponeurosis or capsulopalpebral is critical in many eyelid surgical procedures.

THE PREAPONEUROTIC FAT POCKETS

The preaponeurotic fat pockets in the upper eyelid and the pre-capsulopalpebral fat pockets in the lower eyelid are anterior extensions of extraconal orbital fat. These eyelid fat pockets are surgically important landmarks and help identify a plane immediately anterior to the major eyelid retractors. In the upper eyelid there are typically two fat pockets, a medial pocket, and a central one. Laterally, the lacrimal gland may be mistaken for a third fat pocket. In the lower eyelid there are three pockets, medial, central, and lateral.

THE MAJOR EYELID RETRACTORS

The retractors of the upper eyelid consist of the levator palpebrae and Müller's muscles. The levator palpebrae superioris muscle arises from the lesser sphenoid wing just above the

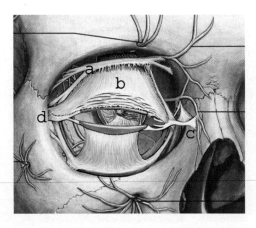

Figure 7 Anterior orbital fascial system. **a.** Whitnall's ligament; **b.** levator aponeurosis; **c.** medial canthal tendon; **d.** lateral canthal tendon.

annulus of Zinn. The muscle runs forward in the superior orbit just above the superior rectus muscle. Near the superior orbital rim a condensation is seen along the muscle sheath (9), that attaches medially and laterally to the orbital walls and soft tissues. This is the superior transverse orbital ligament of Whitnall. Its exact role remains a matter of controversy, but it appears to provide some support for the fascial system that maintains spatial relationships between a variety of anatomic structures in the superior orbit.

From Whitnall's ligament the muscle passes into its aponeurosis (Fig. 7). This sheet continues downward 14 to 20 mm to its insertion near the marginal tarsal border. The aponeurotic fibers are most firmly attached at about 3 to 4 mm above the eyelid margin (10,11). Beginning near the upper edge of tarsus, the aponeurosis also sends numerous delicate interconnecting slips forward and downward to insert onto the interfascicular septa of the pretarsal orbicularis muscle and subcutaneous tissue. These multilayered slips maintain the close approximation of the skin, muscle, aponeurosis, and tarsal lamellae, thus integrating the distal eyelid as a single functional unit. This relationship defines the upper eyelid crease of the western eyelid.

As the levator aponeurosis passes into the eyelid from Whitnall's ligament it broadens to form the medial and lateral "horns." The lateral horn forms a prominent fibrous sheet that indents the posterior aspect of the lacrimal gland, defining its orbital and palpebral lobes. It inserts through numerous slips onto the lateral orbital tubercle of the zygomatic bone, at the lateral retinaculum. The medial horn is less well developed. It blends with the intermediate layer of the orbital septum and inserts onto the posterior crus of the medial canthal tendon and the posterior lacrimal crest. Together, the two horns serve to distribute the forces of the levator muscle along the aponeurosis and the tarsal plate.

In the lower eyelid the capsulopalpebral fascia is a fibrous sheet arising from Lockwood's ligament and the sheaths around the inferior rectus and inferior oblique muscles. It passes upward and generally fuses with fibers of the orbital septum about 4 to 5 mm below the tarsal plate. From this junction a common fascial sheet continues upward and inserts onto the lower border of tarsus. Fine fibrous slips pass forward from this fascial sheet to the orbicularis intermuscular septae and subcutaneous tissue, forming the lower eyelid crease and uniting the anterior and posterior lamellae into a single functional unit.

THE SYMPATHETIC EYELID RETRACTORS

Smooth muscles innervated by the sympathetic nervous system are present in both upper and lower eyelid and serve as accessory retractors (12). In the upper eyelid, the supratarsal muscle of Müller originates abruptly from the under surface of the levator muscle just anterior to Whitnall's ligament (13). It runs downward, posterior to the levator aponeurosis to which it is adherent and inserts onto the anterior edge of the superior tarsal border. In the lower eyelid, the sympathetic muscle is less well defined. Fibers run behind the capsulopalpebral fascia to insert onto the lower border of tarsus, although they may end 2 to 5 mm below tarsus (14).

Disruption of sympathetic innervation to these muscles results in Horner's syndrome. This is characterized by the classic triad of ptosis, miosis, and ipsilateral anhidrosis of the face. Specific clinical findings vary according to the location of the lesion along the polysynaptic pathway. The upper eyelid ptosis and elevation of the lower eyelid result from loss of sympathetic smooth muscle tone and accessory retraction.

THE TARSAL PLATES

The tarsal plates consist of dense fibrous tissue approximately 1 to 1.5 mm thick that give structural integrity to the eyelids. Each measures about 25 mm in horizontal length, and is gently curved to conform to the contour of the anterior globe. The central vertical height of the tarsal plate is 8 to 12 mm in the upper eyelid and 3.5 to 4.0 mm in the lower. Medially and laterally they taper to 2 mm in height as they pass into the canthal tendons. As these tarsal plates approach the canthal tendons, they broaden slightly toward the margin and narrow toward the proximal surface, thus assuming a more triangular cross-section. Within each tarsus are the Meibomian glands, approximately 25 in the upper lid and 20 in the lower lid. These are holocrine-secreting sebaceous glands not associated with lash follicles. Each gland is multilobulated and empties into a central ductule that opens onto the posterior eyelid margin behind the gray line. They produce the lipid layer of the precorneal tear film.

THE CANTHAL TENDONS

Medially the tarsal plates pass into fibrous bands that form the crura of the medial canthal tendon. These lie between the orbicularis muscle anteriorly and the conjunctiva posteriorly. The superior and inferior crura fuse to form a stout common tendon that inserts via three limbs (Fig. 7) (2). The anterior limb inserts onto the orbital process of the maxillary bone in front of and above the anterior lacrimal crest. It provides the major support for the medial canthal angle. The posterior limb arises from the common tendon near the junction of the superior and inferior crura, and passes between the canaliculi. It inserts onto the posterior lacrimal crest just in front of Horner's muscle. The posterior limb directs the vector forces of the canthal angle backward to maintain close approximation with the globe. The superior limb of the medial canthal tendon arises as a broad arc of fibers from both the anterior and posterior limbs. It passes upward to insert onto the orbital process of the frontal bone. The posterior head of the preseptal orbicularis muscle inserts onto this limb and the unit forms the soft-tissue roof of the lacrimal sac fossa. This tendinous extension may function to provide vertical support to the canthal angle (15), but also appears to play a significant role in the lacrimal pump mechanism.

Laterally the tarsal plates pass into fibrous strands that become the crura of the lateral canthal tendon. The lateral canthal tendon is a distinct entity separate from the orbicularis muscle. It measure about 1 mm in thickness, 3 mm in width, and approximately 5 to 7 mm in length (16). Insertion of these fibers extends posteriorly along the lateral orbital wall where it blends with strands of the lateral check ligament from the sheath of the lateral rectus muscle.

THE CONJUNCTIVA

The conjunctiva is a mucous membrane that covers the posterior surface of the eyelids and the anterior surface of the globe except for the cornea. The palpebral portion is closely applied to the posterior surface of the tarsal plate and the sympathetic tarsal muscle of Müller. It is continuous around the fornices above and below where it joins the bulbar conjunctiva. Small accessory lacrimal glands are located within the submucosal connective tissue.

At the medial canthal angle is a small mound of tissue called the caruncle. This consists of modified skin containing hairs, sebaceous glands, and sweat glands. Just lateral to the caruncle there is a vertical fold of conjunctiva, the plica semilunaris. The submucosa of this tissue contains adipose cells and smooth muscle fibers resembling the nictitating membrane of lower vertebrates. This likely represents a vestigial structure that has been modified to allow enough horizontal slack at the shallow medial fornix for rotation of the globe.

NERVES TO THE EYELIDS

The motor nerves to the orbicularis muscle derive from the facial nerve (N. VII) through its temporal and zygomatic branches (Fig. 8). The facial nerve divides into two divisions, an upper temporofacial division and a lower cervicofacial division (17). The upper division further subdivides into the temporal and zygomatic branches that innervate the frontalis and orbicularis muscles. The lower cervicofacial division gives rise to the buccal, mandibular, and cervical branches innervating muscles of the lower face and neck. There can be considerable variation in the branching pattern of these nerves, and in some individuals extensive anastomoses interconnect all these peripheral branches.

The sensory nerves to the eyelids derive from the ophthalmic and maxillary divisions of the trigeminal nerve. Sensory input from the upper lid passes to the ophthalmic division through its main terminal branches, the supraorbital, supratrochlear, and lacrimal nerves. The infratrochlear nerve receives sensory information from the extreme medial portion of both upper and lower eyelids. The zygomaticotemporal branch of the lacrimal nerve innervates the lateral portion of the upper eyelid and temple. These branches also innervate portions of the adjacent brow, forehead, and nasal bridge. The lower eyelid sends sensory impulses to the maxillary division via the infraorbital nerve. The zygomaticofacial branch from the lacrimal nerve innervates the lateral portion of the lower lid and part of the infratrochlear branch receives input from the medial lower lid.

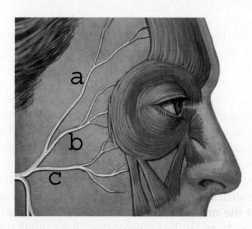

Figure 8 Motor branches of the seventh cranial nerve to the eyelid and brow muscles. **a.** Frontal branch; **b.** zygomatic branch; **c.** buccal branch.

VASCULAR SUPPLY TO THE EYELIDS

Vascular supply to the eyelids is extensive. The posterior eyelid lamellae receive blood through the palpebral arterial arcades (Fig. 9). In the upper eyelid a marginal arcade runs about 2 mm from the eyelid margin and a peripheral arcade extends along the upper border of tarsus between the levator aponeurosis and Müller's muscle. These vessels are supplied medially by the superior medial palpebral vessels from the terminal ophthalmic artery, and laterally by the superior lateral palpebral vessel from the lacrimal artery. The lower lid arcade receives blood from the medial and lateral inferior palpebral vessels.

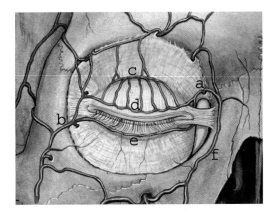

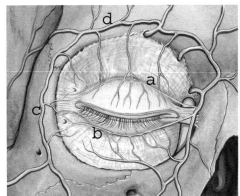

Figure 9 Arterial supply to the eyelids.
a. Medial palpebral artery; **b.** lateral palpebral
artery; **c.** superior peripheral arcade; **d.** superior
marginal arcade; **e.** inferior marginal arcade;
f. angular artery.

Figure 10 Venous supply from the eyelids.
a. Superior venous arcade; **b.** inferior venous
arcade; **c.** transverse facial vein; **d.** superior
palpebral vein.

The venous drainage system is somewhat less well defined than the arterial system. Drainage is primarily into several large vessels of the facial system (Fig. 10). Lymphatic drainage from the eyelids is restricted to the region anterior to the orbital septum. Drainage from the lateral two-thirds of the upper eyelid and the lateral one-third of the lower eyelid is inferior and lateral into the deep and superficial parotid and submandibular nodes. Drainage from the medial one-third of the upper eyelid and the medial two-thirds of the lower eyelid is medially and inferiorly into the anterior cervical nodes. Extensive excision of subcutaneous eyelid tissues or deep incisions in the inferolateral eyelid or in the deep fornix area can result in lymphedema due to disruption of these vessels.

THE EYEBROWS AND FOREHEAD

The eyebrows lie at the junction between the upper eyelid and the forehead. They consist of thickened skin overlying the supraorbital torus and support short, course hairs that emerge from the skin surface at an oblique angle. The complex movements of the brows is provided by the interdigitation of five striated muscles which insert partially along the brow: the frontalis, procerus, depressior supercilii, corrugator, and orbicularis muscles (Fig. 11). All are innervated by the seventh cranial nerve.

The frontalis muscle fibers are oriented vertically on the forehead. They begin superiorly at about the level of the coronal suture line and extend toward the supraorbital rim. The galea aponeurotica splits into a thin superficial portion overlying the frontalis muscle, and a deep thicker layer that extends beneath the muscle to insert onto the supraorbital rim at the arcus marginalis. Beneath the muscle a deep fat layer separates the frontalis muscle from the underlying deep fascia along the orbital rim. This sub-brow fat pad may continue into the upper eyelid where is can be confused with the preaponeurotic fat pockets. It is responsible for the thick full upper lids seen in some patients.

The procerus muscle is a small rectangular muscle that arises by tendinous fibers from the fascia covering the lower portion of the nasal bone. It passes vertically between the brows to insert on skin over the lower forehead. Contraction draws the medial angle of the brows downward and produces transverse wrinkles over the nasal bridge. The depressor supercilii is a narrow band of fibers just lateral to the procerus. It serves to depress the medial brow. The corrugator muscle forms a coarse pyramidal band of fibers beneath the main portion of the frontalis muscle complex and just lateral to the depressor supercilii. It arises from the medial

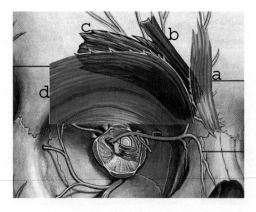

Figure 11 Muscles of the brow. **a.** Procerus muscle; **b.** depressor supercilii muscle; **c.** corrugator muscle; **d.** orbicularis muscle.

end of the frontal bone at the superomedial orbital rim and passes obliquely, superiorly, and laterally where it inserts into the deep fascia of the frontalis muscle along the medial one-third of the brow by two heads, the oblique and the transverse heads.

REFERENCES

1. Hrecko T, Farkas LG, Katic M. Clinical significance of age-related changes in the palpebral fissure between ages 2 and 18 in healthy Caucasians. Acta Chir Plast 1968; 32:194–204.
2. Dutton JJ. Atlas of Clinical and Surgical Orbital Anatomy. Philadelphia: W.B. Saunders, 1994.
3. Ahl NC, Hill JC. Horner's muscle and the lacrimal system. Arch Ophthalmol 1982; 100:488–493.
4. Barker DE. Dye injection studies of orbital fat compartments. Plast Reconstr Surg 1977; 59:82–85.
5. Putterman AM, Urist MJ. Surgical anatomy of the orbital septum. Ann Ophthalmol 1974; 6:290–294.
6. Anderson RL, Dixon RS. The role of Whitnall's ligament in ptosis surgery. Arch Ophthalmol 1979; 97:705–707.
7. Harvey JT, Anderson RL. The aponeurotic approach to eyelid retraction. Ophthalmology 1981; 88:513–524.
8. Meyer DR, Linberg JV, Wobig JL, McCormick S. Anatomy of the orbital septum and associated eyelid connective tissue. Ophthal Plast Reconstr Surg 1991; 7:104–113.
9. Lemke BN, Stasior OG, Rosenberg PN. The surgical relations of the levator palpebrae superioris muscle. Ophthal Plast Reconstr Surg 1988; 4:25–30.
10. Anderson RL, Beard C. The levator aponeurosis. Attachments and their clinical significance. Arch Ophthalmol 1977; 95:1437–1441.
11. Collin JRO, Beard C, Wood I. Experimental and clinical data on the insertion of the levator palpebrae superioris muscle. Am J Ophthalmol 1978; 85:792–801.
12. Manson PN, Lazarus RB, Morgan R, Iliff N. Pathways of sympathetic innervation to the superior and inferior (Müllers) tarsal muscles. Plast Reconstr Surg 1986; 78:33–40.
13. Kuwabara T, Cogan DG, Johnson CC. Structure of the muscles of the upper eyelid. Arch Ophthalmol 1975; 93:1189–1197.
14. Hawes MJ, Dortzbach RK. The microscopic anatomy of the lower eyelid retractors. Arch Ophthalmol 1982; 100:1313–1318.
15. Anderson RL. The medial canthal tendon branches out. Arch Ophthalmol 1977; 95:2951–2952.
16. Gioia VM, Linberg JV, McCormick SA. The anatomy of the lateral canthal tendon. Arch Ophthalmol 1987; 105:529–532.
17. Malone B, Maisel RH. Anatomy of the facial nerve. Am J Otolaryngol 1988; 9:494–504.

Chapter 2

Evaluation of Eyelid Malpositions

A thorough eyelid examination should be included in the documentation of any eyelid malposition. Accurate diagnosis of eyelid dystopia including some determination of its etiology is essential prior to consideration of surgical or nonsurgical correction.

HISTORY

An adequate history can provide useful clues to the cause of the eyelid malposition and may suggest the need for further evaluation. In some cases the history may make immediate surgical intervention unwise.

The time of onset of the malpositioned lid may be congenital or acquired. In the case of ptosis, a careful birth history will uncover the possible use of forceps during delivery, or the occurrence of other birth trauma. Abnormal eyelids in other family members should alert the observer to the possibility of a familial disorder such as blepharophimosis syndrome or craniosynostosis syndrome. The presence of other congenital anatomical deformities or especially neurologic deficiencies may indicate a more serious genetic syndrome, congenital oculomotor nerve palsy, or a central mechanism for the eyelid disorder.

Rapidity of onset should be questioned in all patients. An acute-onset ptosis in an adult may be the result of a metabolic disturbance or compressive lesion. Hemorrhage into a pre-existing, unsuspected eyelid or orbital mass can result in a sudden-onset ptosis especially in children, often associated with some degree of proptosis or motility disturbance. A history of recent trauma with new onset eyelid malposition should raise suspicion not only of scarring and/or levator transection, but also for retained foreign body. Trauma without eyelid laceration is more likely to result in a contusive injury to the levator muscle or its nerve, with a high likelihood of spontaneous recovery. Orbital fractures can be associated with eyelid malpositions; a ptosis that evolves over several days following eyelid trauma may indicate an enlarging hematoma or abscess.

Gradual-onset of an eyelid malposition is more typical of involutional disease, but may occur with a paralytic or cicatricial process. Eyelid changes occurring with other extraocular muscle dysfunction or loss of vision demands investigation of the orbital apex and cavernous sinus. A history of decreased facial movement with associated ocular surface irritation, tearing, or blurred vision may accompany lagophthalmos or paralytic ectropion. A history of changes in the eyelid skin might suggest a chronic inflammatory process, infection, or dermatosis that has led to cicatricial changes in the anterior lamella. Chronic ocular surface disease may result in posterior lamellar scarring (tarsus or conjunctiva), contraction of the conjunctival fornices, or symblepharon formation.

A history of slow progression is not uncommon with most involutional eyelid changes, but this usually occurs over several years. Almost all patients with ptosis or dermatochalasis will report some increase in droopiness late in the day or when tired; this does not usually indicate myasthenia gravis. The occurrence of an eyelid malposition with orbital pain is always worrisome and demands investigation to rule out neoplasm or pseudotumor. Any such association requires radiographic study.

A history of previous eye surgery is important. Eyelid malpositions are not uncommon sequelae of retinal detachment surgery, strabismus surgery or cataract extraction. Ptosis is reported to occur following cataract surgery in 7–8% of cases. Other surgery, especially intracranial or thoracic procedures, may result in central third nerve palsy or Horner's syndrome respectively.

The patient should be questioned carefully about previous episodes of eyelid edema, as with allergic angioneurotic edema or blepharochalasis which can affect eyelid position. This is particularly true in younger patients. A past or present history of systemic diseases that commonly affect the eyelid and orbit such as thyroid ophthalmopathy should be noted. Symptoms of thyroid hormone imbalance should be reviewed since the eyelid manifestations of Graves' disease may precede diagnosis of systemic thyroid dysfunction.

A thorough ocular history should be obtained to attempt to uncover the presence of chronic conjunctivitis or uveitis, or a past or present history of cicatricial diseases such as ocular pemphigoid or Stevens-Johnson syndrome. A history of morning ocular irritation and spontaneous eyelid eversion during sleep, particularly in an obese male, should lead to careful examination of the conjunctiva for papillary conjunctivitis, and of the tarsus for possible floppy eyelid syndrome.

Any prior malignancy should raise the possibility of a mechanical etiology for a malpositioned eyelid from metastatic disease. Previous excision of an eyelid or periocular tumor should alert the observer to the possibility of deep orbital recurrence resulting in distortion of eyelid position.

OBSERVATION

While taking the history the surgeon should observe the patient's eyes and face. It should be noted whether the eyelid position is unilateral or bilateral, and whether there is any associated disorder affecting the brows and midface. The position of the eyelids, canthal angles, and eyelash orientation should be noted (Fig. 1). The presence of concurrent anatomical deformities, such as brow ptosis, diffuse facial laxity, skeletal abnormalities, clefting disorders, or stigmata of Down's syndrome or other genetic disorders should be recorded. Any abnormal eyelid movements with extraocular muscle contraction or with jaw movement should be carefully documented. These may sometimes be quite subtle. A head turn or tilt should lead to careful evaluation of ocular motility to rule out the presence of associated strabismus.

EXAMINATION

For all patients with eyelid malpositions a complete ophthalmic examination is mandatory. Visual acuity with a current refraction is recorded, and especially in children presenting with upper eyelid ptosis, the presence of amblyopia must be ruled-out. In any patient unexplained decrease in vision requires comprehensive investigation. Pupil size and reactivity should be measured, and any asymmetry noted. Corneal examination must evaluate the presence of keratopathy secondary to corneal exposure as a result of the malpositioned eyelid.

A slit lamp examination should include a magnified evaluation of the conjunctiva and eyelid margin (Fig. 2). Thickening of the lid margin or injection of the conjunctiva may represent inflammation or infiltrating neoplasm. Malpositions or misalignments of the eyelashes should be noted.

A Schirmer's test is essential in all older adults to establish the adequacy of tear production (Fig. 3). Ptosis repair or blepharoplasty in a patient over 40 or 50 years with borderline tear function can push them into a symptomatic dry eye syndrome. Some inflammatory diseases or those that involve the lacrimal gland can also be associated with dry eye syndrome.

Extraocular motility is examined in all patients and the presence of an adequate Bell's phenomenon noted. The absence of Bell's phenomenon should lead the surgeon to be more cautious in consideration of elevating the eyelid in patients where lagophthalmos might result. Hypertropia may be responsible for a pseudoptosis, and strabismus surgery may be more

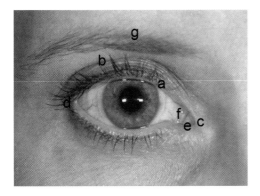

Figure 1 Major features of the normal eyelid. **a.** Eyelid margin with cilia; **b.** upper eyelid crease; **c.** medial canthus; **d.** lateral canthus; **e.** caruncle; **f.** plica; **g.** brow.

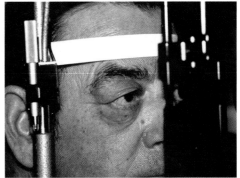

Figure 2 Slit lamp examination of the anterior segment of the eye and the eyelid margins.

appropriate here than ptosis repair. The lack of spontaneous eye or eyelid movements may suggest progressive external ophthalmoplegia.

A pupillary examination should be recorded. The presence of anisocoria should raise the possibility of Horner's syndrome, third nerve palsy, or ocular trauma.

Palpation of the eyelid and anterior orbit may reveal a mass lesion or deep scar responsible for the eyelid malpositon. The upper eyelid should be everted to examine the tarsal plate and palpebral conjunctiva for any irritative lesions or symblepharon formation that could influence the eyelid position. The bulbar conjunctiva should also be examined up to the superior fornix using an eyelid retractor if necessary.

A thorough orbital examination should be recorded and actual or relative proptosis evaluated by Hertel exophthalmometry (Fig. 4). A relatively proptotic globe may give the illusion of eyelid retraction while an enophthalmic globe may give the impression of ptosis. Some eyelid diseases can extend posterior to the orbital septum to involve the orbit. If there are any orbital signs such as proptosis, motility disturbance, palpable masses, or vascular congestion, orbital imaging with CT or MRI should be ordered (Fig. 5).

Simple observation will reveal the presence of entropion or ectropion. If not immediately obvious, asking the patient to squeeze the eyelids closed may trigger spontaneous entropion formation. The snap-back test (pulling outward on the eyelid and observing for spontaneous reapposition to the globe) will often demonstrate excessive eyelid laxity or subtle ectropion (Fig. 6). The eyelids normally maintain enough elasticity to reappose the globe in less than 2 seconds.

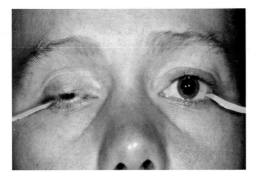

Figure 3 Shirmer's test for tear secretion.

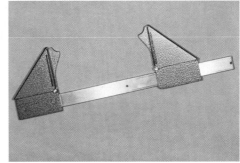

Figure 4 Hertel exophthalmometer for the measurement of proptosis.

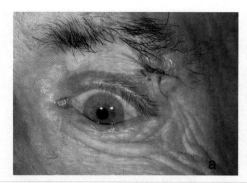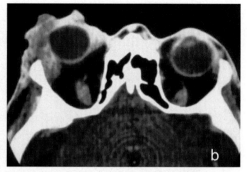

Figure 5 Basal cell carcinoma with extension into the anterior orbit. **a.** Lesion of the left brow; **b.** corresponding CT scan.

Excessive upper or lower eyelid skin and fat herniation (steatoblepharon) should be noted. Hooding of skin over the lashes should be noted and if associated ptosis is suspected this redundant tissue should carefully be lifted to evaluate the position of the upper eyelid margin relative to the pupil.

The interpalpebral fissures are measured vertically with a millimeter ruler at the level of the pupil with eyes in primary position (Fig. 7). The degree to which the eyelid margin covers the superior corneal limbus is also recorded. Additionally, the distance between the upper eyelid margin and the central pupillary reflex, known as the margin to reflex distance (MRD1) is a useful measurement, since total vertical fissure distance may be unreliable in the presence of lower eyelid retraction. The distance between the lower eyelid margin and the central pupillary reflex is sometimes recorded as the MRD2.

Next, the patient is asked to gently close the eyes. Any residual lagophthalmos is measured and recorded. Presence or absence of an eyelid crease gives some indication of the status of the levator aponeurosis and its position above the eyelid margin should be measured. Care must be taken to measure the true crease which may be covered by redundant skin. The absence of a definitive eyelid crease, or a very high position (more than 10 mm), suggests redundancy or dis-insertion of the levator aponeurosis, but is also seen in poor to absent-function myopathic ptosis.

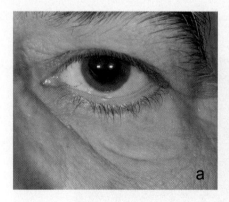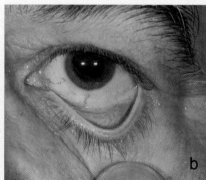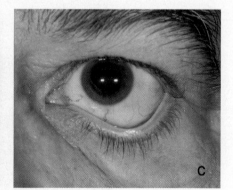

Figure 6 Lower eyelid laxity determined with the snap-back test. **a.** The lid in normal position after a blink; **b.** the lid is pulled forward away from the eye; **c.** before another blink the lax lid fails to snap back against the eye indicating significant laxity.

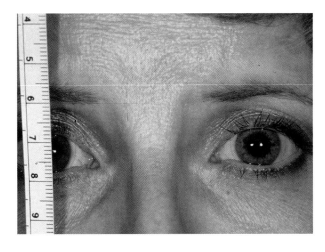

Figure 7 Measurement of vertical palpebral fissure and margin to reflex distance (MRD1).

Levator muscle function is perhaps the single most important measurement made during the preoperative evaluation, and is most predictive of the surgical outcome for ptosis repair following any particular surgical procedure. It must be performed with great care. Function is recorded as maximum eyelid excursion from extreme downgaze (without closing the eyes), to extreme upgaze position. A millimeter ruler is placed in front of the eyelids with the patient looking down as far as possible, and the position of the upper eyelid margin noted against the scale. The patient is asked to look up as far as possible and the eyelid margin position on the scale is again noted (Fig. 8). The difference between the two readings is the total excursion and is recorded as levator function. Contraction of the frontalis muscle can elevate the eyelid by up to 3 to 4 mm so that the examiner must be certain to eliminate any possible contribution form this source. This is done properly by placing a thumb firmly over the brow to immobilize it against the supraorbital rim during measurement. This procedure is critical in patients with poor levator function, since a difference of only 1 or 2 mm in function may influence the choice of a surgical procedure.

All cases of ptosis or eyelid retraction should be tested for a Hering's phenomenon. Because central innervation of the levator muscles is bilaterally equal, an asymmetry in eyelid height may

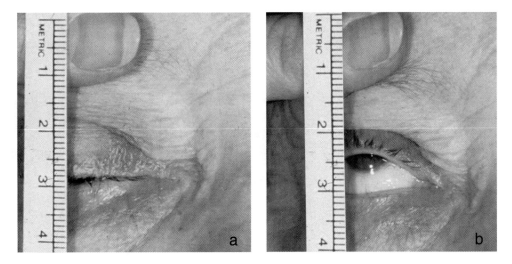

Figure 8 Measurement of levator muscle function. **a.** Extreme downgaze; **b.** extreme upgaze.

result in a central compensatory increase or decrease in motor output to the levator muscles, thus masking an abnormal position of the contralateral eyelid. For example, a patient with bilateral but asymmetric ptosis may have a centrally mediated unconscious increased eyelid height in order to improve visual field. The more ptotic lid still appears ptotic but the less ptotic lid may appear normal. Correction of the apparently unilateral ptosis could uncover the ptosis in the opposite lid requiring additional surgery. In some patients this can be uncovered preoperatively by manually elevating the ptotic lid and seeing the "normal" lid drop (Fig. 9). Conversely, the "normal" lid might actually be retracted, and a decrease in central output might result in both lids being lower, with the contralateral lid now appearing ptotic. In this case depressing the "normal" lid downward could result in the ptotic lid coming up. This so-called Hering's phenomenon is sometimes useful in predicting the results of surgery. However, the results of this test are not always reliable in predicting the behavior of the eyelids after surgical correction.

In congenital myogenic ptosis levator function is usually reduced because of levator fibrosis, with deficient stretching as well as impaired contraction. Typically, the eyelid is ptotic in primary gaze, more ptotic in upgaze, but less ptotic or even relatively retracted in downgaze (Fig. 10). This contrasts with acquired ptosis where the eyelid characteristically shows the same degree of ptosis in all positions of gaze.

Any patient with a history of significant worsening of ptosis late in the day or when tired should be suspected of having myasthenia gravis. This is especially true if the eyelid appears near normal in the morning, or the condition is associated with difficulty in swallowing, generalized weakness, or diplopia. A levator fatigue test can be performed easily without risk. The patient is asked to look upward for several minute without blinking. The position of the eyelid is measured before and immediately after the test. Any increase in ptosis with fatigue of the muscle is suggestive of myasthenia gravis. The definitive diagnostic procedure is the Tensilon test, which should be performed on all patients with a high suspicion of the disease.

Appropriate documentation of all eyelid malpositions with photographs and formal perimetry showing the relative impact of the eyelid on vision have become mandatory by third party payers prior to approval of any surgical intervention for an eyelid malady. A current refraction should be documented since any change in the height or tone of the eyelid can result in a postoperative change in corneal astigmatism. Finally, the patient's expectations for both visual and cosmetic improvement should be carefully elicited as this may impact the technique of surgical repair selected.

Once the nature and etiology of the eyelid malposition has been determined, the appropriate therapy must be selected. When the cause is determined to result from mechanical obstruction to eyelid movement, orbital disease, or ocular irritation initial therapy must be directed towards the source of the pathology. Frequently the malposition may resolve upon treatment of the inciting factor. Surgical correction of eyelid malpositions ranges from simple

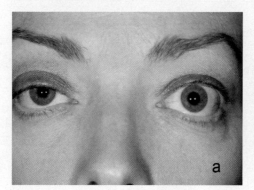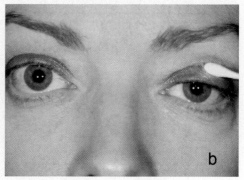

Figure 9 Positive Hering's phenomenon. The right eyelid shows a pseudoptosis resulting from retraction of the left upper lid **a**. When the left lid is held down, the right lid elevates due to Hering's law **b**.

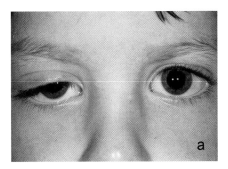 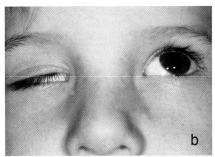 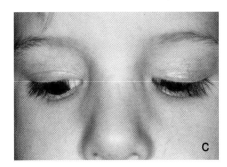

Figure 10 Congenital myogenic ptosis showing fibrosis of the levator muscle. **a.** In primary position the lid shows moderate ptosis; **b.** in upgaze the ptosis increases; **c.** in downgaze the ptosis decreases or even reverses.

to quite complex and may require specialized reconstructive techniques. A description of individual surgical techniques for various eyelid malpositions is beyond the scope of this text, but several generalities are true.

The success of ptosis repair depends a great deal on selecting the most appropriate procedure for each particular patient. In many cases this will be rather easy. All eyelid procedures can be performed on an outpatient basis under minimal intravenous sedation and local infiltrative anesthesia. Extensive reconstructive techniques requiring flaps and grafts may require a greater level of anesthetic control. When surgery is performed while the patient is conscious, it better enables the surgeon to predict the position of the eyelids postoperatively and minimizes the risk of postsurgical complications such as eyelid retraction, lagophthalmos, residual eyelid laxity, and excessive eyelid skin removal.

Perhaps the most dreaded complication of eyelid surgery is vision loss. With proper surgical technique this is an unlikely event. Unrecognized intraoperative or postoperative orbital hemorrhage can lead to compressive optic neuropathy. This risk is minimized by having the patient restrain from any medication that may inhibit the clotting mechanism and determining in advance any patient with a coagulation disorder. The cornea and sclera are at risk for laceration, particularly when laser, electrical, or radiofrequency devices are used by the inexperienced surgeon. Postoperative infection is rare, but severe infection of the orbit or ocular surface may lead to permanent vision loss.

REFERENCES

Dutton JJ. Atlas of Ophthalmic Surgery: Vol. II Oculoplastic, Lacrimal and Orbital Surgery. St. Louis: Mosby-Year Book, 1992.

Hosal BM, Tekli O, Gursel E. Eyelid malpositions after cataract surgery. Eur J Ophthalmol 1998; 8:12–15.

Morax S, Hurbli T. The management of congenital malpositions of eyelids, eyes and orbits. Eye 1988; 2:207–219.

Nowinski T, Anderson RL. Advances in eyelid malpositions. Ophthal Plast Reconstr Surg 1985; 1:145–148.

Zucker JL. Eyelid disorders: recognizing pathologic changes in the older patient. Geriatrics 1993; 48:61–62.

Chapter 3

Evaluation of Eyelid Lesions

INTRODUCTION

The eyelids may be affected by benign and malignant lesions. Most of these are common elsewhere on the body, but when occurring on the eyelid they are often different in character, appearance, and behavior because of the unique characteristics of eyelid skin.

A large number of cutaneous and systemic disorders may be associated with eyelid lesions. In many instances the eyelid findings are quite specific for a particular disorder, at other times they may be rather non-specific. These ocular findings in combination with other cutaneous and systemic abnormalities frequently allow the clinician to make the correct diagnosis. Localized unilateral eyelid lesions most commonly represent benign or malignant neoplasms, infections, or inflammations. Bilateral lesions more frequently represent disseminated systemic conditions such as collagen vascular diseases, metabolic disorders, vesico-bullous diseases, dermatoses, and hypersensitivity disorders.

Eyelid lesions are classified according to the anatomic structures from which they arise. These include the epidermis, dermis, and various cells and adnexal structures within these layers. Eyelid inflammations may present as a localized or diffuse erythematous area. They can be associated with ulceration, induration, eczematous changes, necrosis, edema, or loss of eyelashes. If skin contraction occurs the eyelid margins may be malpositioned manifesting as an ectropion or canthal angle dystopia. Inflammatory lesions may be painful and at times can be associated with lymphadenopathy. Infectious conditions of the eyelid result from viral, bacterial, fungal or parasitic processes and may be primary or secondary. The latter can result as extensions from head and neck foci such as the sinuses or lacrimal sac, or from hematogenous spread from distant sites. The cause of the infection on the eyelid is often evident, such as in a site of trauma or recent surgery. However, when the infection is either atypical or recurrent, a biopsy, smear, or culture may help to exclude the presence of occult malignancy or unusual infectious organism. A systemic evaluation may also be valuable for particularly aggressive infections and those caused by fungi and parasites.

From several recent large series looking at the frequency of eyelid lesions benign processes account for approximately 70% to 75% of all lesions, and malignant neoplasms for 25% to 30% (1–5). Among the benign lesions the most frequent diagnoses are squamous papilloma (26%), nevus (22%), cysts (20%), seborrheic keratosis (13%), vascular lesions (9%), and neural lesions (<1%). The most common malignant tumor on the eyelid is the basal cell carcinoma followed in rapidly descending order by squamous cell carcinoma, sebaceous cell carcinoma, and malignant melanoma. Other rare tumors such as Kaposi's sarcoma, adnexal carcinomas, and Merkel cell tumor are occasionally seen, as are metastatic cancers. One large series of nearly 1100 malignant eyelid tumors from China showed the frequencies of basal cell and sebaceous cell carcinomas to be nearly equal at 38% and 32%, respectively, quite different from the usually quoted values from the Western literature. However, most other studies give the frequency of malignant tumors on the eyelids as 80–85% basal cell carcinoma, 7–9% sebaceous cell carcinoma, 5–10% squamous cell carcinoma, and 1–5% malignant melanoma (1–3,5).

As with diseases elsewhere in the body, the medical history can be very important in the identification of eyelid diseases and should precede the ophthalmic examination. Many congenital eyelid lesions may be associated with other developmental anomalies and systemic conditions requiring pediatric consultation when necessary including possible genetic counseling. In the adult, acquired malpositions and involutional changes usually precipitate or accompany the development of cutaneous lesions. Inflammatory conditions have characteristic clinical findings, but these often overlap with more serious diseases such as malignant tumors. A careful history that focuses on the onset of the eyelid disorder, the time course, presence of concomitant changes or symptoms, travel history, and prior therapy is helpful in narrowing the examination and deciding on any specific ancillary studies.

Current and past illnesses should be reviewed. Of importance in patients presenting with rash-like symptoms is the recognition of atopy (as manifest by hay fever or asthma) as this history is suggestive of atopic dermatitis. Inquiry regarding past allergic reactions to food or medications is essential. Any systemic condition that may suppress the immune system and thus predispose the patient to cutaneous infections or neoplasia (such as HIV and diabetes) should be questioned.

The family history should also be reviewed since the presence of eczema or atopy may be important in pruritic lesions. Many neoplasms such as neurofibromatosis occur as part of heritable illness. A social and travel history is critical. An occupational history is also important as a considerable number of skin reactions are caused by or are worsened by exposure to various chemicals in the work environment.

EXAMINATION

Examination of the eyelid includes examination of the skin, conjunctiva, eyelid margin, and eyelashes. Lesions localized to any one or several of these structures may offer appreciable diagnostic information. The distribution of lesions on the skin itself is equally important. One should first determine whether the distribution is random or whether certain areas are preferentially involved. Finally, certain distributions that suggest participation of underlying nerves or vessels (dermatomal and segmental distributions) point to specific diagnoses such as Herpes infection or oculodermal melanocytosis. Proper evaluation of an eyelid lesion begins with visual recognition and appropriate description. Mastering appropriate terminology will aid in diagnosis and allow the physician to better document the examination.

A *lesion* is any single, small area of skin pathology. Lesions may be solitary or multiple. A *rash* represents the totality of multiple lesions. As such, it is essentially synonymous with the term *eruption*.

TYPES OF LESIONS
Macule

A macule represents a small area of color change. A macule is flat and not palpable. Some macules are slightly depressed below the surface of the skin; these are termed atrophic macules (Fig. 1). Generally, macules are less than 1.5 cm in diameter.

Patch

A patch is an extension of a macule in length and width. By definition a patch is an area of color change that is 1.5 cm or larger in diameter.

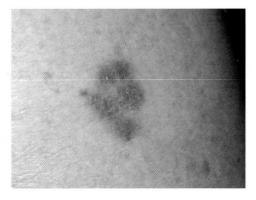

Figure 1 A macule showing a non-palpable flat area of color change.

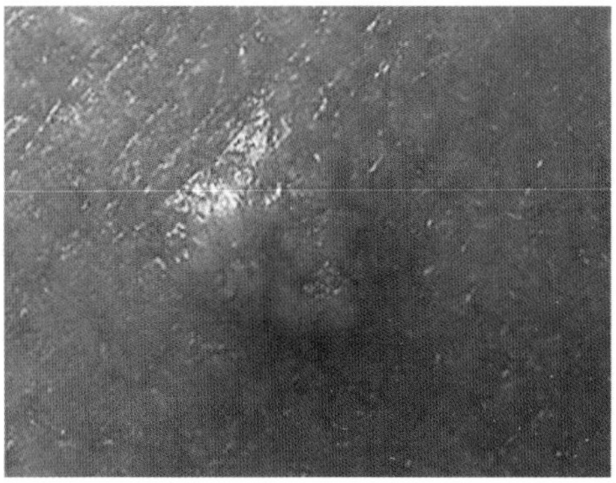

Figure 2 A slightly elevated palpable papule.

Papule

A papule is a small palpable lesion less than 1.5 cm in diameter. Most are elevated, although some papules are visible but not necessarily elevated (Fig. 2). Papules may be of any color and the surface may be smooth or rough. They come in a variety of shapes such as sessile, pedunculated, filliform, and verrucous. A *wheal* is an edematous papule in which the substance of the lesion is made up of nonloculated, interstitial fluid.

Plaque

A plaque is an enlargement of a papule in length and width. As such, it represents a planar enlargement of a papule. Most plaques are elevated but may be palpable without being visibly raised above the skin surface.

Cyst

A cyst is a cavity with a cellular lining derived from glandular, ductal, or epidermal elements (Fig. 3). It is filled with fluid or more consolidated material secreted by these cells.

Vesicle

A vesicle is a small blister less than 0.5 or 1 cm in diameter, depending on the author. It can be considered as a fluid-filled papule in which the fluid is loculated. For this reason, when the roof of a vesicle is incised the fluid runs out and the compartment collapses, in contrast to a wheal which when incised produces a drop of fluid on the surface, but the lesion does not change in size or shape.

Pustule

A pustule is a vesicle that is filled with neutrophils (Fig. 4). For this reason it is white, or yellow-white, in color.

Bulla

A bulla is a blister that is larger than 0.5 or 1 cm in diameter, depending on the author. It is otherwise entirely similar to a vesicle. The fluid in a bulla is usually contained in a single compartment, but occasionally multiple compartments are present.

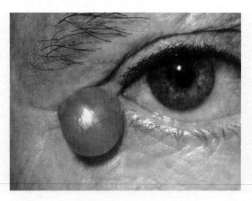

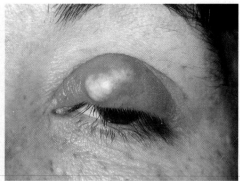

Figure 3 A clear sweat gland cyst, representing a fluid-filled cavity.

Figure 4 A pustule filled with purulent material of neutrophils.

MODIFICATIONS OF LESIONS

Many lesions, regardless of their etiology, can show surface modifications involving their epidermal component. These can sometimes make identification more difficult and in some cases can mask the underlying pathologic process. The epidermis may be palpably thickened (acanthotic) and/or its surface may be scaling (hyperkeratotic). For example, excessive keratin deposition can be seen with many different types of lesions leading to a "cutaneous horn." However this is a descriptive term only and can be seen with numerous benign and malignant lesions. The epidermis may be damaged causing weeping and crusting, or areas of missing epidermis results in areas of erosion or ulceration.

Scale

Scale occurs when there is an abnormal increase in the outermost layer of the epidermis, that is the stratum corneum. A scale is thus made up of flattened keratinized cells that, for one reason or another, are accumulating on the surface of the lesion. This process may be due either to faster than normal creation or slower than normal exfoliation of these cells. Several types of scale are recognized; pityriasis-type scale and lichen-type scale.

Pityriasis-Type Scale

Pityriasis-type scale consists of flakes too small to be individually visualized. For this reason pityrisasis-type scale cannot ordinarily be seen unless the surface of the lesion is scraped. Scraping the surface in this situation results in a small pile of fine white powder. Because of this characteristic, pityriasis-type scales are just barely palpable as a slight roughness on the surface of the lesion.

Lichen-Type Scale

Lichen-type scale is tightly adherent to the surface of the lesion. It is palpable as a slight roughness and, because of reflected light, is visible as a shiny surface (Fig. 5). In order to appreciate this shininess it is often necessary to move the light back and forth over the lesion until just the right angle for reflection is obtained.

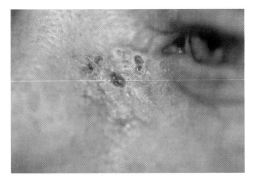

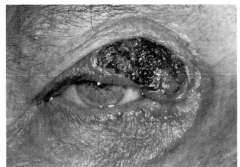

Figure 5   A lichen-type scale showing a shiny reflective surface.

Figure 6   A crust formed from dried blood and exudate.

Crust

Crusts occur when plasma exudes through a damaged or absent epidermis. It represents the dried serum proteins after water has evaporated. A crust is rough on palpation and is visible as amorphous material that is yellow to brown in color (Fig. 6). Where damage to the skin occurs more deeply than the level of the epidermis, blood vessels will be disrupted and there may be a component of dried blood mixed in with the crust. In such situations the color of the crust will be red, violet, or black depending on the amount and freshness of the blood present.

Erosion

An erosion occurs when the epithelial surface of a lesion is absent (Fig. 7). This may occur either because of the breakdown (or removal) of an overlying blister roof or as the result of trauma, especially that from scratching. Erosions formed as a secondary change to blisters are generally round in configuration. They often have an encircling collarette of scale representing the peripheral remnants of the blister roof. On the other hand erosions formed as a result of external trauma generally are angular or linear in configuration and lack the collarette of scale. The visible depth of an erosion is quite shallow since, by definition, no dermal damage is present. The surface of an erosion may be moist (weeping) or may be covered with crust. A fissure is a special type of erosion that forms as a thin crack between adjacent islands of intact epithelium; these fissures form when epithelial cells shrink as a consequence of excessive dryness. They can be conceptualized as similar to the cracks that form in a dry lakebed.

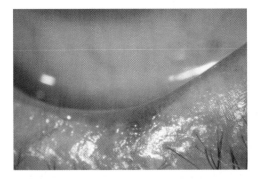

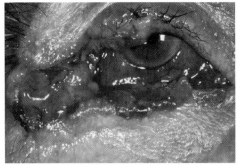

Figure 7   A superficial erosion with missing epithelium.

Figure 8   A deep ulcer involving the epithelium and dermis.

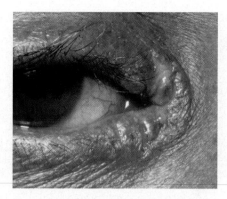

Figure 9 Lichenification with thickening of the epidermis and superficial scales.

Ulcer

An ulcer is similar to an erosion in that the overlying epithelium is absent. However, dermal damage is present, and the resultant defect is visible deeper than that of an erosion (Fig. 8). This dermal damage is almost always accompanied by vessel disruption and bleeding. Hence, the crusts that form within ulcers have red, violet, or blue-black hues, which accompany the presence of blood. The blood also adds fibrin which in turns adds "toughness" and adherence to the curst. This difficult-to-remove dark-colored crust is known as *eschar*.

Lichenification

The epidermis responds to chronic trauma with increased cell proliferation and increased keratin production (Fig. 9). The characteristic morphologic features of lichenification include: palpable thickness of the skin compared to nearby normal skin; accentuation of the normal cross-hatched skin markings; and the presence of lichen-type scale. Lichenification is especially characteristic in the chronic lesions of atopic dermatitis and neuro-dermatitis. It is particularly marked in the variant of these two diseases known as *lichen simplex chronicus*.

ARRANGEMENT

The arrangement of lesions refers to the pattern or relationship of nearby, non-confluent, lesions. Typical arrangement patterns include *clustering* (a grouping of lesions), *beading* (closely set, but not confluent papules in a linear or circular arrangement), *satellitosis* (small peripheral lesions around a central larger lesion), *reticular* (lattice or net-like arrangements), and *linear*.

MORPHOLOGY
Size

A rough estimation of size is indicated by the term chosen for the basic lesion: vesicle versus bulla, macule versus patch, and papule versus plaque. In each of these pairs the point of separation occurs at about 1.5 cm in diameter. However, in most instances an actual measurement of the diameter should be given. Where a lesion is other than round, the shortest and the longest diameter should be stated. Where multiple lesions are present one can determine the size of the most representative lesion and then give the range of sizes.

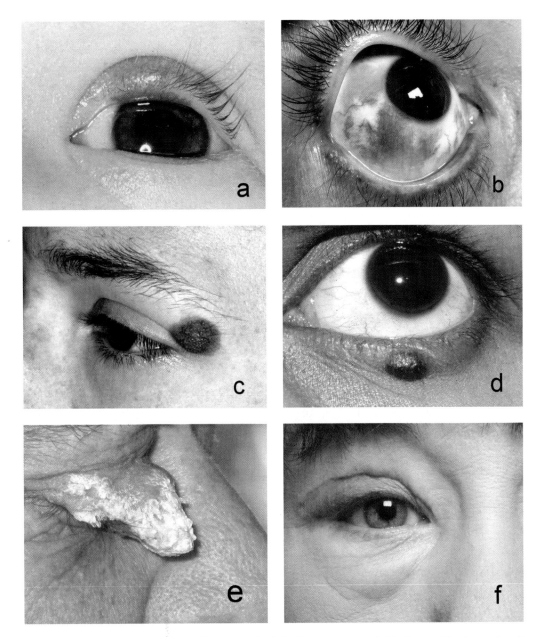

Figure 10 Color variations of eyelid lesions. **a.** Red; **b.** blue; **c.** brown; **d.** black; **e.** white/gray; **f.** yellow.

Color

Color is surprisingly hard to describe accurately. This is partly due to the lack of absolute color standards and partly due to the confounding effect that the patient's normal skin color has on lesional color. One must also discount the color contributed by "secondary" characteristics such as scale or crust. This can usually be accomplished by looking at the peripheral edge of a lesion, since both scale and crust are often less prominent in this location. The basic hues found in skin lesions are red, white, blue, brown, black, yellow, and "skin" color. Each of these colors often gives a clue to the nature of the lesion (Fig. 10).

Color	Diagnostic implication
Pink/red	Vascular or inflammatory
Blue	Blood or pigment, deep within the skin
Brown/black	Melanin bearing cells, or old blood
Gray/white	Accelerated keratin turnover
Yellow	Lipid or fat

Consistency

The consistency of a lesion is stated as being soft, medium, firm, or fluctuant. Soft lesions are easily compressible (lipomas, neurofibromas), medium lesions are slightly compressible (most inflammatory lesions), and firm lesions cannot be compress at all (fibromas). The consistency of cysts is somewhat of an exception to this grading system. A cyst may be somewhat compressible as you first start to squeeze it, but the limits of elasticity of the wall are quickly reached and the lesion then begins to feel quite firm.

Configuration

Configuration represents the shape of the lesion as it is seen from above. Common types of configurations include nummular (coin sized and shaped), gyrate, annular (ring-like border with some degree of clearing in the center), and linear lesions. Most lesions have a circular configuration. A few lesions are oval, notably those of pityriasis rosea, and many others are irregular in shape. Examples of irregular shapes include gyrate and serpigenous lesions, which generally occur due to the melding of adjacent lesions that are enlarging in a centrifugal manner until they reach the point of confluence. Such lesions are frequently found, for example in psoriasis and urticaria. On the other hand, irregular lesions with angular or linear shapes generally occur as a result of external trauma such as scratching or are due to the direct inoculation of antigen (ocular medications) or virus (linear warts). Linear lesions (the shape, not the arrangement of a group of lesions) are special types that occur as part of the Koebner phenomenon. Here, external trauma is followed sometime later by the appearance of lesions in the traumatized site. This phenomenon, also known as the isomorphic response, is a characteristic feature of psoriasis, lichen planus, and a few other less common diseases.

Margination

Margination describes the nature of the transition between the lesion and normal skin. In general margination is said to be either sharp (distinct) or diffuse (Fig. 11). Lesions are considered to be sharply marginated or well circumscribed when the transition from normal to abnormal skin occurs in the space of a millimeter or less, and when this degree of sharpness is maintained around the whole periphery of the lesion. In many cases further description of the transitional zone is helpful. Thus a lesion can have square borders or shoulders (verruca vulgaris, seborrheic keratosis), rolled borders (basal cell carcinoma), or sloped or domed borders (dermatofibroma). In

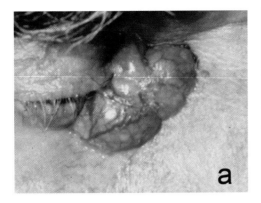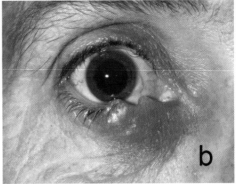

Figure 11　Margin characteristics of eyelid lesions. **a.** Sharply defined; **b.** diffuse.

a general way the shape of the shoulder reflects the depth of the pathology; very superficial lesions tend to be square shouldered and deep lesions tend to have sloped shoulders. Diffuse margination refers to a blending of the lesion into the surrounding skin over several millimeters such that the edges cannot precisely be defined.

SURFACE CHARACTERISTICS

The surface of a lesion provides clues as to its location within the eyelid skin. Lesions arising from the epidermis tend to have more sharply marginated edges. The lesion itself is usually irregular with loss of normal epithelial fine markings and topography. In contrast, dermal lesions tend to elevate and stretch the overlying epidermis which usually retains normal topography, although with large lesions the epithelium may be thin, smooth, and shiny. The edges of dermal lesions are sloped and blend gently into surrounding tissue.

In general, the surface of a lesion is often described as smooth or rough (Fig. 12). Roughness occurs when either scale or crust is present. Differentiation between these two changes is important since scale is usually associated with epithelial hyperplasia, and crust is associated with epithelial damage. Crust is always visible, whereas scale may or may not be visible. Thus roughness in the absence of visible change is always due to the presence of scale. Crust may be of the superficial type (yellow or yellow-brown color) or of the hemorrhagic type (red, violaceous, or black color). The former overlies erosions, and the latter overlies ulcers.

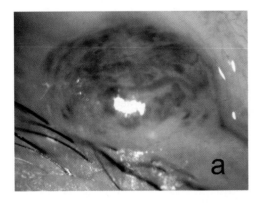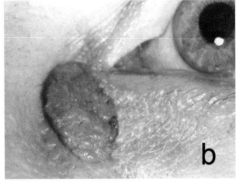

Figure 12　Surface characteristics of eyelid lesions. **a.** Smooth; **b.** rough.

In the evaluation of any eyelid lesion one of the major goals is to rule out malignancy. Most malignant neoplasms arising on the eyelid skin can mimic benign lesions and therefore can easily be missed. Although the large majority of eyelid lesions will be benign, the consequences of misdiagnosis are significant enough so that any undiagnosed lesion or one that does not respond to medical therapy should be biopsied for histopathologic examination.

Information gained from the clinical history may also suggest malignancy. Most important here is progressive growth which may be slow or rapid. Other suggestive findings are irritation, intermittent drainage, bleeding, crusting, and changes in pigmentation.

Certain clinical characteristics often suggest malignancy. (see Table 1 for summary.) These include irregular shape, rolled "pearly" borders, and associated induration (Fig. 13). Malignant lesions often have a "hardened" feel on palpation when compared to the surrounding skin. Erosion is common as is ulceration leading to hemorrhage, exudation, and crust formation.

Table 1 Common Eyelid Malignancies and Lesions with which They Are Most Often Confused

Lesion	Surface	Color	Margins	Other
Acquired melanosis	Flat	Brown	Well defined to diffuse	May be amelanotic
Actinic keratosis	Flat, scaly	Pink, red	Round to irregular	
Apocrine adenoma	Nodular to papillomatous	Yellowish	Well defined	
Basal cell carcinoma	Raised, pearly	Skin colored	Round, well defined	Ulceration, telangiectasias
Blue nevus	Smooth, domed	Blue to black	Round to oval, well defined	Firm
Chalazion			Diffuse	Erythema
Dermatofibroma	Flat to domed	Skin colored to reddish	Round to oval	Hard
Inverted follicular keratosis	Warty	Skin colored to brown	Well defined	
Keratoacanthoma	Smooth, central crater	Skin colored to red	Round, well-defined	Rapid growth and involution
Lentigo maligna	Smooth, flat to nodular	Tan, brown to black	Irregular	
Lentigo senilis	Smooth, flat	Uniform brown	Round to oval	Darken with sun exposure
Lymphoma	Smooth	Pink to red	Diffuse	
Malignant melanoma	Flat to nodular	Patchy brown to black	Diffuse to defined	
Melanocytic nevus	Smooth, flat to elevated	Uniform brown	Round or oval	
Metastatic tumors	Smooth	Skin colored, red, blue	Diffuse	May be ulcerated, telangiectasias
Neurofibroma	Nodular	Skin colored	Round, well defined	
Papilloma	Warty, sessile to pedunculated	Skin colored	Well defined	
Pigmented basal cell carcinoma	Nodular, smooth	Brown to black	Irregular	
Squamous cell carcinoma	Scaly, ulcerated	Skin colored to red	Irregular	Telangiectasias
Trichoepithelioma	Raised, pearly	Skin colored	Round	

Telangiectasias, or fine new vessels, are particularly suggestive of malignancy (Fig. 14). Alterations of normal architecture including obliteration of epithelial folds and lines, loss of lashes (Fig. 15), and absence of meibomian gland orifices is particularly characteristic; benign lesions generally do not invade or distort normal eyelid structures. Malignant lesions frequently are not painful or tender.

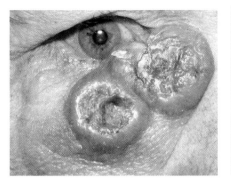

Figure 13 Rolled pearly borders suggestive of malignancy.

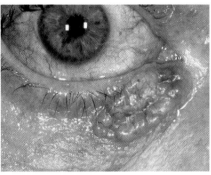

Figure 14 Telangiectasias are fine dilated blood vessels seen within a lesion.

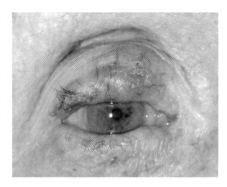

Figure 15 Loss of eyelashes associated with a carcinoma of the eyelid.

Another important warning sign is fixation to deeper tissues or bone. This often suggests infiltration. Regional lymphadenopathy can be seen with infectious lesions, but should also raise suspicion for squamous cell, and especially sebaceous cell carcinoma. Restriction of ocular motility and proptosis suggest deep orbital extension and requires evaluated by means of CT or MRI scanning. If malignancy is suspected, except for basal cell carcinoma, systemic evaluation for metastases should be undertaken.

Features of benign lesions:
- Slow growth over months to years
- Well-demarcated borders
- Intact epithelium
- Even pigmentation when present

Features of malignant lesions:
- Slow growth to rapid growth over weeks to months
- Infiltrative, ill-defined borders
- Epithelium may be ulcerated
- Uneven pigmentation when present, or change in pigmentation

REFERENCES

Abdi U, Tyagi N, Maheshwari V, Gorgi R, Tyagi SP. Tumors of the eyelid: a clinicopathologic study. J Indian Med Assoc 1996; 94:405–416.
Bright DC. Dermatologic conditions of the eyelids and face. Optom Clin 1991; 1:89–102.
Ni Z. Histopathological classification of 3,510 cases with eyelid tumor. Zhonghua Yan Ke Za Zhi 1999; 32:435–437.
Obata H, Aoki Y, Kubota S, Kanai N, Tsuru T. Incidence of benign and malignant lesions of eyelid and conjunctival tumors. Nippon Ganka Gakkai Zasshi 2005; 109:573–579.
Lee SB, Saw SM, Au Euony KG, Chan TK, Lee HP. Incidence of eyelid cancers in Singapore from 1968 to 1995. Br J Ophthalmol 1999; 83:595–597.
Tesluk GC. Eyelid lesions: incidence and comparison of benign and malignant lesions. Ann Ophthalmol 1985; 17:704–707.

Chapter 4

Eyelid Lesions and Tissues of Origin

The plethora of lesions that can occur on the eyelids is rather daunting, not to say confusing, to the average clinician. Many names are similar and while they may be meaningful to the pathologist based on details of microscopic findings, they often add little to the clinical recognition or management of these diseases. Placing such lesions into a more or less organized system based on anatomical tissues of origin may be a useful exercise.

All lesions that involve the eyelids or any other region of the body can be thought of as deriving from two basic sources. Those that arrive in the lids from other more remote sources are *exogenous* lesions. These include metastatic tumors from sites such as the breast or lung. Also included here are infiltrations in the dermis and epidermis of cellular or other materials that secondarily involve eyelid structures. Included here are diseases such as amyloidosis, sarcoidosis, infectious inflammations such as herpes and cellulitis, xanthelamas, acute atopic dermatitis, erythema multiforme, granuloma annulare, and lymphoid and myeloid infiltrates. All exogenous lesions disturb the normal eyelid architechture to some extent, and may be generalized or confined to specific eyelid tissue types.

The majority of lesions seen on the eyelids are derived from normal lid tissues and structures. The epidermis is the source for a large number of lesions that characteristically disturb the fine wrinkles and pores normally seen on the skin surface (Fig. 1). These include most of the common cutaneous malignancies seen on the lids. The basal cell carcinoma arises from basal cells in the deep epidermis. Squamous carcinomas are derived from stratified squamous cells of the epidermis. Malignant melanomas arise from melanocytes that normally reside in the basal epidermis, but some probably arise from dermal nevoid cells.

Of the benign lesions derived from the epidermis many can look rather similar clinically. Some may remain epidermal in location, but many extend into the underlying dermis. Epidermal lesions include the papilloma, actinic keratosis, seborrheic keratosis, inverted follicular keratosis, ichthyosis, keratoacanthoma, lentigo, milia, molluscum contagiosum, and acquired melanosis. When epidermal cells become buried beneath the surface, keratin can accumulate to form an epidermoid cyst.

The dermis is composed largely of collagen with a small amount of elastin. Few lesions arise directly from these materials, but the dermis is frequently involved with infiltrative and other processes (Fig. 2). In angioedema the dermis is edematous with an inflammatory cell infiltrate. White blood cell infiltration also predominates in blepharitis, cellulitis, insect bites, and in cicatricial phemphigoid. Leukemic infiltrates also accumulate within the dermal stroma.

Although melanocytes usually migrate to the epidermis during embryogenesis, they can arrest in the dermis where they form pigmented lesions. These include the junctional and compound nevus located at the epidermal/dermal junction and dermis, respectively, congenital blue nevus and cellular blue nevus within the dermis, and oculodermal melanocytosis. Lymphangiomas arise from lymphatic endothelium within the dermis. A number of lesions occur in the dermis but are of uncertain cellular etiology. The cylindroma may have eccrine relationships but also involves the dermal collagen to a large extent. Dermatofibromas demonstrate some relationship to fibroblasts but their specific etiology remains uncertain. The origin of Merkel cell tumors remains controversial, but they appear to have neuroendocrine relationships. Myxomas have an association with dermal fibroblasts which secrete the surrounding matrix, however their cellular etiology remains unclear. Microcystic adnexal carcinoma is derived from dermal ductal elements, but also includes epidermal relationships.

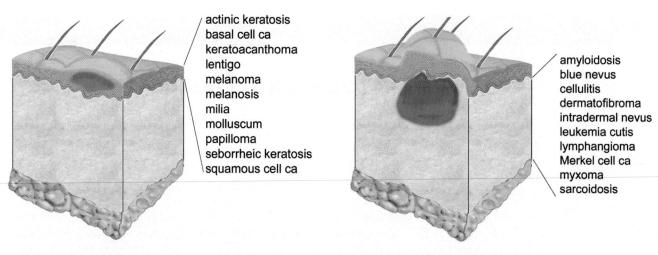

actinic keratosis
basal cell ca
keratoacanthoma
lentigo
melanoma
melanosis
milia
molluscum
papilloma
seborrheic keratosis
squamous cell ca

amyloidosis
blue nevus
cellulitis
dermatofibroma
intradermal nevus
leukemia cutis
lymphangioma
Merkel cell ca
myxoma
sarcoidosis

Figure 1 A lesion of the epithelium with loss of epithelial surface characteristics of fine wrinkles and cellular structure.

Figure 2 Dermal lesions displace the epithelium upward usually without obliterating fine surface features.

The dermis also contains epithelial appendages which are the source for many eyelid lesions. The pilosebaceous unit consists of the hair follicle and associated holocrine sebaceous gland and apocrine sweat gland of Moll. All of these structures can be the site of origin for eyelid lesions. The diverse cellular components of this apparatus can give rise to many different lesions that can look similar clinically. Lesions are grouped into four major categories depending upon differentiation towards sebaceous, hair follicle, apocrine, or eccrine tissues. Within these groups lesions are further subdivided into hyperplasias, hamartomas, adenomas, and carcinomas.

The hair follicle is a tubule with root cells at the base around the papilla and bulb (Fig. 3). Higher up follicular epithelium lines the follicle, and finally cortical cells lay down the outer keratin layers to the hair. Tumors arising from proliferations of cortical cells are termed pilomatrixomas. Solid proliferations of follicular cells manifest as trichofolliculomas, whereas an obstruction of the follicle results in a cystic lesion called a trichilemmal cyst. Solid tumors arising from the basal epithelial bulb are tichoepitheiomas.

Large sebaceous glands empty into the hair follicle. Proliferations of the secretory epithelium produce solid dermal tumors called sebaceous adenomas (Fig. 4). Occasionally the excretory

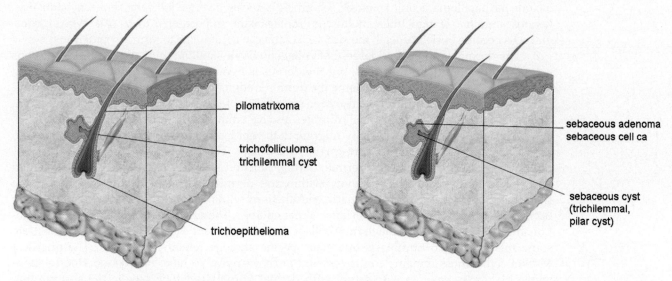

pilomatrixoma

trichofolliculoma
trichilemmal cyst

trichoepithelioma

sebaceous adenoma
sebaceous cell ca

sebaceous cyst
(trichilemmal,
pilar cyst)

Figure 3 Hair follicle lesions.

Figure 4 The hair follicle and associated dermal lesions.

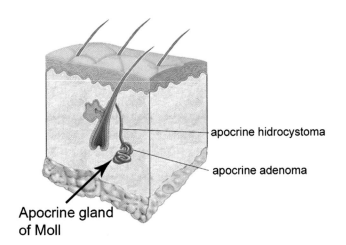

Figure 5 Apocrine glands of Moll.

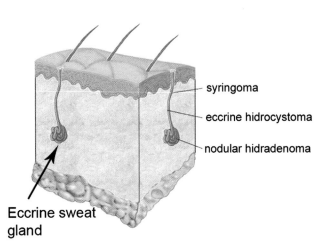

Figure 6 The eccrine sweat gland can be the origin of several dermal lesions.

duct becomes blocked with accumulation of sebum, producing a sebaceous cyst (steatocystoma). More commonly, however, the block is higher up in the follicle and although the cyst is still contains some sebum the epithelial lining adds keratin and leads to the diagnosis of trichilemmal (= tricholemmal) or pilar cyst. Apocrine sweat glands of Moll normally produce a somewhat viscous secretion that empties into the hair follicle (Fig. 5). Solid tumors arising from the secretory epithelium give rise to apocrine adenomas. If the duct becomes obstructed, a cyst results that can have a layered precipitate of cellular debris. These are apocrine hidrocystomas.

Eccrine sweat glands empty directly to the skin surface (Fig. 6). Like the apocrine sweat glands, these can form solid and cystic lesions. Benign tumors arising from the ductal epithelium are called syringomas, whereas those from the tubular secretory epithelium are nodular hidradenomas. An obstruction of the secretory duct will result in an eccrine hidrocystoma filled with a clear fluid. Clinically, the eccrine and apocrine cysts may not always be distinguishable.

Vascular elements are present in the dermis and can give rise to a number of important eyelid lesions (Fig. 7). These include hemangiomas and angiosarcomas derived from endothelial cells, and hemangiopericytomas arising from the endothelial pericyte. Arteriovenous hemangiomas or malformations are abnormal vascular channels. Nerves are another component of the dermis and are the tissues of origin for neural tumors such as neurofibromas.

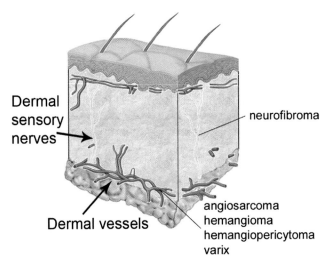

Figure 7 Blood vessels and nerves in the dermis and subcutaneous tissues serve as the sites of origin for several vascular and neural lesions.

In addition to cutaneous layers and their included adnexal appendages eyelid lesions can arise from other eyelid structures. Most important in this group are the tarsal plate meibomian glands. These are modified holocrine sebaceous glands arranged as tubules, with about 25 to 30 in the upper eyelid and 20 in the lower lid. They are not associated with the eyelashes or a pilosebaceous unit, although they can occasionally revert to such a structure where they can be related to the development of abnormal hairs called distichiasis. An obstruction of the meibomian duct can result in an infected cyst called a chalazion. In contrast, a similar infection involving small isolated sebaceous glands (glands of Zeis) or those associated with the skin pilosebaceous units results in a more acute and superficial process called a hordeolum. Any of these sebaceous glands can also give rise to a malignant tumor, the sebaceous cell carcinoma.

Chapter 5

Histopathologic Terminology

The use of descriptive terms in histopathology is a valuable method for standard communication which allows both the pathologist and the clinician to understand specific histologic characteristics of biological materials. One or more of these characteristics may be specific for certain lesions, thus allowing a more precise diagnosis. In some cases, knowledge of such characteristics can also help the clinician make a provisional diagnosis that might allow therapeutic decisions such as to biopsy or not, or to treat medically or to observe.

In the following pages we describe and illustrate the more common descriptive terms in histopathologic diagnosis, which are used throughout this book.

Acantholysis

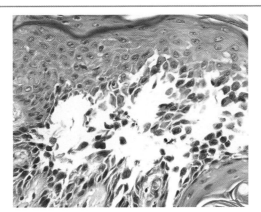

Acantholysis is the loss of cohesion between epidermal (or epithelial) cells leading to the formation of intraepidermal clefts, vesicles, or bullae. Primary acantholysis results from dissolution or separation of the desmosomes between unaltered cells. Secondary acantholysis occurs between damaged cells such as during viral infection. An example of primary acantholysis in pemphigus vulgaris is shown.

Acanthosis

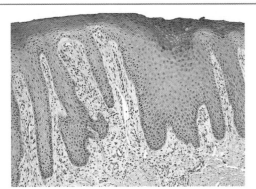

Acanthosis is an increase in the thickness of the squamous cell layer (stratum spinosum) of the epidermis. Acanthosis often results in elongated projections of the epidermis into the dermis, as shown in this example.

Actinic Elastosis

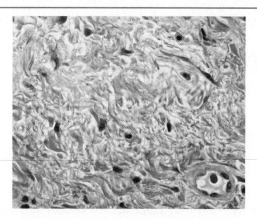

Actinic elastosis, also referred to as solar elastosis, is characterized by lightly basophilic, irregular, thickened elastic fibers in the dermis. Individual fibers are sometimes not evident, and there may be only an amorphous mass of lightly basophilic material in the dermis. Elastic tissue stains may be used to highlight actinic elastosis.

Apoptosis

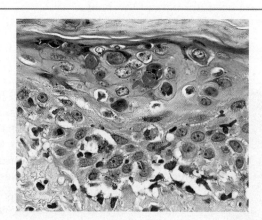

Apoptosis is programmed cell death recognizable morphologically by chromatin condensation, cell shrinkage, and hypereosinophilia. Apoptotic cells with no remaining nucleus appear as homogenous, eosinophilic, round structures termed colloid bodies or cytoid bodies. Apoptosis requires energy, transcription of new genes, and protein synthesis.

Ballooning Degeneration of the Epidermis

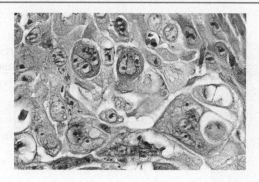

In ballooning degeneration of the epidermis, marked intracellular edema leads to acantholysis and subsequent formation of an intraepidermal vesicle or bulla. Ballooning degeneration is characteristic of cutaneous viral infections.

Birefringence

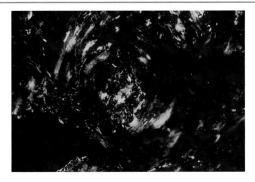

Birefringence is the splitting of a light wave into two waves that have perpendicular polarizations and speed of travel. Birefringence results from a substance having different indexes of refraction, and is thus also referred to as double refraction. Birefringent objects appear as shining bodies on a dark background when viewed with polarized light. Birefringent objects are usually white or yellow in sections stained with hematoxylin and eosin. Collagen and hair are normal structures in the skin that are birefringent, while foreign bodies are the most frequent extraneous birefringent materials. Amyloid is birefringent when stained with Congo red, as shown here.

Bulla

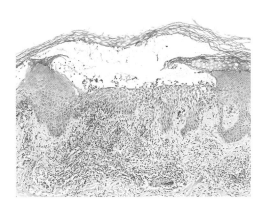

A bulla is a fluid-filled blister greater than 0.5 or 1 cm in diameter, depending on the author. Bullae may be subcorneal (shown), intraepidermal, suprabasilar, or subepidermal.

Colloid Body

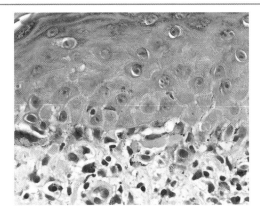

Colloid bodies are also known as cytoid bodies, Civatte bodies, hyalin bodies, and apoptotic bodies. They are apoptotic epidermal cells (keratinocytes) lacking nuclei and appear as homogeneous, eosinophilic, and round structures. Colloid bodies are not specific for any disease, but they are commonly seen in lupus erythematosus, lichen planus, and graft-versus-host disease.

Decapitation Secretion

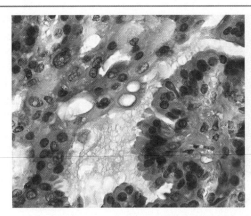

Decapitation secretion is characteristic of apocrine cells. During decapitation secretion, portions of the apical eosinophilic cytoplasm of the cells is pinched off into the lumina lined by the apocrine cells.

Dyskeratosis

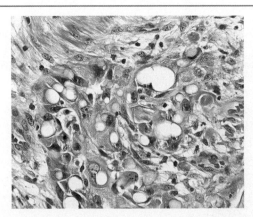

The meaning of the term dyskeratosis varies depending on the disease. In acute graft-versus-host disease, lichen planus, and lupus erythematosus, dyskeratotic cells are cells undergoing apoptosis and are smaller than adjacent epidermal keratinocytes, have brightly eosinophilic cytoplasm, and shrunken hyper-basophilic nuclei (*see* Apoptosis). In acantholytic dermatosis, the dyskeratotic cells are also termed "corps ronds" and have a central, basophilic, pyknotic nucleus surrounded by a clear halo and enveloped within a basophilic or eosinophilic rim. Neoplastic dyskeratosis is manifest as brightly eosinophilic bodies, sometimes with remnants of nuclei, within a tumor (shown). These bodies represent neoplastic cells undergoing apoptosis.

Epidermotropism

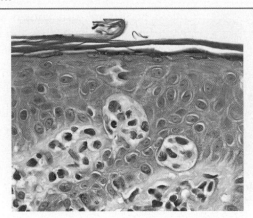

Epidermotropism is the presence of atypical lymphocytes in the epidermis *without spongiosis* and is characteristic of mycosis fungoides. The atypical lymphocytes in the epidermis may occur singly surrounded by a clear halo or they may form small clusters referred to as Pautrier microabscesses.

Epithelioid Cells

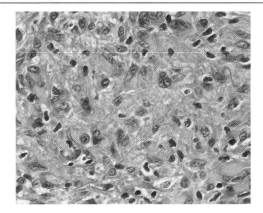

Epithelioid cells are activated macrophages that have an epithelial-like appearance. They are large cells with oval to elongated nuclei, eosinophilic cytoplasm, and indistinct cell borders. They occur singly or may form groups termed granulomas.

Exocytosis

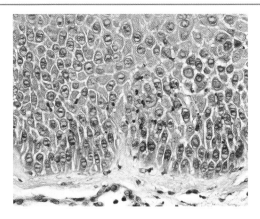

Exocytosis refers to the presence of inflammatory cells within the epidermis in conjunction with spongiosis. Exocytosis is characteristic of inflammatory dermatoses.

Fibrinoid Degeneration (Necrosis)

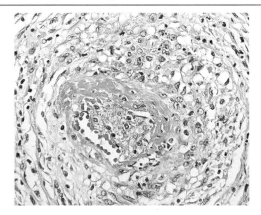

Fibrinoid degeneration, also referred to as fibrinoid necrosis, is manifest by the deposition of fibrin within vessel walls or dermal collagen. Fibrin is homogeneous and eosinophilic in sections stained with hematoxylin and eosin. In the skin, fibrinoid necrosis of vessel walls is seen in leukocytoclastic vasculitis, while fibrin deposition in dermal collagen is seen in rheumatoid nodules and sometimes in lupus erythematosus, especially the systemic variant. An orbital vessel in a patient with Wegener's granulomatosis is shown.

Foam Cell

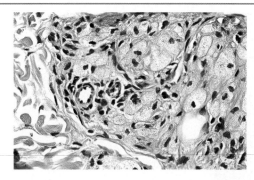

A foam cell is a macrophage laden with lipid, causing it to have vacuolated, bubbly-appearing cytoplasm.

Foreign Body Giant Cell

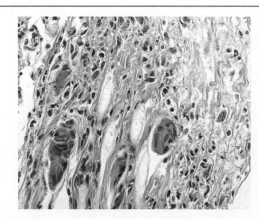

A foreign body giant cell is a multinucleated giant cell derived from fusion of epithelioid cells (activated macrophages). Foreign body giant cells are characterized by their large size and haphazardly arrayed nuclei.

Granulation Tissue

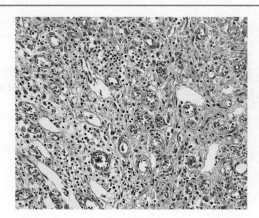

Granulation tissue is the hallmark of wound healing, and the term comes from the soft, pink, granular appearance when viewed from the surface of a wound. Histologically, granulation tissue consists of a proliferation of small blood vessels and fibroblasts, often accompanied by edema.

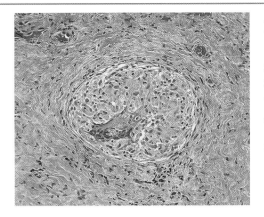

A granuloma is a microscopic aggregate containing varying proportions of activated macrophages (epithelioid cells), multinucleated giant cells resulting from fusion of epithelioid cells, and other mononuclear leukocytes (lymphocytes, plasma cells, monocytes, and macrophages). *Foreign body granulomas* are reactions to relatively inert particles and typically have multinucleated giant cells, macrophages, and usually only small numbers of epithelioid cells. *Immune or allergic granulomas* are a response to insoluble particles that can induce a cell-mediated immune response; they may result from foreign substances such as zirconium, beryllium, or dyes used for tattoos, or microbes such as *Mycobacterium tuberculosis* and fungi. Immune/allergic granulomas typically contain abundant epithelioid cells and variable numbers of multinucleated giant cells. Other descriptors used for granulomas are *sarcoidal, tuberculoid,* and *palisading. Sarcoidal granulomas*, also termed *naked granulomas*, have epithelioid cells and multinucleated giant cells with only a sparse periphery of lymphocytes (shown). Sarcoidal granulomas are characteristic not only of sarcoidosis, but they also are seen in some infections, granulomatous rosacea, orofacial granulomatosis (including the Melkersson-Rosenthal syndrome), and as a response to some foreign materials. *Tuberculoid granulomas* have epithelioid cells, multinucleated giant cells (especially Langhans' giant cells), and a moderate to dense periphery of lymphocytes. Central necrosis ("caseation necrosis") may or may not be present. Tuberculoid granulomas are characteristic not only of *Mycobacterium tuberculosis* infection but are also seen in other infectious diseases. *Palisading granulomas* in the skin have a central zone of degenerated collagen (termed "necrobiosis") surrounded by macrophages, palisading epithelioid cells, lymphocytes, and variable numbers of multinucleated giant cells. Palisading granulomas are characteristic of granuloma annulare, necrobiosis lipoidica, rheumatoid nodules, and necrobiotic xanthogranuloma.

Horn Cyst

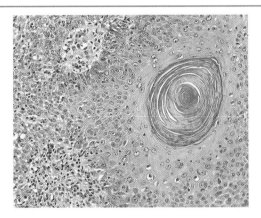

A horn cyst is a circumscribed, round, intraepidermal accumulation of keratin. Keratin-filled invaginations of the epidermis are referred to as "pseudo-horn cysts." Both horn cysts and pseudo-horn cysts are characteristic of seborrheic keratoses, though they may also be seen in other neoplasms of the skin.

Hydropic Degeneration of Basal Layer

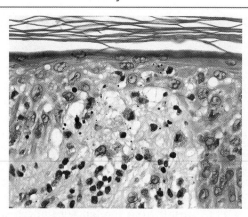

Hydropic degeneration of the basal layer, also termed vacuolar degeneration and liquefactive degeneration, refers to degeneration of the basal cell layer characterized by formation of clear spaces (vacuoles) beneath the basal layer. It is a histological feature prominent in lupus erythematosus, erythema multiforme, graft-versus-host disease, as well as other dermatological diseases not common to the eyelids.

Hyperkeratosis

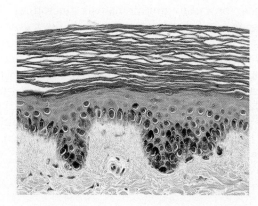

Hyperkeratosis is increased thickness of the stratum corneum (horny layer) of the epidermis. Hyperkeratosis may result from orthokeratosis, parakeratosis, or a combination of these two. Refer to Orthokeratosis and Parakeratosis (below).

Keratohyalin

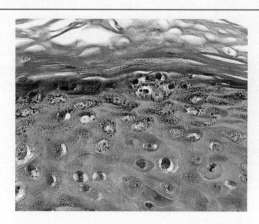

Keratohyalin is seen as darkly basophilic granules found in keratinocytes of the granular layer (stratum granulosum) of the epidermis. Keratohyaline granules form matrix that cements cytokeratin tonofibrils together resulting in increased strength and stability.

Koilocyte

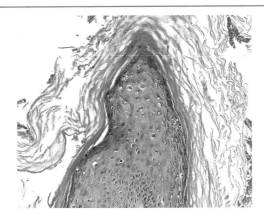

Koilocytes are vacuolated keratinocytes with eccentrically placed, basophilic, shrunken nuclei surrounded by clear halos. They are found in the upper spinous and granular cell layers of the epidermis in human papillomavirus infections (verruca vulgaris, in the eyelid).

Langhans' Giant Cell

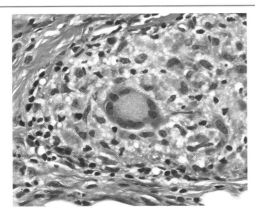

Langhans' giant cells are multinucleated giant cells derived from fusion of epithelioid cells (activated macrophages). They are large cells with their nuclei arranged along the periphery of the cell forming an arc. Langhans' giant cells are non-specific, and they may be seen in both immune-type granulomas (such as sarcoidosis and tuberculosis) and foreign body granulomas.

Lichenoid Inflammation

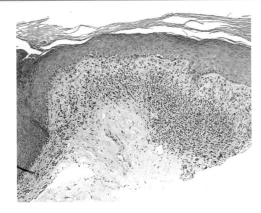

Lichenoid inflammation or lichenoid reaction pattern refers to a dense band of lymphocytes clustered around the interface between the epidermis and dermis, often causing it to be obscured. Lichenoid inflammation is common to many dermatological conditions, though only a few, such as erythema multiforme and graft-versus-host disease, are seen in the eyelids.

Melanophage

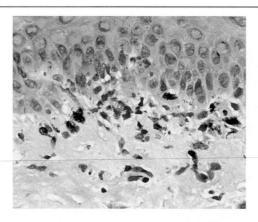

A macrophage containing phagocytized melanin is referred to as a melanophage. Melanin granules are dark brown and non-refractile in sections stained with hematoxylin and eosin. Melanophages are seen in the dermis in inflammatory conditions affecting the epidermis, as well as in neoplasms such as seborrheic keratosis, blue nevus, and melanomas.

Necrobiosis

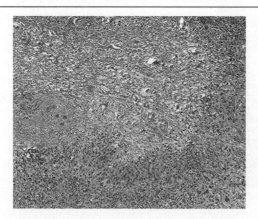

Necrobiosis refers to death of cells or tissue due to aging or overuse. Zones of smudged or homogenized dermal collagen characterize it histologically. Necrobiosis is often seen as the center of a palisading granuloma. In granuloma annulare, the necrobiotic zone contains mucin, while in rheumatoid nodules there is usually fibrin within the necrobiotic area. The photomicrograph shows a zone of necrobiosis at the top left, surrounded by palisading epithelioid cells in a case of granuloma annulare involving the eyelid.

Orthokeratosis

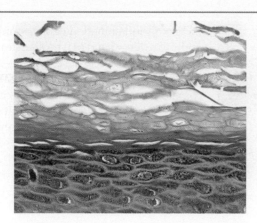

Orthokeratosis is an increased thickness of the horny layer (stratum corneum) by anucleate (i.e., normal appearing) cells. Orthokeratosis my be compact, laminated, or have a basket-weave configuration.

Papillomatosis

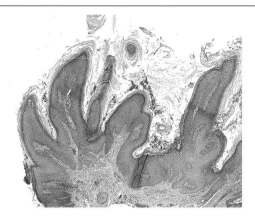

Papillomatosis is characterized histologically by abnormally elongated epidermis and papillary dermis resulting in irregular undulation of the epidermal surface. Papillomatosis is seen most commonly in seborrheic keratosis and verruca vulgaris (shown).

Parakeratosis

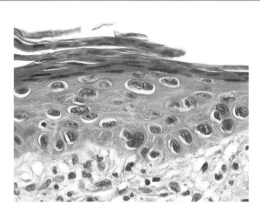

Parakeratosis is an increased thickness of the horny layer (stratum corneum) by nucleated cells. Parakeratosis represents a defect in cellular differentiation and is usually associated with a thinned or absent granular layer. An example of parakeratosis in a specimen with actinic keratosis is shown here.

Pigment Incontinence

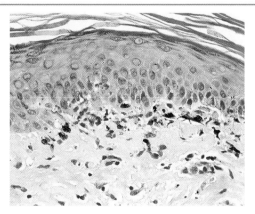

Pigment incontinence refers to the release of melanin granules from the epidermis and its resulting deposition in the upper dermis either free or within macrophages (melanophages).

Pseudocarcinomatous (Pseudoepitheliomatous) Hyperplasia

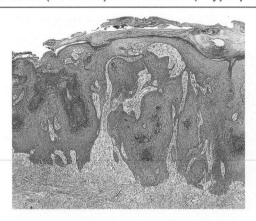

Pseudocarcinomatous hyperplasia is a histopathological reaction pattern manifest as irregular hyperplasia of the epidermis with prominent acanthotic downgrowth of the epidermis. The epidermal proliferation occurs in response to a wide range of stimuli including chronic irritation, trauma, and dermal fungal infections. Pseudocarcinomatous hyperplasia differs from squamous cell carcinoma by having minimal cytological atypia and fewer mitoses.

Psoriasiform Dermatitis

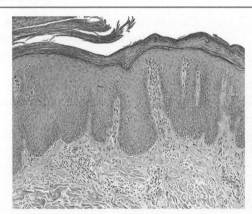

Psoriasiform dermatitis, also known as superficial dermatitis with psoriasiform proliferation, refers to a form of epidermal thickening with uniform elongation of rete ridges that extend downward into the dermis. Parakeratosis is common. The nature of the inflammatory cells in the dermis, the presence and degree of spongiosis, and the presence of exocytosis are features that aid in rendering a more specific diagnosis.

Shadow Cell

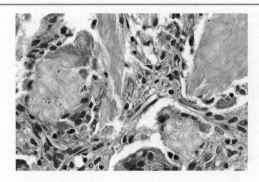

Shadow cells, also known as ghost cells, are characteristic of pilomatrixomas. They are pale, eosinophilic cells with a clear area in place of the nucleus.

Spongiosis

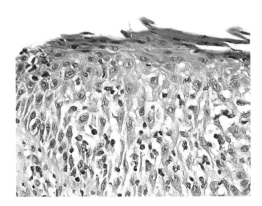

Spongiosis is intercellular edema between squamous cells of the epidermis. It is characteristic of acute dermatitis and may lead to micro- and macro-vesicles (spongiotic blisters). Intracellular edema may accompany severe spongiosis, resulting in bursting of epidermal cells and formation of multilocular bulla.

Squamous Eddies

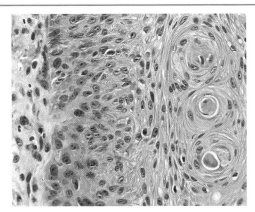

Squamous eddies are whorled onionskin-like foci of brightly eosinophilic keratinocytes. They are a typical feature of irritated seborrheic keratoses.

Touton Giant Cell

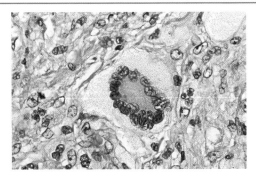

Touton giant cells are multinucleated giant cells derived from fusion of epithelioid cells (activated macrophages). They have a ring of nuclei surrounding eosinophilic non-vacuolated cytoplasm centrally and lipid-filled foamy cytoplasm peripherally. They are characteristic of xanthogranulomas.

Vesicle

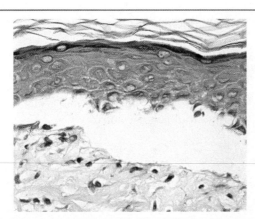

A vesicle is a small blister, generally less than 0.5 cm in diameter. A subepidermal blister is shown.

Chapter 6

Surgical Management of Eyelid Lesions

Some eyelid lesions can be identified by their history and clinical appearance, and then treated appropriately. However, many benign lesions can be confused with more aggressive malignant tumors from which they must be differentiated. When doubt exists as to a specific diagnosis, a biopsy should be obtained and submitted for histopathologic evaluation. Based on the findings a more directed therapeutic approach can then be planned. In some cases such as inflammatory lesions medical therapy alone might be indicated. But for malignant and premalignant neoplasms or for benign lesions that are of cosmetic or functional concern further surgery is often necessary.

When biopsy is necessary for diagnosis there are several techniques that are useful depending upon the lesion and location. In some cases representative tissue only is obtained with most of the lesion left behind. In other techniques an attempt is made to remove the entire lesion.

BIOPSY TECHNIQUES
Shave Biopsy

For elevated lesions of uncertain etiology, especially those on the lid margin, the shave biopsy is a useful procedure. It provides a representative sample of tissue for the pathologist without risking lash loss, eyelid deformity or other complications. In this procedure a scalpel is used to shave off the elevated portion of the lesion flat with the surrounding eyelid (Fig. 1). Light cautery or pressure is applied, with care taken not to injure eyelash follicles. If the lesions is benign or can be treated medically, then no further surgery is necessary. However, if the results require complete excision then a more definitive wedge resection can be performed, preferably under frozen section control.

Incisional Biopsy

For large lesions that cannot be removed as an initial procedure or for which a simple shave is not appropriate, a small segment of the tumor can be excised and submitted for histopathologic exam. As with the shave biopsy, some tumor is intentionally left behind to be managed by further surgery or ancillary therapy once a definitive diagnosis is available. The incisional biopsy should include a representative portion of the tumor plus a segment of the margin to show some adjacent normal tissue (Fig. 2).

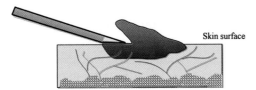

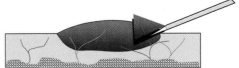

Figure 1   Technique of shave biopsy where a portion of the lesion is shaved flush with the surrounding eyelid skin.

Figure 2   Incisional biopsy with a representative sample of the lesion is excised leaving most of the lesion behind.

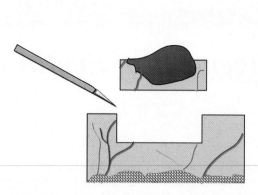 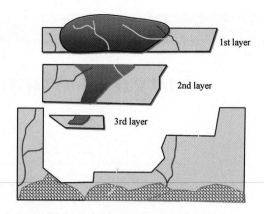

Figure 3 In the excisional biopsy the entire lesion is removed with a small zone of normal tissue.

Figure 4 The Mohs microsurgical technique employs a sequential tangential layered excision procedure with histologic examination of all margins.

Excisional Biopsy

When the lesion is small enough so that it can likely be completely removed at an initial procedure the excisional biopsy is best. This is especially true if a benign tumor is suspected so that clear margins are of less concern. A small rim of normal tissue is taken around the margins of the lesion and care is taken to remain deep to the involved tissue (Fig. 3). For suspected malignant tumors or for benign lesions with a high recurrence rate when incompletely removed, excision should be performed under frozen section control.

Mohs Microsurgical Excision

For all malignant tumors around the eyelids the Mohs procedure gives the highest cure rate, generally in the 99.0–99.5% range. Sequential tangential layers are cut and all surfaces are marked for identification. Histologic examination of the entire cut surface is performed by a trained Mohs surgeon and detailed maps are made to note the precise location of any residual tumor. Additional layers are then cut in areas where residual pathology is noted (Fig. 4). The procedure is continued until all margins are free of tumor. In most cases the defect will require reconstruction using local tissue flaps or grafts. For small defects on non-mobile areas such as the nasal bridge, cheek, or temple, it can sometimes be left to granulate spontaneously.

EYELID RECONSTRUCTION TECHNIQUES
Primary Layered Closure

For smaller defects involving the non-marginal skin and muscle, or full-thickness marginal eyelid, repair can be accomplished by directly re-approximating the individual layers. Non-marginal skin defects can be excised with an elliptical incision (Fig. 5). Muscle and skin are then closed in separate layers. Some undermining of edges may be needed for slightly larger defects. For marginal eyelid defects in younger patients where tissues show less laxity, a 25% lid defect can usually be closed without difficulty. In older patients it may be possible to close 40–50% or more. With modification of the basic technique by cutting the lateral canthal tendon, even larger defects can often be closed primarily. It is important to align the lid margin and lash line first, and then the tarsus, orbicularis, and skin in separate layers to avoid any cosmetic deformity (Fig. 6).

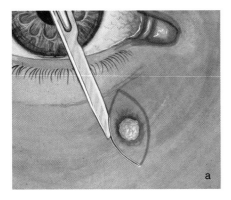 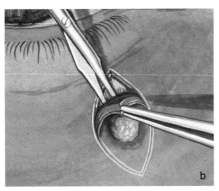 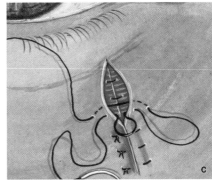

Figure 5 The elliptical excision is used for small lesions where the defect can be closed primarily. *Source*: From Dutton JJ. Atlas of Ophthalmic Surgery, Volume II. Oculoplastic, Lacrimal, and Orbital Surgery. St. Louis: Mosby Year Book, 1992.

Free Tarsoconjunctival Graft

For full thickness defects that are too large to close primarily, a graft taken from the posterior surface of the ipsilateral or contralateral upper eyelid will provide both conjunctiva and tarsus to reconstruct the posterior lamella. The donor site is left to granulate. The graft is sutured to the residual tarsus or canthal tendons in the recipient site and then covered by a sliding myocutaneous flap to reconstruct the anterior lamella (Fig. 7). This technique works equally well for the lower or upper eyelid.

Rhombic Flap

The rhombic flap is a rotational type flap for repair of small quadrangular defects in the para-orbital region. It can be designed from any of four quadrants around the defect by marking out a V-shaped cut from one of the corners (Fig. 8). When closed, tension is concentrated across the arms of the V so that the flap can be planned to avoid vertical tension that might distort the eyelid. Once the V is closed there is no residual tension on the flap. The procedure yields excellent cosmetic and functional results.

Cutler-Beard Procedure

When a total or near total upper eyelid is missing the Cutler-Beard procedure is one of the major techniques available for reconstruction. A full-thickness horizontal blepharotomy is cut 4 to 5 mm below the lower lid lash line across the entire lid, and the incisions are then extended vertically to the inferior fornix to create a flap (Fig. 9). This leaves a bridge of marginal eyelid supported

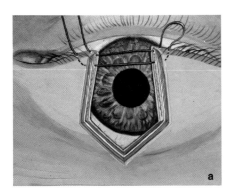 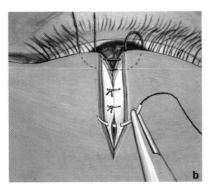 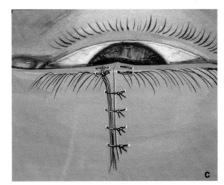

Figure 6 Primary layered closure is used for full-thickness marginal defects where all tissues are re-apposed in layers. *Source*: From Dutton JJ. Atlas of Ophthalmic Surgery, Volume II. Oculoplastic, Lacrimal, and Orbital Surgery. St. Louis: Mosby Year Book, 1992.

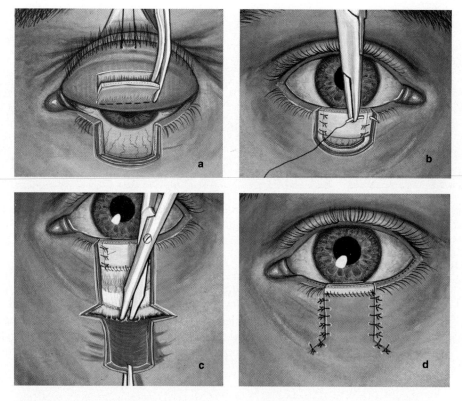

Figure 7 For full-thickness partial lid defects a free tarso-conjunctival graft from upper to lower lid is then covered with a myocutaneous flap. *Source*: From Dutton JJ. Atlas of Ophthalmic Surgery, Volume II. Oculoplastic, Lacrimal, and Orbital Surgery. St. Louis: Mosby Year Book, 1992.

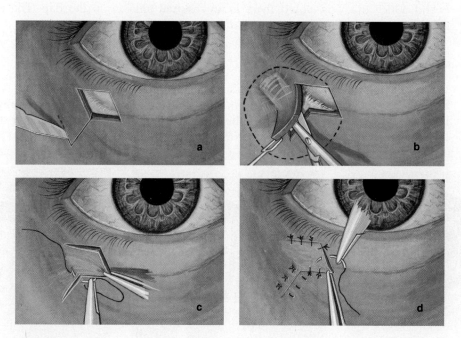

Figure 8 The rhombic flap is useful for non-marginal lesions where vertical tension on the eyelids can be avoided. *Source*: From Dutton JJ. Atlas of Ophthalmic Surgery, Volume II. Oculoplastic, Lacrimal, and Orbital Surgery. St. Louis: Mosby Year Book, 1992.

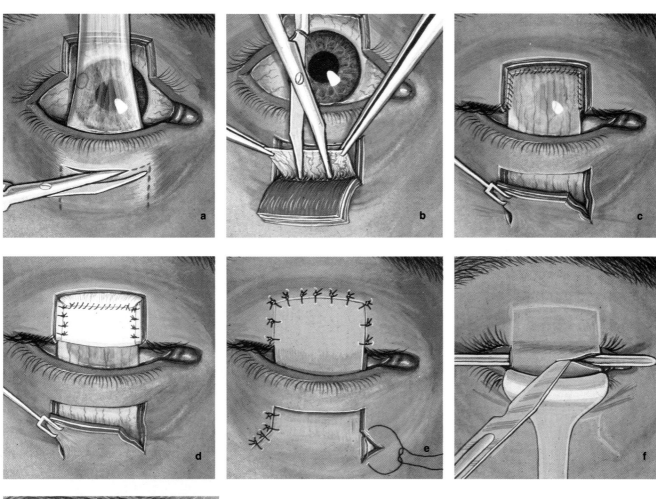

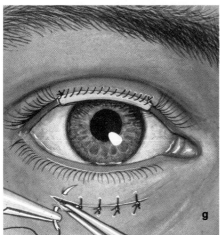

Figure 9 The Cutler-Beard procedure is used for near total upper eyelid defects. *Source*: From Dutton JJ. Atlas of Ophthalmic Surgery, Volume II. Oculoplastic, Lacrimal, and Orbital Surgery. St. Louis: Mosby Year Book, 1992.

by the medial and lateral palpebral arteries. Layers of the flap are advanced beneath the bridge and sutured to corresponding layers in the upper lid defect. Sclera or other material can be placed between the conjunctiva and orbicularis muscle and attached to the levator aponeurosis to approximate the tarsus. After three weeks the flap is cut at an appropriate length and the lower lid is repaired by reattaching the marginal bridge. Although lashes are lacking on the new reconstructed upper lid, the procedure gives an excellent functional and cosmetic result.

Hughes Tarsoconjunctival Flap Procedure

The Hughes procedure is a two-staged operation for reconstruction of total or near total lower eyelid defects. As with the free tarsoconjunctival graft, a block of tarsus and conjunctiva is marked out on the ipsilateral upper lid. However, the upper border is left attached superiorly and a conjunctival flap is dissected off of the underlying Müller's muscle to the superior fornix (Fig. 10). The tarsal flap is advanced down into the lower lid defect and sutured to residual tarsus or canthal tendons and the lower lid retractors. The anterior lamella is reconstructed with a skin graft or myocutaneous flap. After three weeks the conjunctival flap is cut off along the new lower lid margin.

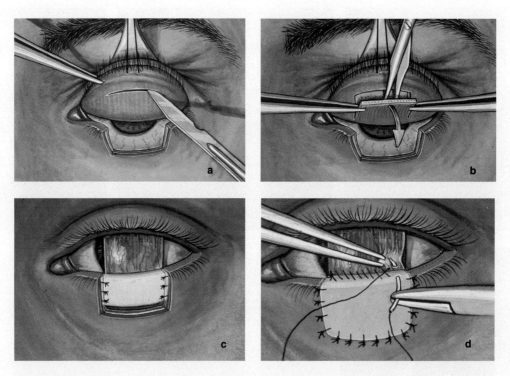

Figure 10 The Hughes tarso-conjunctival flap is the major procedure for total lower eyelid reconstruction. *Source*: From Dutton JJ. Atlas of Ophthalmic Surgery, Volume II. Oculoplastic, Lacrimal, and Orbital Surgery. St. Louis: Mosby Year Book, 1992.

REFERENCES

Dutton JJ. Atlas of Ophthalmic Surgery. Vol. II. Oculoplastic, Lacrimal, and Orbital Surgery. St. Louis: Mosby Year Book, 1992.

Nerad JA. Oculoplastic Surgery. Krachmer JH (ed). The Requisites in Ophthalmology. St. Louis: Mosby Year Book, 2001.

Chapter 7

Atlas of Eyelid Malpositions

Ankyloblepharon
Blepharochalasis
Blepharophimosis Syndrome
Blepharoptosis
Brow Ptosis
Chronic Progressive External
  Ophthalmoplegia
Coloboma
Cryptophthalmos
Dermatochalasis
Distichiasis
Ectropion
Entropion
Epiblepharon
Epicanthal Folds
Essential Blepharospasm

Euryblepharon
Floppy Eyelid Syndrome
Hemifacial Spasm
Horner's Syndrome
Madarosis
Marcus-Gunn Jaw Winking
  Syndrome
Microblepharon
Oromandibular Dystonia
Prolapsed Orbital Fat
Retraction of the Eyelid
Steatoblepharon
Tarsal Kink Syndrome
Telecanthus
Trichiasis

Ankyloblepharon

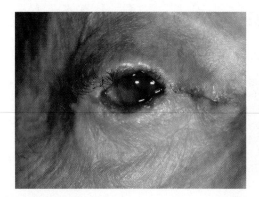 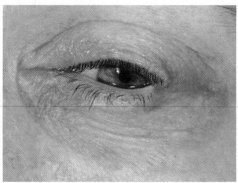

INTRODUCTION   Ankyloblepharon is a condition where the eyelid margins are fused together to varying degrees. In congenital ankyloblepharon the fused eyelids fail to completely separate during embryogenesis. It can occur as a sporadic isolated finding or in association with diverse chromosomal and syndromic conditions characterized by failure of separation of apposed tissues suggesting a common defect in the mechanisms that regulate tissue fusion. It has also been associated with trisomy 18. The condition may be complete, partial, or interrupted. In the latter, called ankyloblepharon filiforme, multiple epithelial bands are present between the upper and lower lid margins. More commonly, in partial ankyloblepharon, the horizontal palpebral fissure is shortened. Ankyloblepahron can also be seen following trauma, chemical burs, cicatrizing diseases such as Stevens-Johnson syndrome or cicatricial ocular phemphigoid, or inflammations such as ulcerative blepharitis or herpes simplex.

CLINICAL CHARACTERISTICS   In simple congenital ankyloblepharon the eyelid margins are usually fused laterally, and less commonly medially. The condition frequently accompanies other developmental anomalies such as anophthalmos, microphthalmos, ptosis, or cleft lip. In many cases the lateral canthal angle is displaced downward giving an antimongaloid slope to the palpebral fissure. The lateral canthal tendon is lax or not developed so that there is also significant laxity of the lower eyelids. In ankyloblepharon filiforme adnatum one or more narrow epithelial bands connect the central upper and lower eyelid margins. These vary from 0.5 to 5 mm in width, and may range from 1 to 10 mm in length. The zone of attachment is between the eyelashes and the meibomian gland orifices. In cases of total ankyloblepharon lacrimal secretions may accumulate beneath the lids forming a large fluid cyst. Ankyloblepahron is most commonly confused with euryblepharon since in both cases the lateral portion of the lid may be lax and displaced downward. However, in ankyloblepharon the eyelid margins are fused together for some distance giving a shorter horizontal fissure, whereas in euryblepharon the fissure is longer than normal.

TREATMENT   Treatment of ankyloblepharon is surgical and is indicated for improvement of visual field or for cosmetic improvement. A lateral canthoplasty with widening of the palpebral fissure by tightening the lateral canthal tendon will help in mild cases. In more extensive cases where the horizontal fissure is very narrow, a lateral canthotomy is performed with reconstruction of the eyelid margins by folding over the conjunctiva to cover the marginal tarsus. In ankyloblepharon filiforme simple lysis of the epithelial bands is sufficient.

REFERENCES

Bacal DA, Nelson LB, Zackai EH, et al. Ankyloblepharon filiforme adnatum in trisomy 18. J Pediatr Ophthalmol Strabismus 1993; 30:337–339.

Bajaj MS, Pushker N, Balasubramanya R. Massive tear fluid cysts as a sequel of acquired ankyloblepharon. Clin Experiment Ophthalmol 2003; 31:452–453.

Canpanella PC, Rosenwasser GO, Sassani JW, Goldberg SH. Herpes simplex blepharoconjunctivitis presenting as complete acquired ankyloblepharon. Cornea 1997; 16:360–361.

Insler MS, Helm CJ. Ankyloblepharon associated with systemic 5-fluorouracil treatment. Ann Ophthalmol 1987; 19:374–375.

Jain S, Atkinson AJ, Hopkisson B. Ankyloblepharon filiforme adnatum. Br J Ophthalmol 1997; 81:708.

Kumar P, Punnoose SE, Jain V. Grade I ankyloblepharon following chemical burn. Plast Reconstr Surg 2005; 116:1175–1176.

Ozyazgan I, Eskitascoglu T, Dundar M, Karac S. Hereditary isolated ankyloblepharon filiforme adnatum. Plast Reconstr Surg 2005; 115:363–364.

Patil BB, Mohammed KK. Ankyloblepharon filiforme adnatum. Eye 2001; 15:813–815.

Weiss AH, Riscile G, Kousseff BG. Ankyloblepharon filifome adnatum. Am J Med Genet 1992; 42:369–373.

Blepharochalasis

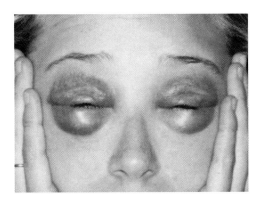 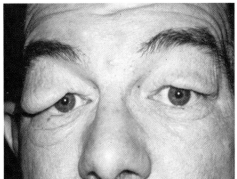

INTRODUCTION   Blepharochalasis is a rare disorder that usually affects the upper eyelids of young individuals less than 20 years old. The etiology is unknown. IgA deposits have been found within the periorbital tissues suggesting an underlying immune mechanism. Elastin mRNA expression is not decreased in affected eyelids compared to normal control fibroblasts suggesting that environmental or other matrix components of elastin are involved in the loss of elastin fibers. A few cases show an autosomal dominant pattern of inheritance. Blepharochalasis can be associated with other skin disorders such as dermatomyositis.

CLINICAL CHARACTERISTICS   Blepharochalasis begins with an early active phase characterized by recurrent episodes of mild, transient, painless eyelid edema. There then follows a later quiescent phase where the eyelid skin becomes redundant and baggy, with atrophic thinning and wrinkling. The upper eyelid skin hangs loosely in folds over the eyelid margin. There may be areas of dehiscence in the orbital septum with fat prolapse into the baggy skin. The levator aponeurosis can be stretched resulting in ptosis, and the lacrimal gland may prolapse into the lateral eyelid. Secondary blepharophimosis, ectropion, and pseudoepicanthal folds may be seen. As the patient ages these changes are exacerbated by normal aging.

Blepharochalasis (Contd.)

TREATMENT
Treatment is surgical and may require multiple procedures. Excess eyelid skin is excised as for a standard blepharoplasty and ptosis is corrected with levator aponeurosis advancement. When there is associated fat atrophy, fat grafts may be appropriate. Lacrimal gland prolapse is repaired by refixation to the orbital rim.

REFERENCES

Bergin DJ, McCord CD, Berger T, Friedberg H, Waterhouse W. Blepharochalasis. Br J Ophthalmol 1988; 72:863–867.

Braakenburg A, Nicolai JP. Bilateral eyelid edema: cutis laxa or blepharochalasis? Ann Plast Surg 2000; 45:538–540.

Collin JR. Blepharochalasis. A review of 30 cases. Ophthal Plast Reconstr Surg 1991; 7:153–157.

Custer PL, Tenzel RR, Kowalczyk AP. Blepharochalasis syndrome. Am J Ophthalmol 1985; 99:424–428.

Dozsa A, Karolyi ZS, Degrell P. Bilateral blepharochalasis. J Eur Acad Dermatol Venerol 2005; 19:725–728.

Dutton JJ. Atlas of ophthalmic surgery. Vol. II. Oculoplastic, Lacrimal, and Orbital Surgery. St Louis: Mosby Year Book, 1992:36–59.

Huemer GM, Schoeller T, Wechselberger G, et al. Unilateral blepharochalasis. Br J Surg 2003; 56:293–295.

Hundal KS, Mearza AA, Joshi N. Lacrimal gland prolapse in blepharochalasis. Eye 2004; 18:429–430.

Jordan DR. Blepharochalasis syndrome: a proposed pathophysiologic mechanism. Can J Ophthalmol 1992; 27:10–15.

Kaneoya K, Momota Y, Hatamouchi A, et al. Elastin gene expression in blepharochalasis. J Dermatol 2005; 32:26–29.

Langley KE, Patrinely JR, Anderson RL, Thiese SM. Unilateral blepharochalasis. Ophthalmic Surg 1987; 18:594–598.

Schaeppi H, Emberger M, Wieland U, et al. Unilateral blepharochalasis with IgA-deposits. Hautarzt 2002; 53:613–617.

Blepharophimosis Syndrome

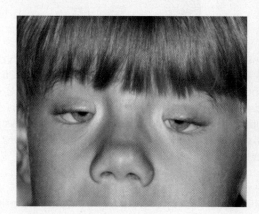 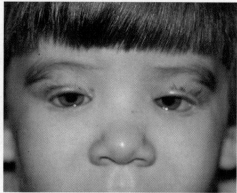

INTRODUCTION
This is a group of related congenital eyelid deformities with a strong autosomal dominant hereditary etiology although sporadic cases also occur. Blepharophimosis refers to a horizontal narrowing of the palpebral fissure, and the syndrome (known as BPES) is characterized by blepharophimosis, ptosis, and epicanthus inversus. Depending upon the presence (type I) or absence (type II) of premature ovarian failure, two clinical forms have been described. Both forms have been mapped to chromosome 3q23 and are due to mutations of a forkhead

transcription factor FOXL2 gene. Intelligence is not affected and there are no associated systemic abnormalities. The condition is always bilateral and symmetrical. Blepharophimosis is also seen as a part of other syndromes including Michels syndrome (blepharophimosis plus cleft lip and-palate, and mental retardation), Carnevale syndrome (blepharophimosis plus abnormal ears, strabismus, and umbilical diastasis), OSA syndrome (blepharophimosis plus humeroradial synostosis and spinal abnormalities), van den Ende-Gupta syndrome (blepharophimosis plus arachnodactyly and congenital contractures), the Schwartz-Jampel syndrome (blepharophimosis plus ptosis and blepharospasm), and Ohdo syndrome (blepharophimosis plus mental retardation, dental hypoplasia, and partial deafness).

CLINICAL CHARACTERISTICS   There is a wide variation in the range and degree of features seen in this disorder. The classical appearance is of reduced horizontal length of the palpebral fissures, flattening of the supraorbital ridges, and arching of the eyebrows. The upper lids show varying degrees of myogenic ptosis that may be so severe as to result in marked backward head tilt. The upper eyelid crease is usually absent. Epicanthus inversus is present and may be mild to severe. A manifest strabismus is seen in 20% of children, mostly esotropia, and 35% have refractive errors enough to warrant corrective lenses. Forty percent of children will have some degree of amblyopia. Telecanthus may be present but the extent is variable. Rare cases have been described associated with other ophthalmic abnormalities including Duane syndrome, microphthalmos, and ocular colobomas. Acquired blepharophimosis is associated with laxity or disinsertion of the lateral canthal tendon.

TREATMENT   Treatment is indicated when visual function is threatened or for improved cosmesis. When the ptosis is severe enough to cause amblyopia, repair must be undertaken at an early age. When levator muscle function is poor or absent a frontalis suspension procedure will be required. Correction of the epicanthus and telecanthus are best delayed until the child is at least two years old in order to allow for tissues around the nose to develop enough to make surgery easier. In most cases any telecanthus does not have to be repaired since correction of the epicanthus will give adequate cosmetic results. The epicanthus is repaired with a Y to V procedure or a more complicated four-flap technique that combines a Y to V with multiple Z-plasties. When telecanthus is to be corrected, medial displacement of the canthal tendons with or without resection of bone will usually be required.

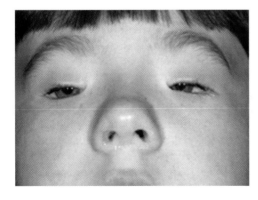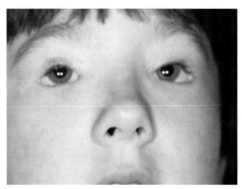

REFERENCES

Beaconsfield M, Walker JW, Collin JR. Visual development in the blepahrophimosis syndrome. Br J Ophthalmol 1991; 75:746–748.

Beckingsale PS, Sullivan TJ, Wong VA, Oley C. Blepharophimosis: a recommendation for early surgery in patients with severe ptosis. Clin Experimental Ophthalmol 2003; 31:138–142.

Custer PL, Tenzel RR, Kowalczyk AP. Blepharophimosis syndrome. Am J Ophthalmol 1985; 99:424–428.

Dawson EL, Hardy TG, Collin JR, Lee JP. The incidence of strabismus and refractive error in patients with blepahrophimosis, ptosis and epicanthus inversus syndrome (BPES). Strabismus 2003; 11:173–177.

Lee LR, Sullivan TJ. Blepharophimosis syndrome: association with colobomatous microphthalmos. Aust NZ J Ophthalmol 1995; 23:145–147.

Mauriello JA Jr, Caputo AR. Treatment of congenital forms of telecanthus with custom designed titanium medial canthal screws. Ophthal Plast Reconstr Surg 1994; 10:195–199.

Nowinski TS. Correction of telecanthus in the blepharophimosis syndrome. Int Ophthalmol Clin 1992; 32:157–164.

Panidis D, Rousso D, Vavilis D, Skiadopoulos S, Kalogeropoulos A. Familial blepharophimosis with ovarian dysfunction. Human Reprod 1994; 9:2034–2037.

Stromme P, Sandboe FR. Blepharophimosis-ptosis-epicanthus inversus syndrome (BPES). Acta Ophthalmol Scand 1996; 74:45–47.

Zlotogora J, Sagi M, Cohen T. The blepharophimosis, ptosis, and epicanthus inversus syndrome: delineation of two types. Am J Hum Genet 1983; 35:1020–1027.

Blepharoptosis

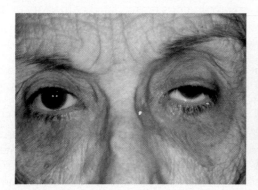 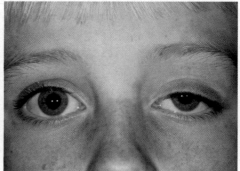

INTRODUCTION   Blepharoptosis, or ptosis, is a drooping of the upper eyelid such that the eyelid margin rests lower with respect to the superior corneal limbus. There are numerous causes for ptosis and these can be classified according to mechanistic etiologies. Aponeurotic ptosis is caused by defects in the levator aponeurosis, either redundancy or frank disinsertion. This can be seen from trauma or surgery, or as an involutional phenomenon which is the most common form of adult acquired ptosis. Myogenic ptosis results from myopathic or myogenic diseases affecting the levator muscle. It most commonly occurs as a congenital developmental defect, but can be associated with chronic progressive external ophthalmoplegia, myotonic dystrophy, oculopharyngeal dystrophy, myasthenia gravis, trauma, or toxins. In neurogenic ptosis there is an interruption of nervous innervation to the levator muscle. Etiologies include vascular lesions, ischemia, multiple sclerosis, toxins, infections, tumors, and trauma. Depending upon the site of neural injury there may be an associated palsy of other extraocular muscles innervated by the oculomotor nerve. Also included in this group are the so-called synkinetic syndromes such as the Marcus Gunn Jaw Wink, and misdirected third nerve fibers. Horner's syndrome resulting from loss of sympathetic innervation to Müller's accessory sympathetic muscle is also grouped under the neurogenic ptoses. Mechanical ptosis refers to a physical restriction to eyelid opening by an orbital or eyelid mass or scarring.

CLINICAL PRESENTATION   In all forms of ptosis the eyelid margin lies more than two millimeters below the superior corneal limbus. The condition may be unilateral or bilateral. The ptosis may be mild or severe, and often results in significant loss of superior visual field. In severe bilateral congenital myogenic ptosis a backward head tilt is often seen. Levator muscle function is typically good to excellent (8 or more mm) in aponeurotic, but is usually reduced in myogenic or neurogenic ptosis. In unilateral aponeurotic ptosis the degree of lid droop in the affected eyelid remains constant with respect to the normal opposite eye in all positions of vertical gaze. Typically, the ptosis becomes worse at night or when the patient is tired. In unilateral myogenic ptosis the degree of lid droop increases in upgaze, but decrease in downgaze or the affected lid may even be relatively retracted. This is because of fibrosis of the levator muscle that does not contract or stretch very well. Mechanical ptosis is usually associated with eyelid scars or masses, or with concurrent orbital disease.

TREATMENT   The goal of treatment for ptosis is to elevate the eyelid margin to a more normal position and to restore superior visual field. When levator muscle function is good or excellent correction simply requires a tightening or reattachment of the aponeurosis to the tarsal plate. This is achieved through a skin or transconjunctival incision. Surgery is best performed under local anesthesia to allow for patient cooperation in elevating the lid during surgery. When levator muscle function is only fair (5–8 mm) aponeurotic advancement alone will usually be inadequate. Shortening of the levator muscle above the level of Whitnall's ligament will allow greater degrees of shortening and a better result. For poor levator function cases (4 mm or less), the only reliable method of elevating the lid is with a frontalis suspension procedure using a silicone rod or other suspensory material.

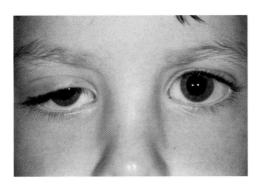 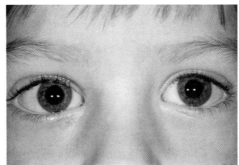

REFERENCES

Anderson RL, Dixon RS. Aponeurotic ptosis surgery. Arch Ophthalmol 1979; 97:1123–1128.

Anderson RL, Gordy DD. Aponeurotic defects in congenital ptosis. Ophthalmology 1979; 86:1493–1500.

Anderson RL, Jordan DR, Dutton JJ. Whitnall's sling for poor function ptosis. Arch Ophthalmol 1990; 108: 1628–1632.

Ben Simon GJ, Lee S, Schwartz RM, McCann JD, Goldberg RA. External levator advancement vs Muller's muscle-conjunctival resection for correction of upper eyelid involutional ptosis. Am J Ophthalmol 2005; 140:426–432.

Ben Simon GJ, Macedo AA, Schwartz RM, Wang DY, McCann JD, Goldberg RA. Frontalis suspension for upper eyelid ptosis: evaluation of different surgical designs and suture material. Am J Ophthalmol 2005; 140:877–885.

Bernardini FP, de Consiliis C, Devoto MH. Frontalis suspension sling using a silicone rod in patients affected by myogenic blepharoptosis. Orbit 2002; 21:195–198.

Bowyer JD, Sullivan TJ. Management of Marcus Gunn Jaw winking synkinesis. Ophthal Plast Reconstr Surg 2004; 20:92–98.

Burnstine MA, Putterman AM. Management of myopathic ptosis. Ophthalmology 2002; 109:1023–1031.

Callahan M, Beard C. Beard's Ptosis, 4th Edition. Birmingham, England: Aesculapius, 1990.

Dutton JJ. A Color Atlas of Ptosis: A Practical Guide to Evaluation and Management. Singapore: PG Publishing, 1988.

Dutton JJ. Atlas of Ophthalmic Surgery. Vol. II, Oculoplastic, Lacrimal, and Orbital Surgery. St Louis: Mosby Year Book, 1992: 70–93.

Erb MH, Kersten RC, Yip CC, Hudak D, Kulwin DR, McCulley TJ. Effect of unilateral blepharoptosis repair on contralateral eyelid position. Ophthal Plast Reconstr Surg 2004; 20(6):418–422.

Frueh BR. The mechanistic classification of ptosis. Ophthalmology 1980; 87:1019–1021.

Jordan DR. Correcting aponeurotic ptosis. Ophthalmology 2006; 113(1):163–164.

Lee AG. Ocular myasthenia gravis. Curr Opin Ophthalmol 1996; 7:39–41.

Mauriello JA, Wagner RS, Caputo AR, Natale B, Lister M. Treatment of congenital ptosis by maximum levator resection. Ophthalmology 1986; 93:466–469.

Putterman AM, Urist MJ. Mueller muscle-conjunctival resection. Technique for treatment of blepharoptosis. Arch Ophthalmol 1975; 93:619–623.

Weinstein GS, Buerger GF Jr. Modification of the Mueller's muscle-conjunctival resection operation for blepharoptosis. Am J Ophthalmol 1982; 93:647–651.

Brow Ptosis

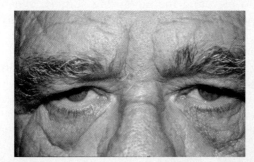 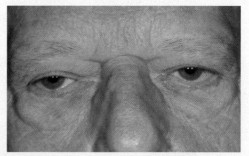

INTRODUCTION   Brow ptosis results from sagging of forehead skin and loss of fascial support of the eyebrows to the frontal bone. It is a common deformity in the aging face and frequently accompanies laxity of other periorbital structures, such as eyelid skin and canthal tendons. A downward displacement of the eyebrows can accentuate the degree of redundancy in upper eyelid skin and result in significant loss of superior visual field. The ptosis may be general, involving the entire width of the brow, or more exaggerated medially, or more commonly, laterally. Often associated with brow ptosis is descent of the sub-brow fat pad producing a thickened upper eyelid. Failure to recognize brow ptosis as a contributing factor in upper eyelid surgery can lead to a disappointing result from ptosis repair and/or blepharoplasty alone.

CLINICAL CHARACTERISTICS   In the normal face the brows typically lie at about the level of the orbital rim medially and above the rim centrally and laterally. The male brow has a flatter contour especially medially, whereas the female brow usually shows a greater arc. When brow ptosis is present part or all of the brow lies below the superior orbital rim. The sub-brow fat pad frequently descends into the upper eyelid and excess skin hangs down to simulate or exacerbate dermatochalasis. Laterally, excess skin may hang in cascading folds that cover the lateral canthal angle and may extend onto the temple. With medial brow ptosis the glabellar skin forms horizontal folds over the bridge of the nose. Brow ptosis may result in a pseudoblepharoptosis which cannot be adequately repaired with standard aponeurotic advancement techniques.

TREATMENT Several procedures are available for the correction of brow ptosis. The choice depends upon a number of factors: (*i*) the sex of the patient and, therefore, the desired brow contour; (*ii*) the relative position of the brows; (*iii*) the density of the brow cilia; (*iv*) the presence of associated deformities such as "crow's feet" and prominent transverse glabellar folds; and (*v*) the height of the scalp hair line or presence of male-pattern baldness. Each procedure has its advantages and disadvantages, and selecting the most appropriate operation must be individualized for each patient. The brow pexy is the simplest technique where the deep fascia of the frontalis muscle is fixed to periosteum to prevent the action of gravity from pulling the brows downward. More recently the trans-blepharoplasty Endotine (Coapt) has made this procedure more effective. In the direct brow lift an ellipse of skin is removed from above the brow, leaving a fine scar just above the brow hairs. However, this tends to arch the brow contour more than in a normal male brow. When there is associated forehead ptosis a forehead elevation can be achieved through an endoscopic lift or via a coronal lift. In all cases of brow ptosis repair, the brows should be repositioned before excision of residual dermatochalasis.

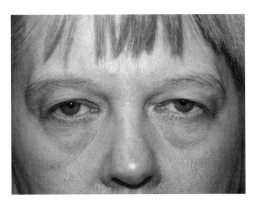 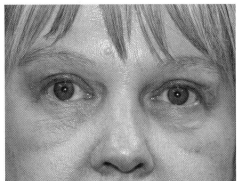

REFERENCES

Booth AJ, Murray A, Tyers AG. The direct brow lift: efficacy, complications, and patient satisfaction. Br J Ophthalmol 2004; 88:688–691.

Brennan HG. Correction of the ptotic brow. Otolaryngol Clin North Am 1980; 13:265–273.

Carruthers J. Brow lifting and blepharoplasty. Dermatol Clin 2001; 19:531–533.

Chen AH, Frankel AS. Altering brow contour with botulinum toxin. Facial Plast Surg Clin North Am 2003; 11:457–464.

Connell B. Brow ptosis–local resections. In: Aston SJ, ed. Third International Symposium of Plastic and Reconstructive Surgery of the Eye and Adnexa. Baltimore: Williams and Wilkins, 1982.

Dailey RA, Saulny SM. Current treatments for brow ptosis. Curr Opin Ophthalmol 2003; 14:260–266.

Goldstein SM, Katowitz JA. The male eyebrow: a topographic anatomic analysis. Ophthal Plast Reconstr Surg 2005; 21:285–291.

Holck DE, Ng JD, Wiseman JB, Foster JA. The endoscopic browlift for forehead rejuvenation. Semin Ophthalmol 1998; 13:149–157.

Johnson CM Jr, Anderson JR, Katz RB. The brow-lift. Arch Otolaryngol 1978; 105:124–126.

Niechajev I. Transpalpebral browpexy. Plast Reconstr Surg 2004; 113:172–180.

Paul MD. The evolution of the brow lift in aesthetic plastic surgery. Plast Reconstr Surg 2001; 108:1409–1424.

Tower RN, Dailey RA. Endoscopic pretrichial brow lift: surgical indications, technique and outcomes. Ophthal Plast Reconstr Surg 2004; 20:268–273.

Watson SW, Niamtu J 3rd, Cunningham LL Jr. The endoscopic brow and midface lift. Atlas Oral Maxillofac Surg Clin North Am 2003; 11:145–155.

Yeatts RP. Current concepts in brow lift surgery. Curr Opin Ophthalmol 1997; 8:46–50.

Chronic Progressive External Ophthalmoplegia

INTRODUCTION   Chronic progressive external ophthalmoplegia (CPEO) is a mitochondrial myopathy characterized by slowly progressive paralysis of the extraocular muscles. Although it can be seen in the absence of other clinical manifestations, CPEO is often associated with skeletal muscle weakness. It is a disorder of mitochondrial DNA where deletions of various lengths result in mitochondrial dysfunction. Since mtDNA codes for major components of cellular respiration tissues with a high oxidative demand, such as muscle, brain, and heart, are particularly affected. The extraocular muscles contain a higher than average amount of mitochondria so that these muscles are preferentially weakened. CPEO can occur as a sporadic mutation, as a point mutation of maternal mitochondrial tRNA, or as an autosomal dominant or autosomal recessive deletion of mtDNA. Kearns-Sayre syndrome (KSS) is a related mitochondrial myopathy characterized by early onset CPEO, pigmentary retinopathy, and cardiac conduction defects.

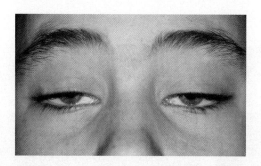

CLINICAL PRESENTATION   CPEO begins in young adulthood with bilateral and symmetrical ptosis as the first clinical sign. Ophthalmoplegia follows months to years later and with progression the patient adopts a chin-up head posture with contraction of the frontalis muscles to help elevate the upper lids. Ultimately the globes are frozen in the midline. Exposure keratopathy and loss of superior visual field are major complications. Because the muscle weakness is symmetric, patients do not complain of diplopia. Rarely, ophthalmoplegia can be seen in the absence of ptosis. Weakness of facial, neck, and shoulder muscles may also be seen giving the patient a flat facial appearance. Occasionally neurological abnormalities may be associated including cerebral ataxia or pendular nystagmus. In KSS the retina shows a salt and pepper pattern of pigment degeneration. The ophthalmoplegia generally precedes the cardiac defects.

TREATMENT   In most cases the major problem is loss of visual field due to poor function ptosis. This is treated with taping the lids up initially. In more advanced cases surgery will be needed. Since levator muscle function is poor, repair is usually by a very conservative frontalis suspension using a silicone rod. Care must be used since the Bells' phenomenon is extinguished. We prefer to simultaneously recess the lower lid upward to maintain a small palpebral fissure centralized over the pupil. Strabismus surgery can be useful in selected patients who experience diplopia. In all cases of CPEO a cardiac evaluation is essential to rule out KSS and conduction defects. Muscle biopsy shows ragged red fibers with abnormal aggregates of subsarcolemmal mitochondria. If present it may be managed with a pacemaker.

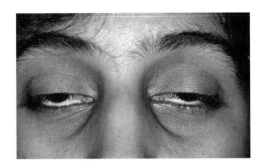 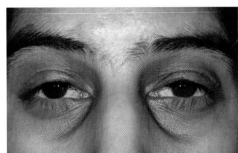

REFERENCES

Cohen JM, Waiss B. Combination ptosis crutch and moisture chamber for the management of chronic progressive external ophthalmoplegia. J Am Optom Assoc 1997; 68:663–667.

Danta G, Hilton RC, Lynch PG. Chronic progressive external ophthalmoplegia. Brain 1975; 98:473–492.

Fassati A, Bordoni A, Amboni P, et al. Chronic progressive external ophthalmoplegia: a correlative study of quantitative data and histochemical and biochemical profile. J Neurol Sci 1994; 123:140–146.

Gross-Jendroska M, Schatz H, McDonald HR, Johnson RN. Kearns-Sayre syndrome: a care report and review. Eur J Ophthalmol 1992; 2:15–20.

Kersten RC, Bernardini FP, Khouri L, et al. Unilateral frontalis sling for the surgical correction of unilateral poor-function ptosis. Ophthal Plast Reconstr Surg 2005; 21:412–416.

Kim JS, Kim CJ, Chi JG, Myung HJ. Chronic progressive external ophthalmoplegia (CPEO) with "ragged red fibers"—a case report. J Korean Med Sci 1989; 4:91–96.

Lee AG, Brazis PW. Chronic progressive external ophthalmoplegia. Curr Neurol Neurosci Rep 2002; 2:413–417.

Mitsumoto H, Aprille JR, Wray SH, Nemni R, Bradley WG. Chronic progressive external ophthalmoplegia (CPEO): clinical, morphologic, and biochemical studies. Neurology 1983; 33:452–461.

Phanthumchinda K, Sinswaiwong S, Jonpiputvanich S. Chronic progressive external ophthalmoplegia. J Med Assoc Thai 1997; 80:791–794.

Spina G, Capone A. A patient with Kearns-Sayre syndrome. Klin Monatsbl Augenheilkd 1994; 204:462–464.

Coloboma

INTRODUCTION   Coloboma refers to a condition where part of the eyelid is missing. It may be acquired from trauma or surgery. However, the term usually refers to a congenital developmental condition. Coloboma may be seen as an isolated defect or as part of craniofacial anomalies such as Goldenhar's syndrome and Tessier craniofacial cleft syndromes. They may also be seen with amniotic band syndrome where they result from a mechanical pressure of the band on the fetal eyelid. Alternatively, coloboma can result from failure of fusion of the embryonic eyelid folds, or when mesoderm fails to migrate into the developing eyelid.

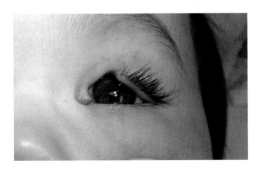

CLINICAL CHARACTERISTICS   The eyelid defect may vary from a small marginal notch to nearly complete absence of the lid. Colobomas are most commonly located in the medial to central upper lid. The edges are rounded and the defect tends to have a triangular shape. Full-thickness tissue is missing, but adjacent adnexal structures tend to be relatively normal. Occasionally colobomas may be bilateral without other ocular or facial anomalies.

TREATMENT   When of significant size colobomas cause corneal exposure. Initial management is with topical lubrication to protect the cornea until the child is old enough to undergo definitive repair. For small defects less than one-third of the eyelid length, surgical correction can be delayed until the child is 8 to 12 months old. However, for larger defects there is a significant threat to visual development and early surgical intervention is justified. Constant monitoring for refractive errors and corneal changes is required. When repair is undertaken lesions less than 25% of the lid width are closed directly by excising the edges and re-approximating them in anatomic layers. If the defect is larger it may require additional horizontal tissue by cutting the lateral canthal tendon or utilizing a Tenzel-type flap or tissue expansion. When most of the lid is missing a lid sharing operation, such as a Cutler-Beard procedure, must be used if the coloboma does not involve both upper and lower eyelids.

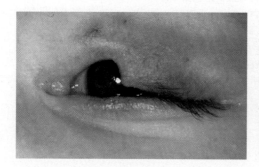 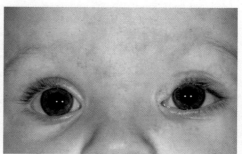

REFERENCES

Adegbehingbe BO, Olabanji JK, Adeoye AO. Isolated bilateral upper lid coloboma—a case report. Niger J Med 2005; 14:224–226.

Ankola PA, Abdel-Azim H. Congenital bilateral upper eyelid coloboma. J Perinatol 2003; 23:166–167.

Collin JR. Congenital upper lid coloboma. Aust N Z J Ophthalmol 1986; 14:313–317.

Miller MT, Deutsch TA, Cronin C, Keys CL. Amniotic bands as a cause of ocular anomalies. Am J Ophthalmol 1987; 15:270–279.

Nouby G. Congenital upper eyelid coloboma and cryptophthalmos. Ophthal Plast Reconstr Surg 2002; 18:373–377.

Seah LL, Choo CT, Fong KS. Congenital upper lid colobomas: management and visual outcome. Ophthal Plast Reconstr Surg 2002; 18:190–195.

Yeo LM, Willshaw HE. Large congenital upper lid coloboma—successful delayed conservative management. J Pediatr Ophthalmol Strabismus 1997; 34:190–192.

INTRODUCTION Cryptophthalmos syndrome is a rare congenital anomaly that manifests with varying degrees of completeness. It can be unilateral or bilateral. The condition occurs as an isolated anomaly in 20% of cases, whereas about 40% are familial. Cryptophthalmos can be seen with multiple congenital systemic malformations such as in Fraser syndrome where it is seen in 80% of affected individuals. Here it is associated with renal agenesis, laryngeal atresia, pulmonary hypoplasia, syndactyli, and low set ears. Such cases have been referred to as cryptophthalmos syndrome. They usually show an autosomal recessive pattern of inheritance, although several cases of dominant inheritance have been reported.

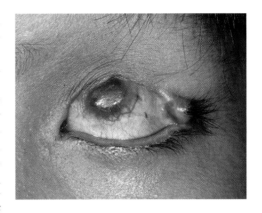

CLINICAL CHARACTERISTICS In cryptophthalmos the palpebral fissures are missing to varying degrees. The underlying globe is incompletely developed, showing early arrest in development of the anterior segment. The cornea is opaque. Various internal structural elements of the eyelid, such as tarsus, orbicularis, levator aponeurosis, and conjunctiva, as well as the brows may be missing. Several types of cryptophthalmos have been described showing different degrees of eyelid formation. In complete cryptophthalmos the lids and brows are absent and a sheet of skin extends over the disrupted eyes from forehead to cheeks. In incomplete cryptophthalmos the palpebral fissure may be partially formed while portions of the lids are not developed and fused to the globes. In abortive cryptophthalmos (congenital symblepharon) the lids and fissure are better developed but partially fused to the globe.

TREATMENT Infants with the syndromic form of cryptophthalmos often die at birth from associated pulmonary and laryngeal malformations. In less severe and isolated cases abnormalities of the eye preclude visual rehabilitation, but surgical repair of the eyelids may be desired for improved cosmesis. Because of the absence of structural elements of the lid, reconstruction is challenging and difficult. Skin and mucous membrane grafts can sometimes lead to an acceptable result. In the symblepharon variant, lysis of the adhesions with a mucous membrane or amniotic membrane graft may restore function to the lid.

REFERENCES

Brazier DJ, Hardman-Lea SJ, Collin JR. Cryptophthalmos: surgical treatment of the congenital symblepharon variant. Br J Ophthalmol 1986; 70:391–395.

Coulon P, Lan PT, Adenis JP, Verin P. Bilateral complete cryptophthalmos. Illustration with a case. Review of the literature. J Fr Ophthalmol 1994; 17:505–512.

Ghose S, Sihota R, Dayal Y. Symmetrical partial lateral "cryptophthalmos." A new concept of its embryological pathogenesis. Ophthalmic Paediatr Genet 1988; 9:67–76.

Gunduz K, Gunalp I. Congenital symblepharon (abortive cryptophthalmos) associated with meningoencephalocele. Ophthal Plast Reconstr Surg 1997; 13:139–141.

Momma WG, Biermann B. Cryptophthalmos: symptoms and treatment of a rare deformity. A case report. J Maxillofac Surg 1977; 5:208–210.

Thomas IT, Frias JL, Felix V, et al. Isolated and syndromic cryptophthalmos. Am J Med Genet 1986; 25:85–98.

Dermatochalasis

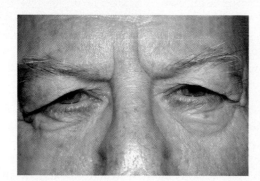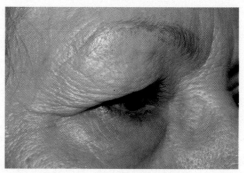

INTRODUCTION   Dermatochalasis refers to a laxity of eyelid skin and loss of muscle tone. It is a common condition that primarily affects persons over the age of 50 years, although it may occasionally be seen in younger individuals. It can affect both upper and lower eyelids and is frequently associated with fat prolapse, or steatoblepharon due to laxity of the orbital septum. As the condition advances the fascial adhesions between the anterior and posterior eyelid lamellae stretch, exacerbating the clinical symptoms. Brow and forehead ptosis are frequent accompanying aging conditions which can mechanically depress the upper eyelid skin and therefore simulate or exacerbate upper eyelid dermatochalasis. Also often seen with brow ptosis is a descent of the sub-brow fat pad into the upper eyelid, simulating steatoblepharon. Excess skin and eyelid fat can also be seen in association with systemic diseases such as Graves' orbitopathy and in inflammatory conditions such as blepharochalasis. A number of genetic connective tissue disorders can also be associated with excess eyelid skin. These include cutis laxa, pseudoxanthoma elasticum, and lipoid proteinosis cutis. An acquired form of cutis laxa without predisposing factors has been described.

CLINICAL PRESENTATION   Dermatochalasis may be of cosmetic importance only. When more severe in the upper eyelid the anterior skin-muscle lamella can overhang the eyelid margin and obstruct superior and temporal visual fields. In some cases the skin will rotate the lid margin downward so that the eyelashes contact the cornea. When associated with steatoblepharon there will be protrusion of fat pockets within the excess folds of skin. When the lacrimal gland descends due to laxity of its suspensor ligaments it causes a bulge in the lateral upper eyelid. In the lower eyelid dermatochalasis appears as horizontal and often cascading folds of skin more prominent laterally. It is frequently associated with horizontal eyelid laxity from lateral canthal tendon and the malar suspensory ligament stretching, resulting in lateral eyelid droop or even frank ectropion. As with the upper lid, concurrent steatoblepharon causes a forward protrusion of lower lid fat pockets.

TREATMENT   Mild degrees of dermatocholasis may be managed with laser skin resurfacing or chemical peels that tighten the skin and encourage new collagen formation. In most cases, however, surgical excision of skin and muscle will be required to achieve an acceptable cosmetic and functional result. If there is significant loss of connection between the anterior and posterior lamellae, the eyelid crease should be reestablished at the same time to prevent an acquired epiblepharon. When there is concomitant brow ptosis, the brow should be repositioned first since some or even all of the excess skin will be corrected with this procedure. Any excess skin in the lid can then be removed. In the lower eyelid tension must be kept in the horizontal direction to prevent retraction, scleral show, and ectropion. Care must be taken not to put excessive tension on fat pockets especially in the lower lid since cases of blindness have been reported from deep orbital hemorrhage, typically within the first three to four hours after surgery. If necessary, the lateral canthal tendon should be tightened or repositioned in a posterior direction at the same time. Care should also be taken to avoid injury to the inferior oblique muscle which lies very superficially between the medial and central fat pockets in the lower lid. Suture canthpexy to reestablish the orbitomeatal ligament will help the lower eyelid contour. In patients with significant dry eyes care should be taken to preserve the orbicularis muscle and its innervation in the upper lid.

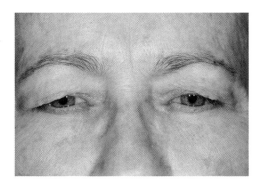 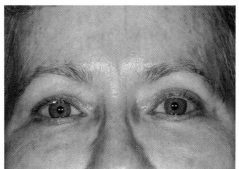

REFERENCES

Bosniak S. Reconstructive upper lid blepharoplasty. Ophthalmol Clin North Am 2005; 18:279–289.

Castro E, Foster JA. Upper lid blepharoplasty. Facial Plast Surg 1999; 15:173–181.

DeAngelis DD, Carter SR, Seiff SR. Dermatochalasis. Int Ophthalmol Clin 2002; 42:89–101.

Dutton JJ. Atlas of ophthalmic surgery. Oculoplastic, Lacrimal, and Orbital Surgery. Vol. II. St. Louis: Mosby Year Book, 1992:36–59.

Glassman ML, Hornblass A. The lateral canthus in cosmetic surgery. Facial Plast Surg Clin North Am 2002; 10:29–35.

Hass AN, Penne RB, Stefanyszyn MA, Flanagan JC. Incidence of postblepharoplasty orbital hemorrhage and associated visual loss. Ophthal Plast Reconstr Surg 2004; 20:426–432.

Lessner AM, Fagien S. Laser blepharoplasty. Semin Ophthalmol 1998; 13:90–102.

McCord CD, Boswell CB, Hester TR. Lateral canthal anchoring. Plast Reconstr Surg 2003; 112:222–237.

Morgenstern KE, Foster JA. Advances in cosmetic oculoplastic surgery. Curr Opin Ophthalmol 2002; 13:324–330.

Ruban JM, Baggio E. Examination and surgical indications for blepharoplasty. J Fr Ophthalmol 2004; 27:635–643.

Distichiasis

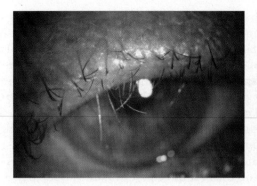 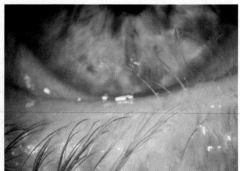

INTRODUCTION   Distichiasis is a congenital or acquired condition in which there is an accessory row of eyelash cilia behind the normal row. The disorder may be familial with an autosomal dominant pattern of inheritance, but may also follow severe inflammatory or traumatic injury. It is believed that these abnormal lashes develop as a result of metadifferentiation of primary epithelial germ cells originally intent upon meibomian gland development. The meibomian glands are modified sebaceous glands that are not associated with the eyelashes or other hairs. In the skin sebaceous glands are usually associated with a hair follicle and an apocrine sweat gland to form a pilosebaceous unit. Under some circumstances it is believed that the meibomian gland can undergo differentiation into a primitive pilosebaceous unit producing an abnormal distichitic eyelash.

CLINICAL CHARACTERISTICS   The eyelid margin is typically normal with respect to the globe and the normal eyelashes are oriented appropriately. Extra, often very fine cilia are seen arising in association with the meibomian gland orifices. These abnormal lashes are directed backward toward the corneal surface where they produce ocular surface symptoms of foreign body sensation, conjunctival injection, corneal abrasion, and reflex epiphora. Distichiasis can be focal with only a few abnormal lashes, or diffuse where they can extend across the entire eyelid margin.

TREATMENT   Mechanical epilation of the offending distichitic lashes will provide temporary relief of symptoms, but the cilia will usually re-grow within three to four weeks. For a permanent cure ablation of the lash follicles is required. Electrolysis, radiosurgery, or cryosurgery are all equally effective. However, unlike trichitic lashes, in distichiasis the cilium shaft may run a circuitous course from the bulb to the lid surface making destruction with an epilating needle more unpredictable. Internal lash resection beneath a skin muscle flap or using a lid-splitting technique is effective, but because the bulbs lie within the tarsus, finding them can be difficult.

REFERENCES

Anderson RL. Surgical repair for distichiasis. Arch Ophthalmol 1977; 95:169.

Byrnes GA, Wilson ME. Congenital distichiasis. Arch Ophthalmol 1991; 109:1752–1753.

Chi MJ, Park MS, Nam H, Moon HS, Baek SH. Eyelid splitting with follicular extirpation using a monopolar cautery for the treatment of trichiasis and distichiasis. Graefes Arch Clin Exp Ophthalmol 2007; 245:637–640.

Choo PH. Distichiasis, trichiasis, and entropion: advances in management. Int Ophthalmol Clin 2002; 42:75–87.

Frueh BR. Treatment of distichiasis with cryotherapy. Ophthalmic Surg 1981; 12:100–103.

O'Donnell BA, Collin JR. Distichiasis: management with cryotherapy to the posterior lamella. Br J Ophthalmol 1993; 77:289–292.

Scheie HG, Albert DM. Distichiasis and trichiasis: origin and management. Am J Ophthalmol 1966; 61:718–720.

Vaughn GL, Dortzbach RK, Sires BS, Lemke BN. Eyelid splitting with excision or microhyfrecation for distichiasis. Arch Ophthalmol 1997; 115:282–284.

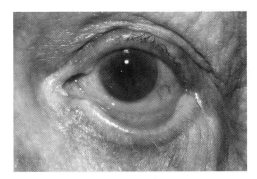 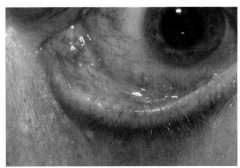

INTRODUCTION   In ectropion the eyelid margin is turned outward away from the globe. This leads to inadequate corneal protection due to lack of apposition to the corneal surface. Chronic ocular discomfort results and ultimately exposure causes epithelial and stromal injury. Tear drainage dysfunction results from eversion of the puncta, and with time the puncta become occluded. The causes of ectropion are numerous. Involutional ectropion is the most common type occurring in older patients, resulting from horizontal laxity of the tarsus and/or canthal tendons. Ectropion is associated with larger than average tarsal plates which when combined with laxity and degenerative histologic changes associated with aging, may have a causal relationship. In cicatricial ectropion there is a shortening of the anterior eyelid lamella from scarring or chronic skin disorders. Paralytic ectropion is caused by loss of orbicularis muscle tone from seventh nerve dysfunctions following surgery or Bell's palsy. An unusual cause of ectropion is the Floppy Eyelid Syndrome, which can sometimes involve the lower eyelids.

CLINICAL PRESENTATION   Ectropion almost always involves the lower eyelid. The lid margin is away from the globe and the conjunctival surface is generally injected and thickened with varying degrees of keratinization and inflammation. There is usually an increased tear lake and some evidence of corneal dryness from exposure is typical. The inferior punctum often becomes stenotic, and it may even be occluded with a superficial membrane from disuse resulting in epiphora. In involutional ectropion horizontal laxity may be diffuse, involving the entire lid margin including tarsus, or confined to the canthal tendons, usually the lateral. In paralytic ectropion there is also loss of orbicularis muscle tone and facial droop on the involved side. Brow ptosis is also usually present with secondary dermatochalasis, and lagophthalmos is a major problem contributing to significant corneal exposure. With cicatricial ectropion the cause is usually obvious by the presence of cutaneous scarring, cicatrizing skin changes, or tumors. An unusual cause of everting eyelid malposition is mechanical ectropion where there is a mass lesion of the conjunctiva displacing the eyelid margin outward.

TREATMENT   Repair of ectropion is generally required because of the corneal exposure, foreign body symptoms, and epiphora. In cases of involutional laxity or seventh nerve weakness, a horizontal lid tightening will give good results. In most cases reconstruction of the lateral canthal tendon with a tarsal strip procedure works best. Occasionally the medial canthal tendon will be lax requiring a tuck of the posterior crus via a transcaruncular incision. For medial punctal eversion a medial spindle resection from the posterior lamella works well. For more generalized tarsal laxity without significant stretching of the canthal tendons a pentagonal wedge

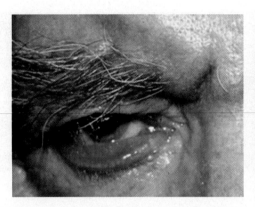
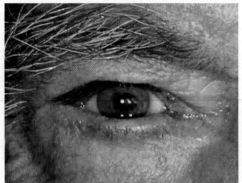

resection at the junction of the central and lateral thirds of the lid is preferred. In cases of paralytic ectropion, repair of the lower lid is usually not sufficient in itself to prevent the chronic corneal exposure. If there is significant facial droop, a vertical midface SMAS lift will help maintain eyelid position. Correction of the lagophthalmos with a gold weight implant, encircling silicone rod, or a lateral tarsorrhaphy may have to be added. Cicatricial ectropion when mild can often be repaired with a simple horizontal tightening procedure. For moderate ectropion combining horizontal shortening with a cheek elevation gives better results. When there is severe skin shortening, however, a full-thickness skin graft or myocutaneous flap will be needed. For mechanical ectropion attention to management of the conjunctival lesion is required, but additional eyelid shortening may be needed if the lid has become stretched.

REFERENCES

Bashour M, Harvey J. Causes of involutional ectropion and entropion—age related tarsal changes are the key. Ophthal Plast Reconstr Surg 2000; 16:131–141.

Benger RS, Frueh BR. Involutional ectropion: a review of the management. Ophthalmic Surg 1987; 18:136–139.

Clement CI, O'Donnell BA. Medial canthal tendon repair for moderate to severe tendon laxity. Clin Experiment Ophthalmol 2004; 32:170–174.

Crawford GJ, Collin JR, Moriarty PA. The correction of paralytic medial ectropion. Br J Ophthalmol 1984; 68:639–641.

Dutton JJ. Atlas of ophthalmic surgery. Oculoplastic, Lacrimal, and Orbital Surgery. Vol. II. St Louis: Mosby Year Book, 1992: 94–113.

Frueh BR, Su CS. Medial tarsal suspension: a method of elevating the medial lower eyelid. Ophthal Plast Reconstr Surg 2002; 18:133–137.

Leatherbarrow B, Collin JR. Eyelid surgery in facial palsy. Eye 1991; 5:585–590.

Mittelviefhaus H. Cicatricial ectropion in progressive skin diseases. Orbit 2001; 20:91–99.

Neuhaus RW. Anatomical basis of "senile" ectropion. Ophthal Plast Reconstr Surg 1985; 1:87–89.

Nowinski TS, Anderson RL. The medial spindle procedure for involutional ectropion. Arch Ophthalmol 1985; 103: 1750–1753.

Schellini SA, Sampaio Junior Ade A. Subperiosteal midface lift: an alternative to correct the cicatricial eyelid ectropion. Arq Bras Oftalmol 2005; 68:527–531.

Stasior OG. Involutional ectropion. Clin Plast Surg 1978; 5:593–596.

Stefanyszyn MA, Hidayat AA, Flanagan JC. The histopathology of involutional ectropion. Ophthalmology 1985; 92: 120–127.

Sullivan TJ, Collin JR. Medial canthal resection: an effective long-term cure for medial ectropion. Br J Ophthalmol 1991; 75:288–291.

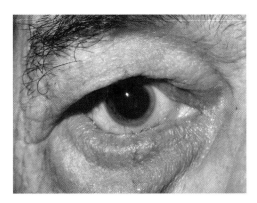 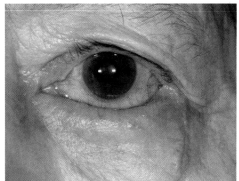

INTRODUCTION   Entropion is a turning inward of the eyelid margin. Like ectropion, the causes are numerous, but unlike the latter the results may be far more devastating to the eye. Occasionally entropion can be seen as a congenital malposition, usually associated with deformities of the eyelid and tarsus, such as the tarsal kink syndrome. Involutional entropion is the most common form seen in older individuals related to aging with horizontal and vertical laxity of eyelid suspensory structures, particularly the capsulopalpebral fascia. Entropion is more common when the tarsal plate is narrow allowing it to rotate inward. Cicatricial entropion is seen with shortening of the conjunctival surface from diseases such as cicatricial pemphigoid, Stevens-Johnson syndrome, trachoma, or from chemical burns. In mechanical entropion there may be a mass lesion that rotates the eyelid margin inward. Epiblepharon is sometimes included as a special type of entropion that is more mechanical than anything else. Here, the lower lid crease is not well formed and there is an upward override of the anterior lamella resulting in the entropion. Epiblepharon can also be an acquired deformity following trauma or surgery. Spastic entropion is anatomically similar to epiblepharon and is sometimes seen following ocular surgery associated with ocular irritation. Here there is associated loss of fixation between the anterior and posterior lamellae combined with eyelid laxity. With contraction of the orbicularis muscle the anterior lamella rides up and mechanically rotates the lid inward.

CLINICAL PRESENTATION   Whatever the specific etiology of entropion the mucocutaneous border of the eyelid and the lashes are directed towards the globe. In some cases, as with cicatricial ocular pemphigoid, distortion of eyelid tissues may include a true trichiasis. However, in most cases the lashes are in a normal position relative to the lid margin, and the resulting corneal touch is secondary to the lid malposition. The clinical spectrum of entropion may vary from a mild, intermittent backward tilting of the marginal tarsus associated with only occasional corneal touch, to severe 180 degree inversion of the entire eyelid with the lashes and skin in full contact with the globe. The resulting ocular surface irritation is associated with conjunctival injection, reflex lacrimation and epiphora, and ocular discomfort from corneal epithelial disruption. Corneal abrasion and even frank ulceration may evolve if the condition is not corrected. A secondary blepharospasm is frequently present which exacerbates the condition.

TREATMENT   The surgical correction of involutional entropion is directed at repair of the primary anatomical defect. If eyelid horizontal laxity is the only significant finding repair is achieved with simple horizontal lid shortening. When vertical lid laxity is a contributing factor, tightening or reattachment of the capsulopalpebral fascia either alone or in combination with horizontal tightening is required. Simultaneous reformation of the eyelid crease with internal sutures is an important part of this procedure. Correction of cicatricial entropion is aimed at restoration of the deficient posterior lamella. If minimal, this can be achieved by advancement of a skin and muscle flap or with full-thickness eyelid rotating sutures. If the tarsus is deformed an interpositional graft of tarsus from another lid or with cartilage, hard palate, or donor sclera will help reposition the lid margin. An effective procedure is marginal rotation by resecting a horizontal V-groove from the anterior tarsal face. For contraction of conjunctiva, mucous membrane or amniotic membrane grafting will release the cicatrix and allow realignment of the lid margin. Epiblepharon is corrected with eyelid sutures in infants, but in older children resection of an ellipse of skin and muscle with reformation of the lid crease gives more permanent results. Spastic entropion will sometimes resolve spontaneously. Temporary correction can be attained with botulinum toxin, 5–10 units into the pretarsal muscle. Surgical repair requires tucking of the retractors with crease reformation.

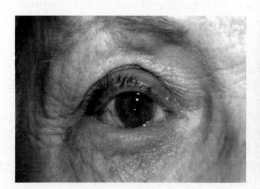 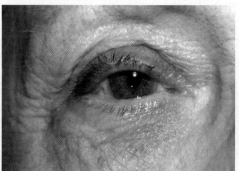

REFERENCES

Barnes JA, Bunce C, Olver JM. Simple effective surgery for involutional entropion suitable for the general ophthalmologist. Ophthalmology 2006; 113:92–96.

Boboridis K, Bunce C, Rose GE. A comparative study of two procedures for repair of involutional lower lid entropion. Ophthalmology 2000; 107:959–961.

Danks JJ, Rose GE. Involutional lower lid entropion: to shorten or not to shorten? Ophthalmology 1998; 105:2065–2067.

Dutton JJ. Atlas of ophthalmic surgery. Oculoplastic, Lacrimal, and Orbital Surgery. Vol. II. St Louis: Mosby Year Book, 1992: 114–143.

Ho SF, Pherwani A, Elsherbiny SM, Reuser T. Lateral tarsal strip and quickert sutures for lower eyelid entropion. Ophthal Plast Reconstr Surg 2005; 21:345–348.

Khan SJ, Meyer DR. Transconjunctival lower eyelid involutional entropion repair: long-term follow-up and efficacy. Ophthalmology 2002; 109:2112–2127.

Levine MR, Enlow MK, Terman S. Spastic entropion after cataract surgery. Ann Ophthalmol 1992; 24:195–198.

Meadows AE, Reck AC, Gaston H, Tyers AG. Everting sutures in involutional entropion. Orbit 1999; 18:177–181.

Rougraff PM, Tse DT, Johnson TE, Feurer W. Involutional entropion repair with fornix sutures and lateral tarsal strip procedure. Ophthal Plast Reconstr Surg 2001; 17:281–287.

Shiu M, McNab AA. Cicatricial entropion and trichiasis in an urban Australian population. Clin Experiment Ophthalmol 2005; 33:582–585.

Steel DH, Hoh HB, Harrad RA, Collins CR. Botulinum toxin for the temporary treatment of involutional lower lid entropion: a clinical and morphological study. Eye 1997; 11:472–475.

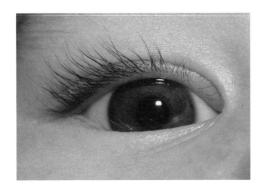 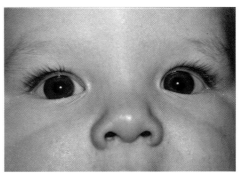

INTRODUCTION   Epiblepahron is a congenital bilateral condition in which the anterior skin-muscle lamella of the eyelid rides up over the eyelid margin, turning it inward toward the globe. While this simulates entropion in appearance and consequences, it is quite different in its etiology. Epiblepharon is caused by the absence of the lower eyelid crease and the fascial attachments that unite together the anterior and posterior lamellae at that point. With contraction of the orbicularis muscle the anterior lamella rides upward over the lid margin, rotating the lashes inward. The entropion is typically worse in downgaze. Epiblepharon is more common in the Asian eyelid, especially when there is significant epicanthus, and in those with a high body mass index.

CLINICAL CHARACTERISTICS   Epiblepharon appears as a redundant horizontal fold of pretarsal skin and orbicularis muscle that extends upward over the lower lid margin and lash line. In some patients the lid may appear completely normal in primary gaze, with the condition developing only on downgaze. In more severe cases the condition is manifest even in the primary gaze position. The overriding skin mechanically displaces the lash-bearing mucocutaneous border backward against the cornea. Symptoms include foreign body sensation, irritation, and reflex epiphora. More than half of affected children will have a with-the-rule astigmatism. However, up to 80% of affected children may have minimal or no ocular symptoms. Epiblepharon can also be seen as an acquired condition following trauma or surgery where there is disruption of fascial attachments between the anterior and posterior lamellae. It has also been described as a finding in Graves' eye disease. Rarely epiblepharon can be seen in the upper eyelid as a developmental anomaly.

TREATMENT   In many cases epiblepharon resolves spontaneously by the age of six or seven years, as the face elongates with growth. Treatment may be required, however, for significant ocular symptoms. This can be achieved in young children with the placement of full-thickness eyelid sutures of the Quickert-Rathbun type. This creates a scar band between the anterior and posterior lamellae that simulates the normal eyelid crease. In older children or where the fold is large, excision of an ellipse of skin with reformation of the crease will give better results.

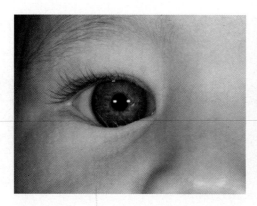 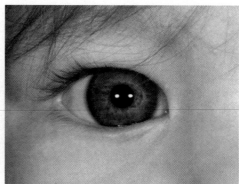

REFERENCES

Chang EL, Hayes J, Hatton M, Rubin PA. Acquired lower eyelid epiblepharon in patients with thyroid eye disease. Ophthal Plast Reconstr Surg 2005; 21:192–196.

Choo C. Correction of oriental epiblepharon by anterior lamellar reposition. Eye 1996; 10:545–547.

Choo CT, Chan CM, Fong KS. Surgical management of upper lid epiblepharon. Eye 1998; 12:623–626.

Dutton JJ. Atlas of ophthalmic surgery. Oculoplastic, Lacrimal, and Orbital Surgery. Vol. II. St Louis: Mosby Year Book, 1992:118–121.

Hayasaka Y, Haysaka S. Epiblepharon with inverted eyelashes and high body mass index in Japanese children. J Pediatr Ophthalmol Strabismus 2005; 42:300–303.

Jeong S, Park H, Park YG. Surgical correction of congenital epiblepharon: low eyelid crease reforming technique. J Pediatr Ophthalmol Strabismus 2001; 38:356–358.

Jordan R. The lower-lid retractor in congenital entropion and epiblepharon. Ophthalmic Surg 1993; 24:494–496.

Khwarg SI, Choung HK. Epiblepharon of the lower eyelid: technique of surgical repair and quantification of excision according to the skin fold height. Ophthalmic Surg Lasers 2002; 33:280–287.

Khwarg SI, Lee YJ. Epiblepharon of the lower eyelid: classification and association with astigmatism. Korean J Ophthalmol 1997; 11:111–117.

Lemke BN, Stasior OG. Epiblepharon. An important and often missed diagnosis. Clin Pediatr (Phila) 1981; 20:661–662.

O'Donnell BA, Collin JR. Congenital lower eyelid deformity with trichiasis (epiblepharon and entropion). Aust N Z J Ophthalmol 1994; 22:33–37.

Park RI, Meyer DR. Acquired lower eyelid epiblepharon. Am J Ophthalmol 1996; 122:449–451.

Quickert MH, Wilkes TD, Dryden RM. Nonincisional correction of epiblepharon and congenital entropion. Arch Ophthalmol 1983; 101:778–781.

Serafino M, Bottoli A, Nucci P. Correction of congenital entropion of the lower eyelid: incisional versus rotational surgery. Eur J Ophthalmol 2005; 15:536–540.

Woo KI, Yi K, Kim YD. Surgical correction for lower lid epiblepharon in Asians. Brit J Ophthalmol 2000; 84:1407–1410.

Epicanthal Folds

INTRODUCTION

Epicanthal folds are small webs of skin that contour around the medial canthal region. They can be seen as an isolated finding or in association with other facial anomalies such as the blepharophimosis syndrome or Downs syndrome. They can also be seen as a racial variation, particularly in some East Asian and Southeast Asian eyelids, and in Native Americans and the Khoisan of Southern Africa. They can also be seen in young children as a normal finding before the nasal bridge elevates. Epicanthal folds are categorized by anatomic location, and are termed epicanthus inversus, e. palpebralis, e. tarsalis, and e. supraciliaris.

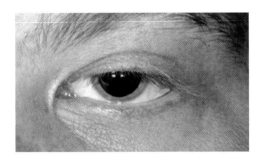 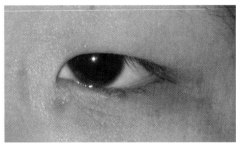

CLINICAL CHARACTERISTICS   Epicanthal folds vary from hardly noticeable to very strongly developed. They usually diminish with age as the nasal bridge changes in height and contour. In epicanthus inversus the fold of skin takes origin from the lower eyelid and extends to the medial canthal angle, covering the canthal angle and caruncle. It confers a rounded contour to the lower eyelid, and the fold often obscures the lid margin medially. It may be associated with a limited from of epiblepharon. In epicanthus palpebralis the skin fold extends from the tarsal region of the upper lid to the margin of the lower lid, giving an abnormal contour to the upper eyelid margin. This type tends to improve with growth of the midface. Epicanthus tarsalis is a fold that extends from the pretarsal upper eyelid skin to the medial canthal angle, and is a normal finding in the Asian eyelid. In epicanthus supraciliaris the fold originates from just below the medial eyebrow and extends to the medial canthus in the region of the lacrimal sac.

TREATMENT   Epicanthal folds are usually only of cosmetic importance, but in some cases they may obscure the medial visual field. When correction is indicated the treatment is surgical. Many different procedures are available, but all rely on tissue rearrangement to lengthen the vertical component of the fold at the expense of the horizontal width. These include the modified Y to V plasty, the Z-plasty, and combinations of Z-plasty and Y to V rearrangements.

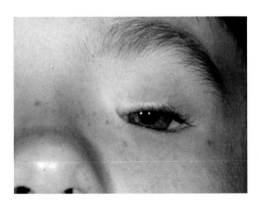 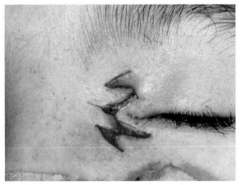

REFERENCES

Cho BC, Lee KY. Medial epicanthoplasty combined with plication of the medial canthal tendon in Asian eyelids. Plast Reconstr Surg 2002; 110:293–300.

de Cunha RP, Moreira JB. Ocular findings in Down's syndrome. Am J Ophthalmol 1996; 122:236–244.

Jordan DR, Anderson RL. Epicanthal folds. A deep tissue approach. Arch Ophthalmol 1989; 107:1532–1535.

Kao YS, Lin CH, Fang RH. Epicanthoplasty with modified Y-V advancement procedure. Plast Reconstr Surg 1998; 102:1935–1841.

McCord CD Jr. The correction of telecanthus and epicanthal folds. Ophthalmic Surg 1980; 11:446–454.

Mustarde JC. The treatment of ptosis and epicanthal folds. Br J Plast Surg 1959; 12:252–258.

Nowinski TS. Epicanthal folds and blepharophimosis: a new technique. Trans PA Acad Ophthalmol Otolaryngol 1988; 40:706–712.

Park JI. Modified Z-epicanthoplasty in the Asian eyelid. Arch Facial Plast Surg 2000; 2:43–47.

Yoo WM, Park SH, Kwang DR. Root Z-epicanthoplasty in Asian eyelids. Plast Reconstr Surg 2003; 111:2476–2477.

Essential Blepharospasm

INTRODUCTION   Essential blepharospasm (EB) is a bilateral focal dystonia of idiopathic origin. The condition usually affects patients in their fifth to sixth decades but can be seen in younger individuals, even in their teens. It is two to three times more common in females. In 33% of cases some familial occurrence of dystonia can be elicited, suggesting a possible genetic predisposition.

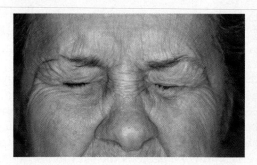 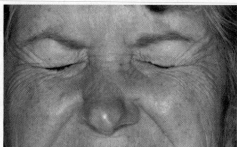

Some evidence suggests a central defect in the coordination of ocular and periocular sensory information and motor response in the orbicularis muscle. EB is usually seen as an isolated finding. However, in many cases it progresses to include adjacent focal dystonias, most commonly oromandibular dystonia. This complex of EB and oromandibular dystonia is referred to as Meige's syndrome. Cervical dystonia is also common in these patients.

CLINICAL CHARACTERISTICS   The disease usually begins insidiously with increased frequency of blinking, and slowly progresses to forceful, sustained eyelid closure. In some cases the disorder may have a sudden onset. The orbicularis muscle shows episodic spasms that vary from mild to extreme. The procerus and corrugator muscles may also be involved. The duration of eye closure may vary from seconds to minutes, and can result in significant visual disability and even functional blindness. Nearly half of affected patients progress to oromandubular dystonia, which includes the mid and lower facial muscles. The association of blepharospasm and oromandubular dystonia is often referred to as Meige's Syndrome. Spasms are exacerbated by stress, and can sometimes be relieved by sensory tricks such as whistling or touching a part of the face.

TREATMENT   The most affective treatment currently available is chemodenervation with botulinum toxin. The latter blocks neuromuscular transmission by inhibiting release of acetyl choline at peripheral nerve endings. Onset is usually within three to five days, and the duration of effect is typically about three months. For the 4% to 5% of patients who do not respond to botulinum toxin type A (Botox®) or who develop resistance to it, botulinum toxin type B (Myobloc®) is also available, and generally works well in most cases. When chemodenervation fails to give adequate results pharmacological agents such as benzodiazepines or anticholinergic agents can be added. For those who do not obtain satisfactory control of spasms on these regimens, surgical myectomy with removal of orbicularis muscle from the upper eyelids combined with brow fixation, will usually produce acceptable results.

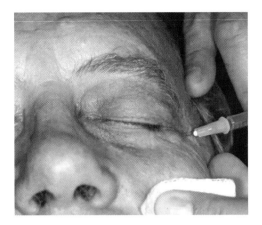

REFERENCES

Anderson RL, Patel BC, Holds JB, Jordan DR. Blepharospasm: past, present, and future. Ophthal Plast Reconstr Surg 1998; 14:305–317.

Aoki KR, Guyer B. Botulinum toxin type A and other botulinum serotypes: a comparative review of biochemical and pharmacological actions. Europ J Neurol 2001; 8(suppl 5):21–29.

Ben Simon GJ, McCann JD. Benign essential blepharospasm. Int Ophthalmol Clin 2005; 45:49–75.

Bradley EA, Hodge DO, Bartley GB. Benign essential blepharospasm among residents of Olmsted County, Minnesota, 1976 to 1995: an epidemiologic study. Ophthal Plast Reconstr Surg 2003; 19:177–181.

Dutton JJ, Buckley EG. Long-term results and complications of botulinum toxin in the treatment of blepharospasm. Ophthalmology 1988; 95:1529–1534.

Dutton JJ. Acute and chronic effects of botulinum toxin in the management of blepharospasm. In Jankovic J, Halleatt M, eds, Therapy With Botulinum Toxin. New York: Marcel Dekker, 1994:199–209.

Dutton JJ. Botulinum-A toxin in the treatment of craniocervical muscle spasms: short- and long-term, local and systemic effects. Surv Ophthalmol 1996; 41:51–65.

Herz NL, Yen MT. Modulation of sensory photophobia in essential blepharospasm with chromatic lenses. Ophthalmology 2005; 112:2208–2211.

Patel BC. Surgical management of essential blepharospasm. Otolaryngol Clin North Am 2005; 38:1075–1098.

Euryblepharon

INTRODUCTION

Euryblepharon is a very rare congenital anomaly of the palpebral fissure. It is distinguished from ankyloblepharon where the lid margins are fused together to varying degrees, and from cryptophthalmos where the eyelids are not formed but skin extends across and over a deformed eye. It may be unilateral or bilateral and is not typically associated with other congenital anomalies or syndromes, nor does there appear to be any familial tendency. It has been suggested that euryblepharon results from a

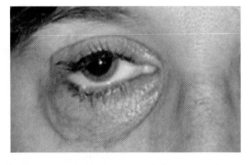

developmental hypoplasia or absence of the palpebral and lacrimal portions of the orbicularis muscle.

CLINICAL CHARACTERISTICS   In euryblepharon the palpebral fissure is elongated horizontally. It may involve the lower and/or upper eyelid, and can be bilateral or unilateral. The lateral portion of the lower eyelid becomes somewhat redundant and ectropic, producing a downward droop giving the patient an antimongaloid slope to the palpebral fissure. The lateral canthal tendon is lax or not developed so that there is also significant laxity of the lower eyelid. The condition can be associated with lagophthalmos and corneal exposure. Rarely, other findings may include a double row of meibomian gland orifices or a lateral displacement of the punctum and canaliculus. Some degree of vertical eyelid skin shortening is also commonly seen.

TREATMENT   Treatment of euryblepharon is surgical and is indicated for exposure symptoms or for cosmetic improvement. A lateral canthoplasty with tightening and repositioning of the lateral canthal tendon is often sufficient. For excessive horizontal lid lengthening, a full-thickness wedge resection maybe needed to correct the ectropion. When vertical shortening causes significant lagophthalmos, skin grafts may be required.

REFERENCES

Keipert JA. Euryblepharon. Br J Ophthalmol 1975; 59:57–58.

D'Esposito M, Magli A, Del Prete A. Genetic study and surgical correction of euryblepharon. Ophthalmologica 1979; 178:396–403.

McCord CD Jr, Chapell J, Pollard ZF. Congenital euryblepharon. Ann Ophthalmol 1979; 11:1217–1224.

Ruban JM, Baggio E. Surgical treatment of congenital eyelid malpositions in children. J Fr Ophthalmol 2004; 27:304–326.

Floppy Eyelid Syndrome

INTRODUCTION   The Floppy Eyelid Syndrome primarily affects obese individuals with a male predominance. The cause of the disease remains unknown and histological examination of the softened and redundant tarsal plate has not suggested any conclusive etiology. A mild chronic inflammatory infiltrate has been reported in some cases, but it is not clear if this was a primary cause or a secondary effect. The tarsal plate and skin show a decreased amount of elastin fibers. The syndrome and its clinical spectrum results from loss of physical integrity of the tarsus, perhaps in part related to habitual sleeping on the involved sides in patients with excessive weight. The condition is also associated with obstructive sleep apnea.

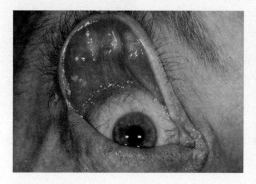 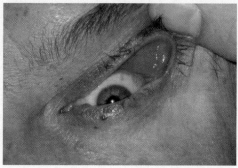

CLINICAL CHARACTERISTICS   More than 75% of patients with Floppy Eyelid Syndrome are males between the ages of 30 and 80 years. Obesity is a nearly constant finding, observed in 96% of cases. A history of sleeping on the face, especially on the involved side is typical. In most cases only the upper eyelid is involved, and in 60% of cases the condition is bilateral. Eyelash ptosis and loss of lash parallelism appear to be constant findings. Associated lower eyelid laxity is seen in 50% of affected patients, and in some a frank floppy lower eyelid will be present. Ocular symptoms include ptosis, ocular irritation, and foreign body sensation, especially upon waking up in the morning. Tear film deficiency is seen in most patients. Conjunctival injection, eyelid swelling, and a mucoid discharge are characteristics resulting from repeated nocturnal eyelid eversion. Chronic papillary conjunctivitis is typical with keratinization and epithelial thickening. Less commonly, superficial punctate keratopathy and a superior pannus result. The tarsus is soft and redundant, and shows marked laxity.

TREATMENT   When the condition is mild topical lubrication combined with taping the eyelids closed at night, or applying an eye shield may provide some relief. In more severe cases, however, surgery will be needed. A full-thickness resection of the eyelid amounting to one-third to one-half of the horizontal length with primary layered closure is curative. This not only prevents spontaneous eyelid eversion during sleep, but also corrects the eyelid ptosis.

REFERENCES

Dufek MA, Shechtman DL. Floppy eyelid syndrome: a diagnostic dilemma. J Am Optom Assoc 1999; 70:450–454.

Dutton JJ. Surgical management of floppy eyelid syndrome. Am J Ophthalmol 1985; 99:557–560.

Klapper SR, Jordan DR. Floppy eyelid syndrome. Ophthalmology 1998; 105:1582.

Langford JD, Lindberg JV. A new physical finding in floppy eyelid syndrome. Ophthalmology 1998; 105:165–169.

Liu DT, Di Pascuale MA, Sawai J, Goa YY, Tseng SC. Tear film dynamics in floppy eyelid syndrome. Invest Ophthalmol Vis Sci 2005; 46:1188–1194.

McNab AA. Reversal of floppy eyelid syndrome with treatment of obstructive sleep apnea. Clin Experiment Ophthalmol 2000; 28:125–126.

McNab AA. Floppy eyelid syndrome and obstructive sleep apnea. Ophthal Plast Reconstr Surg 1997; 13:98–114.

McNab AA. Floppy eyelid syndrome. Ophthalmology 1998; 105:1977–1978.

Periman LM, Sires BS. Floppy eyelid syndrome: a modified surgical technique. Ophthal Plast Reconstr Surg 2002; 18:370–372.

Schlotzer-Schrehardt U, Stojkovic M, Hofmann-Rummelt C, et al. The pathogenesis of floppy eyelid syndrome: involvement of matrix metaloproteins in elastic fiber degeneration. Ophthalmology 2005; 112:694–704.

Valenzuela AA, Sullivan TJ. Medial upper eyelid shortening to correct medial eyelid laxity in floppy eyelid syndrome: a new surgical approach. Ophthal Plast Reconstr Surg 2005; 21:259–263.

Hemifacial Spasm

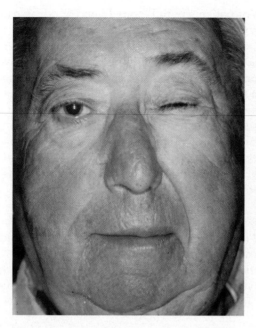 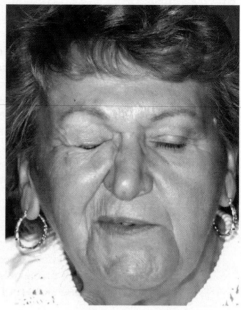

INTRODUCTION   Hemifacial spasm is characterized by involuntary unilateral hyperkinetic tonic and clonic spasms of muscles innervated by the seventh cranial nerve. In contrast with essential blepharospasm, in hemifacial spasm muscle contractions continue during sleep. An anatomic cause appears to be responsible in most cases. In 85% to 90% of cases an abnormal ectatic vascular loop of the vertebral-basilar arterial tree can be seen on MRI compressing the seventh nerve exit root in the cerebellopontine cistern. Most frequently the anteriorinferior cerebellar artery is involved. Rarely, bilateral cases have been described, but the two sides are typically not involved synchronously or to the same degree. In very rare instances compression of the seventh nerve by tumor, aneurysm, or other mass lesions may be the cause. Peripheral seventh nerve injury from trauma or Bell's Palsy can also result in hemifacial spasm following axonal regeneration. A case of hemifacial spasm associated with otitis media has been reported. Arterial hypertension occurs significantly more frequently in patients with hemifacial spasm suggesting a causal relationship. Hemifacial spasm generally occurs in older adults, but rarely can be seen in children.

CLINICAL CHARACTERISTICS   In classic hemifacial spasm contraction of facial muscles often begins with the orbicularis muscle followed by subsequent downward progression over the face. In atypical cases, the onset of symptoms is in the buccal muscles, with upward progression. The difference appears to be caused by the specific vessels involved in the compression. The average age at onset for hemifacial spasm is 45 years with a slight preponderance of females. The condition typically begins with intermittent twitching of one eyelid which progresses over months to years to involve other areas of the ipsilateral facial nerve innervation. In its full-blown state hemifacial spasm involves closure of the eyelids associated with contraction of the entire ipsilateral face and elevation of the mouth.

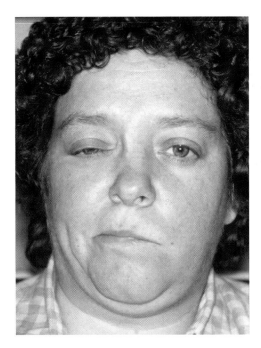 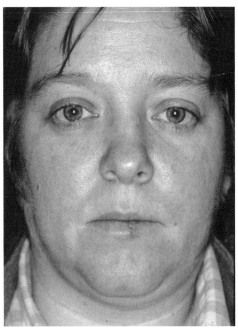

TREATMENT

Anticonvulsants, such as carbamazepine, may be helpful in some cases, as are the short-acting benzodiazepines. But these are useful in only about one-fourth of cases with mild symptoms. The most effective treatment currently available is chemodenervation with botulinum toxin. The latter blocks neuromuscular transmission by preventing degranulation of acetylcholine at peripheral cholinergic nerve endings. The duration of effect is typically three to four months. Complications include transient ptosis, mouth droop, and other muscle weaknesses. Microvascular decompression of the seventh nerve root where it exits the brain stem is an effective surgical treatment in most cases, with about 70% to 89% of cases showing complete relief of spasms. Potential complications include hearing impairment and CSF leak, and the mortality rate is reported at 0.3% to 0.6%. Monitoring of abnormal muscle response intraoperatively may enhance the final result.

REFERENCES

Defazio G, Abbruzzese G, Girlanda P, et al. Botulinum toxin A treatment for primary hemifacial spasm: a 10-year multicenter study. Arch Neurol 2002; 59:418–420.

Dutton JJ. Botulinum-A toxin in the treatment of craniocervical muscle spasms: short- and long-term, local and systemic effects. Surv Ophthalmol 1996; 41:51–65.

Dutton JJ. Treatment of hemifacial spasm and essential blepharospasm with botulinum toxin. In: Wilkins RH, Rengachary SS, eds. Neurosurgery Update I. New York: McGraw Hill, 1990:138–141.

Elgamal EA, Coakham HB. Hemifacial spasm caused by pontine glioma: case report and review of the literature. Neurosurg Rev 2005; 28:330–332.

Frei K, Truong DD, Dressler D. Botulinum toxin therapy of hemifacial spasm: comparing different therapeutic preparations. Eur J Neurol 2006; 13(suppl 1):30–35.

Kalkanis SN, Eskandar EN, Carter BS, Barker FG 2nd. Microvascular decompression surgery in the United States, 1996 to 2000: mortality rates, morbidity rates, and the effects of hospital and surgeon volumes. Neurosurgery 2003; 52: 1251–1261.

Moffat DA, Durvasula VS, Stevens King A, De R. Hardy DG. Outcome following retrosigmoid microvascular decompression of the facial nerve for hemifacial spasm. J Laryngol Otol 2005; 119:779–783.

Oliveira LD, Cardoso F, Vargas AP. Hemifacial spasm and arterial hypertension. Mov Disord 1999; 14:832–835.

Sade B, Mohr G, Dufour JJ. Cerebellopontine angle lipoma presenting with hemifacial spasm: case report and review of the literature. J Otolaryngol 2005; 34:270–273.

Singer C, Papapetropoulos S, Farronay O. Childhood-onset hemifacial spasm: successful treatment with botulinum toxin. Pediatr Neurol 2005; 33:220–222.

Tan EK, Jankovic J. Bilateral hemifacial spasm: a report of five cases and a literature review. Mov Disord 1999; 14:345–349.

Tan EK, Jankovic J. Psychogenic hemifacial spasm. J Neuropsychiatry Clin Neurosci 2001; 13:380–384.

Valls-Sole J, Montero J. Movement disorders in patients with peripheral facial palsy. Mov Disord 2003; 18:1424–1435.

Yuan Y, Wang Y, Zhang SX, Zhang L, Li R, Guo J. Microvascular decompression in patients with hemifacial spasm: report of 1200 cases. Chin Med J 2005; 118:833–836.

Horner's Syndrome

INTRODUCTION

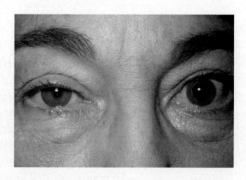

Lesions in either the central or peripheral sympathetic pathways to the eye and face lead to the triad of symptoms known as Horner's syndrome. Loss of sympathetic tone to Müller's accessory eyelid muscle results in upper eyelid ptosis, loss to the dilator muscle of the iris causes pupillary miosis, and absence of sympathetic innervation to facial sweat glands produces anhidrosis. In addition, parasympathetic innervation is unopposed resulting in overaction of parasympathetic stimulation to the iris constrictor muscle, the ciliary muscle, the lacrimal gland, and the salivary glands. The course of the sympathetic fibers from the cervical sympathetic trunk and cervical ganglia divide to follow two separate routes; those to the eye course along the internal carotid artery, while those destined for the sweat glands of the face follow the external carotid system. Thus, the constellation of symptoms may vary depending upon the level of the sympathetic injury. The neurologic deficit may result from ischemia, thoracic trauma, mediastinal neoplasms, enlargement of the thyroid gland, internal carotid dissection, or iatrogenic surgical insults. In children Horner's syndrome may the initial manifestation of neuroblastoma. Horner's syndrome has been reported fairly commonly following lumbar epidural anesthesia. It has also been seen with carotid dissection, Pancoast tumor, and thyroid tumors. The condition can be bilateral in diabetic autonomic neuropathy, amyloidosis, and pure autonomic failure.

CLINICAL SYMPTOMS   Müller's sympathetic eyelid muscles contribute to retraction of both the upper and lower eyelids. In Horner's syndrome there is a minimal ptosis of the upper lid of about 1 to 2 mm, associated with elevation of the lower eyelid. Thus, the interpalpebral fissure is narrowed. The pupil is mildly constricted and there may be loss of sweating on the ipsilateral face and dryness of the mouth. In congenital Horner's syndrome the affected iris is lighter in color resulting in heterochromia. Diagnosis is facilitated by pharmacologic testing with 4% cocaine where the affected pupil does not dilate but he normal pupil does. If the denervation involves the third order neurons between the superior cervical ganglion and the eye, the pupil is supersensitive to epinephrine and will dilate with 1:1000 dilution of epinephrine, a concentration that does not affect the normal pupil.

TREATMENT   In children with congenital Horner's syndrome a history of forceful manipulation of the infant during birth reduces the need for medical work up. In 90% of affected children either trauma or no clearly identifiable cause will be found. However, in 10% an underlying pathology may be uncovered. All cases of acquired Horner's syndrome without a known etiology require extensive evaluation since a high percentage of cases may be associated with a serious underlying condition. In acute cases the eyelid ptosis should be observed. When the ptosis is persistent and visually significant or is of cosmetic concern, surgical correction may be indicated. Since levator function is usually excellent, a conjunctival-Müller's muscle resection or levator aponeurosis advancement procedure will give good results.

REFERENCES

Bell RL, Atweh N, Ivy ME, Possenti P. Traumatic and iatrogenic Horner's syndrome: case reports and review of the literature. J Trauma 2001; 51:400–404.

De la Calle AB, Marin F, Marenco ML. Horner's syndrome following epidural analgesia for labor. Rev Esp Anestesiol Reanim 2004; 51:461–464.

Fetzer SJ. Recognizing Horner's syndrome. J Perianesth Nurs 2000; 15:124–128.

Fields CR, Barker FM 2nd. Review of Horner's syndrome and a case report. Optom Vis Sci 1992; 69:481–485.

George ND, Gonzales G, Hoyt CS. Does Horner's syndrome in infancy require investigation? Br J Ophthalmol 1998; 82:51–54.

Jeffery AR, Ellis FJ, Repka MX, Buncic JR. Pediatric Horner's syndrome. JAAPOS 1998; 2:129–130.

Marx JJ, Thomke F, Birklein F. Horner's syndrome—update on neuroanatomy, topographic diagnosis and etiology. Fortschr Neurol Psychiatr 2005; 73:23–29.

Patel S, Ilsen PF. Acquired Horner's syndrome: clinical review. Optometry 2003; 74:245–256.

Smith SA, Smith SE. Bilateral Horner's syndrome: detection and occurrence. J Neurol Psychiatry 1999; 66:48–51.

Walton KA, Buono LM. Horner syndrome. Curr Opin Ophthalmol 2003; 14:357–363.

Madarosis

INTRODUCTION   Madarosis refers to the loss of eyelashes. It may result from trauma, rubbing the eyelids, or it can follow eyelid surgery with injury to the lash follicles. Madarosis is also associated with systemic diseases such as alopecia areata, but here hair loss is usually seen in other parts of the body as well. Discoid lupus erythematosis involving the eyelids presents with erythema, scarring, and madarosis, but the latter can be the only presenting finding before any other

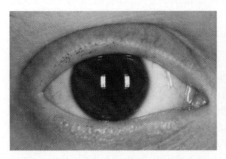 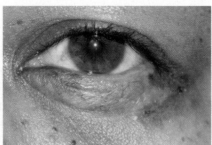 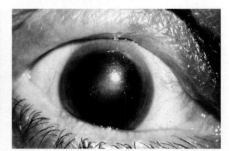

manifestations. Lash loss is also associated with infiltrative lesions such as sarcoidosis, lymphoma, and cutaneous neoplasms. Inflammatory processes including severe blepharitis can cause lashes to fall out, and chronic infections with the mite *Demodex folliculorum*, found in 10% to 15% of normal individuals, can also be associated with madarosis. Loss of lashes and facial hair has been reported as a complication of botulinum toxin for oromandibular dystonia, but this is exceedingly uncommon. Iodine plaque brachytherapy and external beam irradiation for choroidal tumors is a known cause of madarosis. Loss of lashes is a common finding in leprosy and ichthyosis. In some cases the loss of lashes can be factitious or idiopathic.

CLINICAL PRESENTATION   Patients present with absent lashes over some or all of the eyelid margin. In some cases stumps may be seen broken off at or a few millimeters from the skin surface. The lid margin may show evidence of chronic inflammation including erythema, meibomianitis, blepharitis, chalazion, crusting, or ulceration. When the madarosis is localized and associated with lid thickening and telangiectasias, malignancy should be suspected. When associated with excoriations of the facial skin in a young female, a factitious self-inflicted etiology should be considered.

TREATMENT   There is no adequate treatment for madarosis in most cases. Surgical grafting of eyebrow hairs has been used with some success, but often the hairs grow at uncontrolled angles, so that they are cosmetically unattractive or else result in trichiasis. When a specific etiology can be found, such as blepharitis, lid hygiene and topical antibiotics may halt the process. *Demodex* infections are difficult to eradicate, but can be treated with 3% isoptocarbachol or mercury oxide.

REFERENCES

Acharya N, Pineda R 2nd, Uy HS, Foster CS. Discoid lupus erythematosis masquerading as chronic blepahroconjunctivitis. Ophthalmology 2005; 112:e19–e23.

Cru AA, Menezes FA, Chaves E, et al. Eyelid abnormalities in lamellar ichthyosis. Ophthalmology 2000; 107:1895–1898.

Cruz AA, Zenha F, Silva JT Jr, Martinez R. Eyelid involvement in paracoccidiomycosis. Ophthal Plast Reconstr Surg 2004; 20:212–216.

de Gottrau P, Holbach LM, Naumann GO. Palpebral nodule with focal madarosis: neoplasm or chalazion? Apropos of a case. J Fr Ophtalmol 1993; 16:122–124.

Mvogo CE, Bella-Hiag AL, Ellong A, Achu JH, Nkeng PF. Ocular complications of leprosy in Cameroon. Acta Ophthalmol Scand 2001; 79:31–33.

Nowling D. Madarosis and facial alopecia presumed secondary to botulinum a toxin injections. Optom Vis Sci 2005; 82:579–582.

Offret H, Venencie PY, Gregorire-Cassoux N. Madarosis and alopecia areata of eyelashes. J Fr Ophtalmol 1994; 17:486–488.

Rodriguez AE, Ferrer C, Alio JL. Chronic blepharitis and Demodex. Arch Soc Esp Oftalmol 2005; 80:635–642.

Selva D, Chen CS, James CL, Huilgol SC. Discoid lupus erythematosis presenting as madarosis. Am J Ophthalmol 2003; 136:545–546.

Ugurlu S, Bartley GB, Otley CC, Baratz KH. Factitious disease of periocular and facial skin. Am J Ophthalmol 1999; 127:196–201.

Marcus Gunn Jaw Winking Syndrome

INTRODUCTION The Marcus Gunn Jaw Winking Syndrome is a form of congenital synkinetic ptosis that is typically unilateral and non-hereditary, although bilateral and familial cases have been reported. The cause remains unknown, but appears to result from a misdirection of either the efferent motor innervation or the afferent proprioceptive fibers of the third and fifth cranial nerves. This results in inappropriate contraction of muscle fibers of the eye or eyelid during mastication.

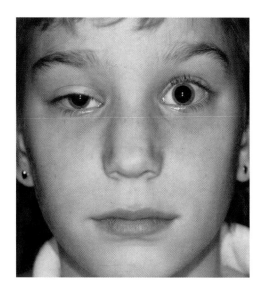
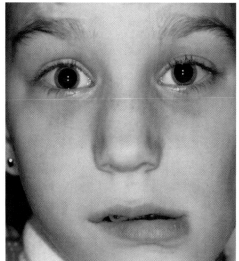

CLINICAL CHARACTERISTICS   The involved upper eyelid typically shows ptosis that may be mild to severe. In most patients the synkinesis is used to reduce the true degree of ptosis which often is greater than appears clinically. With contraction of the masticatory muscles, most commonly the external pterygoid muscle, the ptotic eyelid shows coordinated elevation or even retraction. The characteristic appearance is a "winking" of the eyelid during eating or chewing. The degree of ptosis and the amount of kinetic lid elevation are related proportionately. Aberrant and sometimes bizarre synkinetic movements between the eyelid and other muscles, such as the masseter or temporalis, may be seen. Levator muscle function may be normal or somewhat decreased. Unlike congenital myogenic ptosis, the eyelid crease is usually normal in position. Various types of strabismus may be seen in 25% to 35% of cases, and amblyopia in 35% to 60%. An association between the Marcus Gunn Jaw Winking syndrome and Duane's Retraction syndrome, another neural miswiring disorder, has been reported.

TREATMENT   Therapy is surgical and is often challenging. Preoperatively attention must be paid to any associated strabismus and amblyopia. If the ptosis is the major concern with minimal synkinetic movement, levator surgery alone will usually give good results. For patients with larger amplitude winking, however, it is better to disinsert the levator muscle and elevate the lid with a frontals suspension procedure. There remains some controversy as to the benefit of also disinserting and slinging the contralateral normal eyelid for symmetry. In most cases we prefer unilateral surgery.

REFERENCES

Bowyer JD, Sullivan TJ. Management of Marcus Gunn jaw winking synkinesis. Ophthal Plast Reconstr Surg 2004; 20:92–98.

Davis G, Chen C, Selva D. Marcus Gunn syndrome. Eye 2004; 18:88–90.

Doucet TW, Crawford JS. The quantification, natural course, and surgical results in 57 eyes with Marcus Gunn (jaw-winking) syndrome. Am J Ophthalmol 1981; 92:702–707.

Gogone G, Tomarchio S, Di Pietro M. An atypical case of Marcus Gunn's syndrome. J Fr Ophtalmol 1985; 8:467–470.

Khwarg SI, Tarbet KJ, Dortzbach RK, Lucarelli MJ. Management of moderate-to-severe Marcus Gunn jaw-winking ptosis. Ophthalmology 1999; 106:1191–1196.

Morax S, Mimoun G. Surgical treatment of the Marcus-Gunn syndrome. Indications and results. Apropos of 15 cases. Ophthalmologie 1989; 3:160–163.

Pavone P, Garozzo R, Trifiletti RR, Parano E. Marin-Amat syndrome: case report and review of the literature. J Child Neurol 1999; 14:266–268.

Pratt SG, Beyer CK, Johnson CC. The Marcus Gunn phenomenon. A review of 71 cases. Ophthalmology 1984; 91:27–30.

Rana PV, Wadia RS. The Marin-Amat syndrome: an unusual facial synkinesia. J Neurol Neurosurg Psychiatry 1985; 48:939–941.

Wong JF, Theriault JF, Bouzouaya C, Codere F. Marcus Gunn jaw-winking phenomenon: a new supplemental test in the preoperative evaluation. Ophthal Plast Reconstr Surg 2001; 17:412–418.

INTRODUCTION   Microblepharon is a very rare congenital anomaly that should be distinguished from cryptophthalmos where the eyelids are not formed but skin extends across and over a deformed eye or are fused to a disrupted globe. In microblepharon the eyelid margins are formed and the underlying globe is normal.

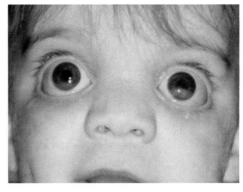

(Courtesy of Richard L. Anderson, M.D.)

CLINICAL CHARACTERISTICS   In microblepharon the eyelid margins are normal but there is a vertical shortening of the lids to varying degrees. The condition may be unilateral or bilateral and can involve both upper and lower eyelids. The shortened lids cause significant lagophthalmos, corneal exposure, and cosmetic deformity. The corneal exposure is associated with symptoms of photophobia, foreign body sensation, and epiphora. If neglected, the cornea can become opaque with dellen formation and even perforation.

TREATMENT   Correction of microphthalmos requires vertical lengthening of the eyelid. The technique will depend upon the degree of eyelid tissue anomaly. For the posterior lamella a hard palate mucosal or chondromucosal graft can be used. For the anterior lamella skin grafts are often needed. Surgery should be timed according to the severity of corneal exposure and the potential development of amblyopia. In severe cases intervention may be indicated within the first few weeks or months of life.

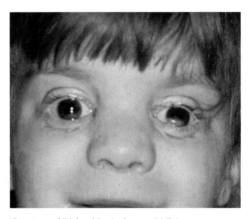

(Courtesy of Richard L. Anderson, M.D.)

REFERENCES

Bernardini FP, Kersten RC, de Conciliis C, Devoto MH. Unilateral microblepharon. Ophthal Plast Reconstr Surg 2004; 20:467–469.

Jordan DR, Hwang IP, Pashby R. Microblepharon: a case report. Ophthalmic Surg Lasers 2000; 31:502–505.

Jordan DR, McDonald H. Microblepharon. Ophthalmic Surg 1992; 23:494–495.

Klauss V, Mnyalla ND, Dechant W, Riedel K. Bilateral congenital microblepharon with ectropion and microphthalmos. Klin Monatsbl Augenheilkd 1981; 179:366–367.

Merriam JC, Stalnecker MC, Merriam GR Jr. Reconstruction of the lids of a child with microblepharon and multiple congenital anomalies. Trans Am Ophthalmol Soc 1988; 86:55–93.

Oromandibular Dystonia

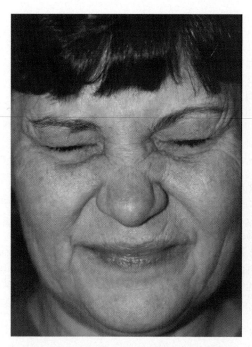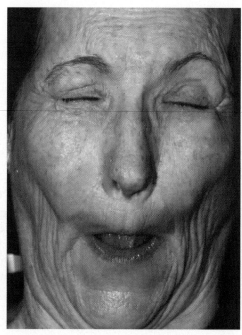

INTRODUCTION   Oromandibular dystonia (OMD) is a focal dystonic movement disorder affecting the mid and lower face, particularly the jaw and tongue. It is characterized by spasms along the sides of the nose, the cheek, mouth, and chin. Uncontrolled spasms make opening and closing of the mouth difficult and can have a profound influence on eating and speaking. Meige's syndrome is a term used for a regional dystonia consisting of the two adjacent focal dystonias, benign essential blepharospasm, and oromandibular dystonia. It is not uncommon for clinical manifestations to begin with orbicularis muscle spasm, later spreading to the lower face and even the neck after months to a few years. The condition can spread further to other focal areas including spastic dysphonia, and cervical dystonia. The etiology is unknown but in the idiopathic form is believed to be related to a neurotransmitter defect possible in the basal ganglia. About 20% of patients with brain injuries develop new onset cervical or oromandibular dystonias. OMD can also result from facial injury and surgery.

CLINICAL PRESENTATION   Symptoms usually begin between the ages of 40 and 70 years and are more common in females. Symptoms begin with mild difficulties opening or closing the mouth and progress to more forceful spasms. Symptoms are often exacerbated by specific activities such as speaking or chewing. Difficulty in swallowing is a common complaint. Spasms of the mid and lower facial muscles occur in an uncontrolled fashion lasting from momentary twitches to sustained forceful and sometimes painful contractions. Occasionally the masseter muscles can be involved with jaw clenching as a major component. Sensory tricks such as humming, singing, or touching the side of the face, chin, or lips, can sometimes reduce the frequency or intensity of spasms.

TREATMENT   Botulinum toxin has become the primary treatment of choice for oromandibular dystonia and essential blepharospasm. More than 90% of patients obtain some relieve of spasms that can last for an average of three months. One to two unit injections of botulinum toxin type A (Botox® or Dysport®) are placed into the involved facial muscles. For patients who become refractory to type A, toxin type B (Myobloc®) can offer some benefit. Complications of botulinum toxin when used in the mid and lower face include bruising, mouth droop, chewing and speaking problems, and dry mouth. Pharmacologic therapy may be useful as an adjunct but is rarely useful as a primary treatment modality. About 20% to 30% of patients will report some benefit from one drug or another. The most important drugs are Clonazepam (Klonopin), trihexyphenidyl (Artane), and baclofen (Lioresal). Unlike blepharospasm, there is no good surgical procedure for oromandibular dystonia.

REFERENCES

Bhidayasiri R, Cardoso F, Truong DD. Botulinum toxin in blepharospasm and oromandibular dystonia: comparing different botulinum toxin preparations. Eur J Neurol 2006; 13:21–29.

Blitzer A, Brin MF, Greene PE, Fahn S. Botulinum toxin injection for the treatment of oromandibular dystonia. Ann Otol Rhinol Laryngol 1989; 98:93–97.

Dutton JJ. Botulinum-A toxin in the treatment of craniocervical muscle spasms: short- and long-term, local and systemic effects. Surv Ophthalmol 1996; 41:51–65.

Erdal J, Werdelin LM, Prytz S, Fuglsang-Frederiksen A, Moller E. Botulinum toxin treatment of patients with oromandibular dystonia. Ugeskr Laeger 2000; 162:6567–6571.

Hanagasi HA, Bilgic B, Gurvit H, Emre M. Clonazepam treatment in oromandibular dystonia. Clin Neuropharmacol 2004; 27:84–86.

Lo SE, Rosengart AJ, Novakovic RL, et al. Identification and treatment of cervical and oromandibular dystonia in acutely brain-injured patients. Neurocrit Care 2005; 3:139–145.

Sankhla C, Lai EC, Jankovic J. Peripherally induced oromandibular dystonia. J Neurol Neurosurg Psychiatry 1998; 65:722–728.

Tan EK, Jankovic J. Botulinum toxin A in patients with oromandibular dystonia: long-term follow-up. Neurol 1999; 53:2102–2107.

Prolapsed Orbital Fat

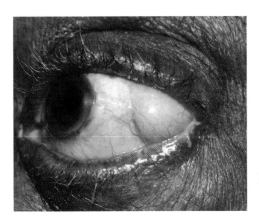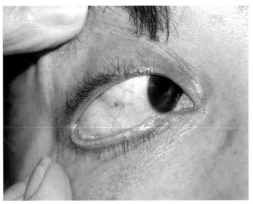

INTRODUCTION   Prolapse of extraconal orbital fat into the eyelids is a common finding generally related to aging phenomena. The fat pockets bulge forward behind a lax orbital septum. That condition is known as steatoblepharon. Prolapse of intraconal orbital fat beneath the conjunctiva is a different phenomenon that presents as a subconjunctival mass rather than a swelling of the

Prolapsed Orbital Fat *(Contd.)*

eyelid. It may be related to trauma, prior eyelid surgery, and has been associated with diseases such as cutis laxa (generalized elastosis). Most often, however, it is seen as an idiopathic condition. It may occur through a dehiscence in Tenon's capsule or the fat can extend into the cowl of Tenon's capsule that extends along an extraocular muscle to its insertion on the sclera. While most patients are older adults, this can be seen in teens and children as well.

CLINICAL PRESENTATION   Prolapse of orbital fat is almost always seen superotemporally where the fat protrudes beneath the lateral part of Whitnall's ligament and palpebral lobe of the lacrimal gland. A soft yellowish-white fat lobule is seen beneath the bulbar conjunctiva just adjacent to the insertion of the lateral rectus muscle or sometimes over it. When small, the lesion may not be visible unless the lid is pulled upward so that the patient may no be aware of it. However, with larger lesions the fat is visible within the palpebral fissure. There is no associated pain or inflammation, and these lesions are usually of cosmetic concern only. Rarely with very large lesions, corneal dryness and even dellen formation can be seen when the lid is lifted off the corneal surface. This condition can be unilateral or bilateral.

TREATMENT   These lesions usually do not require treatment except for cosmetic improvement or when causing corneal exposure. They are easily removed through a conjunctival incision with excision of the prolapsing portion of the fat lobule. Care should be taken not to injure the lateral rectus muscle insertion.

REFERENCES

Daniel CS, Beaconsfield M, Rose GE, et al. Pleomorphic lipoma of the orbit: a case series and review of the literature. Ophthalmology 2003; 110:101–105.

Glover AT, Grove AS. Subconjunctival orbital fat prolapse. Ophthal Plast Reconstr Surg 1987; 3:83–87.

Greaney MJ, Richards AB. Bilateral orbital fat prolapse in cutis laxa. Br J Ophthalmol 1998; 82:713–714.

Jordan DR, Tse DT. Herniated orbital fat. Can J Ophthalmol 1987; 22:173–177.

Jordan DR. Orbital fat prolapse. Arch Ophthalmol 1993; 111:1583.

Liao SB, Ku WC, Song HS, Lin CY. Spontaneous subconjunctival orbital fat prolapse: report of three cases. Chang Gung Med J 2001; 24:399–403.

McNab A. Subconjunctival fat prolapse. Aust N Z J Ophthalmol 1999; 27:33–36.

Monner J, Benito JR, Zayuelas J, et al. Transconjunctival herniation of orbital fat. Ann Plast Surg 1998; 41:658–661.

Retraction of the Eyelid

INTRODUCTION   Eyelid retraction may be seen as a sequel to trauma, surgery, or orbital disease. The most common cause is Graves' disease. This is a systemic autoimmune disease in which the primary target of the immune response is directed toward the TSH receptor of the thyrocyte. Extrathyroidal manifestations principally involve specific fibroblasts of the orbit and of the pretibial dermis. The immune reaction is mediated by anti-TSHR T-cells and results in the release of a Th-1 cytokine profile, proinflammatory mediators, and growth factors that cause deposition of glycosaminoglycans, adipose proliferation, and collagen synthesis with chronic fibrosis. Through the phenomenon of epitope spreading, adjacent tissues become involved, including the extraocular and eyelid muscles, and connective tissue sheaths and fascia.

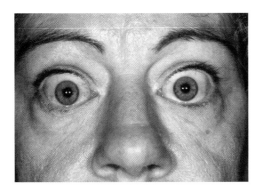 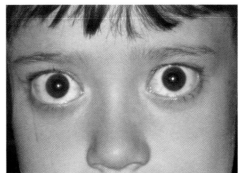

CLINICAL PRESENTATION   In Graves' orbitopathy, the major clinical feature is eyelid retraction. This results in part from the proptosis that accompanies the orbital disease. However, the phenomenon occurs mostly from fibrosis and contraction of the eyelid fascial suspensory system and shortening of the fornix suspensory ligaments of the conjunctiva. There also appears to be some hypertrophy or overaction of the sympathetic muscle of Müller that contributes to eyelid elevation in the upper lid. As retraction becomes worse, scleral show is evident both superiorly and inferiorly. Related to eyelid retraction, on downgaze the upper lid demonstrates a poor ability to follow the globe, such that the superior scleral show becomes worse, a condition known as lid lag. Proliferation and edema of the orbital fat results in prolapse of the fat pockets through the orbital septum, causing the characteristic steatoblepharon of Graves' orbitopathy.

TREATMENT   The management of Graves' orbital and eyelid disease should be medical until the inflammatory component is stable and no longer progressive. It is best to defer treatment of the eyelids until any necessary orbital decompression and strabismus surgery have been completed. Relief of retraction can be temporarily controlled with botulinum toxin injected into the levator muscle. Results last about three months and the procedure can be repeated. Eyelid surgery is indicated for severe retraction, lagophthalmos, and corneal exposure, but also for improved cosmesis. The retracted upper eyelid can be corrected by recession of the levator aponeurosis and Müllers muscle in the upper eyelid, or by a graded blepharotomy of all eyelid layers except for the skin. The lower lid is corrected by recessing the capsulopalpebral fascia, often requiring a scleral or other graft for support. Excessive steatoblepharon is treated with a standard skin and fat blepharoplasty.

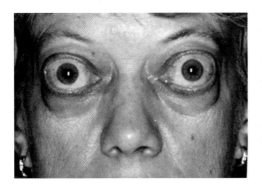 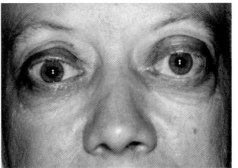

REFERENCES

Biglan AW. Control of eyelid retraction associated with Graves' disease with botulinum toxin A toxin. Ophthal Surg 1994; 25:186–188.

Bodker FS, Putterman AM, Laris A, et al. The effect of hyperthyroidism on Müller's muscle contractility. Ophthal Plast Reconstr Surg 1997; 13:161–167.

Cruz AA, Coelho RP, Baccega A, et al. Digital image processing measurement of the upper eyelid contour in Graves' disease and congenital blepharoptosis. Ophthalmology 1998; 105:913–918.

Dutton JJ. Atlas of ophthalmic surgery. Oculoplastic, Lacrimal, and Orbital Surgery. Vol. II. St Louis: Mosby Year Book, 1992: 144–153.

Elner VM, Hassan AS, Frueh BR. Graded full-thickness anterior blepharotomy for upper eyelid retraction. Trans Am Ophthalmol Soc 2003; 101:67–73.

Feldman KA, Putterman AM, Farber MD. Surgical treatment of thyroid-related lower eyelid retraction: a modified approach. Ophthal Plast Reconstr Surg 1992; 8:278–286.

Grove AS Jr. Levator lengthening by marginal myotomy. Arch Ophthalmol 1980; 98:1433–1438.

Kim JW, Ellis DS, Stewart WB. Correction of lower eyelid retraction by transconjunctival retractor excision and lateral eyelid suspension. Ophthal Plast Reconstr Surg 1999; 15:341–348.

Morton AD, Alner VM, Lemke BN, White VA. Lateral extension of the Muller muscle. Arch Ophthalmol 1996; 114:1486–1488.

Morton AD, Nelson C, Ikada Y, Elner VM. Porous polyethylene as a spacer graft in thee treatment of lower eyelid retraction. Ophthal Plast Reconstr Surg, 2000; 16:146–155.

Mourits MP, Sasim IV. A single technique to correct various degrees of upper lid retraction in patients with Graves' orbitopathy. Br J Ophthalmol 1999; 83:81–84.

Oliver JM, Rose GE, Khaw PT, Colin JR. Correction of lower eyelid retraction in thyroid eye diseases: a randomized controlled trial of retractor tenotomy with adjuvant antimetabolite versus scleral graft. Br J Ophthalmol 1998; 82:174–180.

Ozkan SB, Can D, Soylev MF, Arsan AK, Duman S. Chemodenervation in treatment of upper eyelid retraction. Ophthalmologica 1997; 211:387–390.

Putterman AM. Surgical treatment of thyroid-related upper eyelid retraction. Graded Muller's muscle excision and levator recession. Ophthalmology 1981; 88:507–512.

von Brauchitsch DK, Egbert J, Kersten RC, Kulwin DR. Spontaneous resolution of upper eyelid retraction in thyroid orbitopathy. J Neuroophthalmology 1999; 19:122–124.

Steatoblepharon

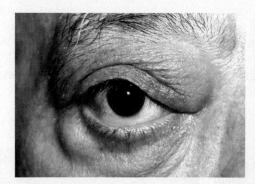 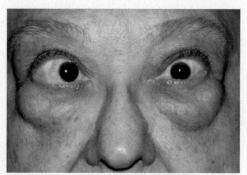

INTRODUCTION   In steatoblepharon the orbital septum becomes weakened and redundant. This allows the extraconal orbital fat pockets to herniate forward into the eyelids. In younger individuals it may be seen as a familial condition, not associated with other signs of aging. However, in most cases steatoblepharon is seen as an involutional phenomenon associated with dermatocholasis, eyelid laxity, and ptosis.

CLINICAL PRESENTATION   The eyelids appear full as the prolapsed orbital fat protrudes beneath the eyelid skin. In the upper eyelid the medial fat pocket is typically the most prominent. Bulging in the lateral upper eyelid is usually not fat, but almost always the result of a prolapsed lacrimal gland. In the lower eyelid there are three compartmentalized fat pockets in 70% of individuals. Other variations include two pockets or even one contiguous pocket. The lateral pocket is typically the most prominent, but fat prolaps often also involves the medial and central fat pockets with a bulging contour across the entire lower eyelid. Steatoblepharon is usually associated with dermatocholasis and in the upper lid may be obscured by extensive overhanging skin folds. Excessive steatoblepharon is typically associated with some systemic disease such as Graves' orbital disease where the fat can be edematous and also increased in volume.

TREATMENT   Treatment is surgical, and often combined with a blepharoplasty. If skin is also to be excised the incision is anterior. For mild fat prolapse the orbital septum can be tightened with light cautery. For more significant degrees of fat prolapse the septum is opened and each fat pocket is isolated, cauterized, and excised. If the lacrimal gland is prolapsed into the lateral upper lid, it is repositioned beneath the superior lateral orbital rim with a suture. In the lower lid when only steatoblepharon is present without dermatochalasis, as in younger patients, a transconjunctival incision can be used. Here the lower capsulopalpebral fascia is opened and the fat pockets excised without disturbing the orbital septum. Care should be taken not to put excessive traction on the fat to avoid possible orbital hemorrhage. When excess skin is also present in the lower lid, a transcutaneous incision is preferred, and the skin is tightened laterally. The modern trend is to reposition most of the fat into the tear trough and beneath the descended malar fat pad.

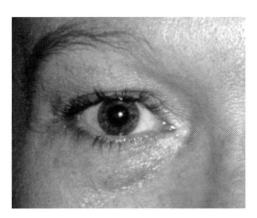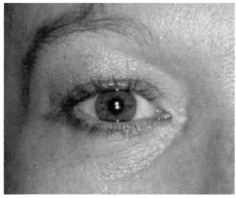

REFERENCES

Bajaj MS, Pushker N, Balasubramanya R. Lower eyelid dermatochalasis with massive postural herniation of orbital fat. Orbit 2004; 23:41–44.

Choo PH, Rathbun JE. Cautery of the orbital septum during blepharoplasty. Ophthalm Plast Reconstr Surg 2003; 19:1–4.

Gladstone HB. Blepharoplasty: indications, outcomes, and patient counseling. Skin Therapy Lett 2005; 10:4–7.

Goldberg RA, Edelstein C, Shorr N. Fat repositioning in lower blepharoplasty to maintain infraorbital rim contour. Facial Plast Surg 1999; 15:225–229.

Goldberg RA, McCann JD, Fiaschetti D, Ben Simon GJ. What causes eyelid bags? Analysis of 114 consecutive patients. Plast Reconstr Surg 2005; 115:1395–1402.

Nassif PS. Lower blepharoplasty: transconjunctival fat repositioning. Facial Plast Surg Clin North Am 2005; 13:553–559.

Persichetti P, Lella F, Delfino S, Scuderi N. Adipose compartments of the upper eyelid: anatomy applied to blepharoplasty. Plast Reconstr Surg 2004; 113:373–378.

Yachouh J, Arnaud D, Jammet P, Goudot P. Transconjunctival inferior blepharoplasty. Rev Stomatol Chir Maxillofac 2005; 106:344–348.

Tarsal Kink Syndrome

INTRODUCTION   The tarsal kink syndrome is a variant of congenital entropion in which there is a horizontal kink or bend in the tarsal plate of the upper eyelid. The cause is unknown, but may be related to *in utero* environmental factors.

CLINICAL PRESENTATION   Typically seen in newborn infants, the eye is red and there may be corneal abrasion. Frank corneal ulceration is not an uncommon sequel, and if not managed early, amblyopia may ensue. The upper eyelid is swollen, with entropion of the lash-bearing margin. The horizontal lid crease is absent, exacerbating the entropion, and there may also be some degree of ptosis. A horizontal ridge representing the tarsal kink may be felt on palpation 3 to 4 mm from the lid margin. Reflex blepharospasm is not uncommon as a result of the corneal irritation. On eversion of the upper eyelid a kink is seen on the tarsus as a concavity just beneath the conjunctiva. The condition is frequently misdiagnosed and treated as conjunctivitis, thus prolonging corneal injury.

TREATMENT   Prompt recognition and treatment of this condition is essential to prevent significant corneal injury and amblyopia. Treatment depends upon the severity of the tarsal deformity. In some cases simple everting eyelid sutures may cure the condition, as will resection of a horizontal strip of skin and orbicularis muscle. In more marked cases a horizontal blepharotomy incision in the region of the kink combined with sutures may be needed. A full marginal rotation procedure through a skin incision will permanently reshape the tarsus in even the most severe situations.

REFERENCES

Bosniak S, Hornblass A, Smith B. Re-examining the tarsal kink syndrome: considerations of its etiology and treatment. Ophthalmic Surg 1985; 16:437–440.

Dutton JJ, Tawfik HA, DeBacker CM, Lipham WJ. Anterior V-wedge resection for cicatricial entropion. Ophthal Plast Reconstr Surg 2000; 16:126–130.

Lucci LM, Fukumoto WK, Alvarenga LS. Trisomy 13: a rare case of congenital tarsal kink. Ophthal Plast Reconstr Surg 2003; 19:408–410.

McCarthy RW. Lamellar tarsoplasty—a new technique for correction of horizontal tarsal kink. Ophthalmic Surg 1984; 15:859–860.

Salour H, Owji N, Razavi ME, Zeaei H. Tarsal kink syndrome associated with congenital corneal ulcer. Ophthal Plast Reconstr Surg 2003; 19:81–83.

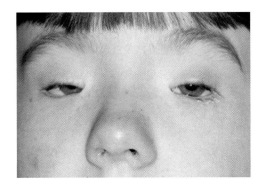 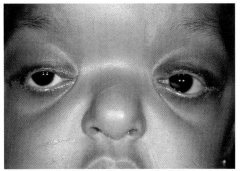

INTRODUCTION   Telecanthus refers to an abnormally wide separation of the medial canthi, with a normal interpupillary distance. The nasal bones are typically normal. This is in contrast to hypertelorism in which there is an increase in the interpupillary distance. The condition can be congenital, where it may be associated with other developmental anomalies such as the Blepharophimosis syndrome, Toriello-Carey syndrome, Blepharo-naso-facial syndrome, Knobloch syndrome, Short syndrome, Smith-Magenis syndrome, and others. Telecanthus can also be an acquired condition resulting from high mid-facial fractures or midline craniofacial lesions such as frontoethmoid meningoencephaloceles.

CLINICAL CHARACTERISTICS   Clinically the eyes as measured by the interpupillary distance are spaced normally apart, but the nasal bridge distance between the medial canthal angles is wide. As a result the eyes may appear somewhat esotropic since the amount of visible medial sclera is less than that laterally. In congenital forms of this anomaly there are associated findings such as ptosis, epicanthus, ocular abnormalities, abnormal ears, nasal defects, arched palate, etc., depending upon the specific syndrome. In traumatic telecanthus there may be associated palpable bony fractures or a soft tissue medial canthal angle dystopia, and the horizontal displacement of the canthal angle may be unilateral or bilateral. With traumatic telecanthus there may be associated lacrimal drainage dysfunction.

TREATMENT   Surgical management by transnasal wiring, screw or miniplate fixation will improve telecanthus. This may be performed for either bilateral or unilateral conditions. For congenital cases repair of associated deformities may require additional procedures. In traumatic telecanthus, early primary repair gives the best chances for a good functional and cosmetic result. Associated injuries, such as to the eyelids and lacrimal drainage systems, can be repaired at the same time.

REFERENCES

Fink SC, Gocken DJ, Oh AK, Hardesty RA. Transnasal canthoplasty. J Craniomaxillofac Trauma 1997; 3:43–48.

Kalavrezos ND, Graetz KW, Eyrich GK, Sailer HF. Late sequelae after high midface trauma. J R Coll Surg Edinb 2000; 45:359–362.

Kos M, Luczak K, Godzinski J, Rapala M, Klempous J. Midfacial fractures in children. Eur J Pediatr Surg 2002; 12:218–225.

Krastinova D, Jasinski MA. Orbitoblepharophimosis syndrome: a 16-year perspective. Plast Reconstr Surg 2003; 111:987–999.

Mathog RH. Posttraumatic telecanthus. Facial Plast Surg 1988; 5:261–267.

Mauriello JA Jr, Caputo AR. Treatment of congenital forms of telecanthus with custom-designed titanium medial canthal tendon screws. Ophthal Plast Reconstr Surg 1994; 10:195–199.

Merkx MA, Freihofer HP, Borstlap WA, van't Hoff MA. Effectiveness of primary correction of traumatic telecanthus. Int J Oral Maxillofac Surg 1995; 24:344–347.

Nowinski TS. Correction of telecanthus in the blepharophimosis syndrome. Int Ophthalmol Clin 1992; 32:157–164.

Shore JW, Rubin PA, Bilyk JR. Repair of telecanthus by anterior fixation of cantilevered miniplates. Ophthalmology 1992; 99:1133–1138.

Trichiasis

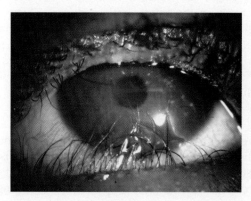 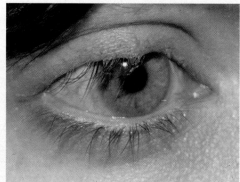

INTRODUCTION   Trichiasis is an acquired condition in which the eyelash cilia are turned backward toward the globe. The lid margin is usually oriented normally with respect to the eye, but the lashes are directed at various angles. Trichiasis usually results from inflammation or scarring of the eyelid following eyelid surgery, trauma, chalazion, or severe blepharitis. It is frequently associated with chronic cicatricial diseases such as ocular pemphigoid, trachoma, and Stevens-Johnson syndrome.

CLINICAL PRESENTATION   The eyelid margin may be normal in position, or it may be associated with entropion. The trichitic lashes arise from the normal lash row, but they are oriented backward towards the cornea. Patients complain of foreign body sensation and chronic ocular surface irritation. Corneal abrasion, conjunctival injection, mucoid discharge, and reflex epiphora are typical findings. In severe cases, frank corneal ulceration may be seen.

TREATMENT   When only a few lashes are involved mechanical epilation will produce temporary relief. Regrowth is usual within three to four weeks. A more permanent cure requires destruction of the offending lash follicles. This is achieved by direct bulb excision, electrolysis, or radiosurgery. When larger areas of the lid margin are involved, cryosurgery may be more effective and less destructive of the lid. Laser ablation of lash follicles has also been reported to be useful. In most cases retreatment is necessary over several sessions in order to completely eliminate the offending lashes. When entropion is also present, the lid margin should be corrected in addition to removing the trichitic lashes since skin against the cornea can also be damaging to corneal epithelium.

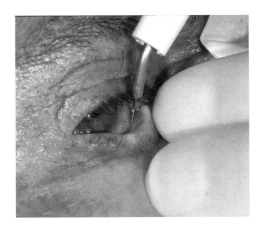

REFERENCES

Basar E, Ozdemir H, Ozkan S, Cicik E, Mirzatas C. Treatment of trichiasis with argon laser. Eur J Ophthalmol 2000; 10:273–275.

Burton MJ, Bowman RJ, Faal H, et al. Long term outcome of trichiasis surgery in the Gambia. Br J Ophthalmol 2005; 89:575–579.

Chi MJ, Park MS, Nam DH, Moon HS, Baek SH. Eyelid splitting with follicular extirpation using a monopolar cautery for the treatment of trichiasis and distichiasis. Graefes Arch Clin Exp Ophthalmol 2005; 17:1–4.

Choo PH. Distichiasis, trichiasis, and entropion: advances in management. Int Ophthalmol Clin 2002; 42:75–87.

Dutton JJ, Tawfik HA, DeBacker CM, Lipham WJ. Direct internal eyelash bulb extirpation for trichiasis. Ophthal Plast Reconstr Surg 2000; 16:142–145.

Elder MJ, Bernauer W. Cryotherapy for trichiasis in ocular cicatricial pemphigoid. Br J Ophthalmol 1994; 78:769–771.

Rosner M, Bourla N, Rosen N. Eyelid splitting and extirpation of hair follicles using radiosurgical techniques for treatment of trichiasis. Ophthalmol Surg Lasers Imaging 2004; 35:116–122.

West ES, Munoz B, Imeru A, et al. The association between epilation and corneal opacity among eyes with trachomatous trichiasis. Br J Ophthalmol 2006; 90:171–174.

Wilcsek GA, Francis IC. Argon laser and trichiasis. Br J Ophthalmol 2003; 87:375.

Chapter 8

Atlas of Eyelid Lesions

Abscess
Acquired Melanosis
Actinic Keratosis
Amyloidosis
Angioedema and Urticaria
Angiosarcoma
Apocrine Adenoma
Apocrine Hidrocystoma
Arteriovenous Hemangioma/
   Malformation
Atopic Dermatitis
Basal Cell Carcinoma
Blepharitis
Blue Nevus
Capillary Hemangioma
Cavernous Hemangioma
Cellular Blue Nevus
Cellulitis
Chalazion and Hordeolum
Chondroid Syringoma
Cicatricial Pemphigoid
Cutaneous Horn
Cylindroma
Dermatofibroma
Dermoid Cyst
Dermolipoma
Eccrine Hidrocystoma
Eccrine Nodular Hidradenoma
Epibulbar Osseous Choristoma
Epidermoid Cyst
Erysipelas
Erythema Multiforme/Stevens-Johnson
   Syndrome/Toxic Epidermal Necrolysis
   Disease Spectrum
Granuloma Annulare
Hemangiopericytoma
Herpes Simplex
Herpes and Varicella Zoster
Ichthyosis
Impetigo
Insect Bite
Intravascular Papillary Endothelial
   Hyperplasia
Intravascular Pyogenic Granuloma
Inverted Follicular Keratosis
Juvenile Xanthogranuloma
Kaposi's Sarcoma
Keloid

Keratoacanthoma
Lentigo Maligna
Lentigo Senilis
Leukemia Cutis
Lupus Erythematosus
Lymphangioma
Lymphoma
Malignant Melanoma
Melanocytic Nevus
Merkel Cell Tumor
Metastatic Tumors
Microcystic Adnexal Carcinoma
Milia
Molluscum Contagiosum
Mucoepidermoid Carcinoma
Mucormycosis
Mycosis Fungoides
Myxoma
Necrobiotic Xanthogranuloma
Necrotizing Fasciitis
Neurofibroma
Nevus Flammeus
Nodular Fasciitis
Oculodermal Melanocytosis
Papilloma
Pemphigus Vulgaris
Phakomatous Choristoma
Pilomatrixoma
Plasmacytoma
Plexiform Neurofibroma
Primary Mucinous
   Carcinoma
Pyogenic Granuloma
Rosacea
Sarcoidosis
Sebaceous Adenoma
Sebaceous Cell Carcinoma
Seborrheic Keratosis
Squamous Cell Carcinoma
Syringoma
Trichilemmal (Sebaceous) Cyst
Trichoepithelioma
Trichofolliculoma
Varix
Verruca Vulgaris
Xanthelasma
Xanthogranuloma

Abscess

INTRODUCTION An abscess is a collection of pus within a cavity formed in soft tissue or bone. It is usually associated with an infection caused by bacteria or parasites that gain access via a break in the skin or sometimes through hematogenous spread. Sometimes a sterile abscess can be induced by retained foreign material. Local tissue cells are destroyed by bacterial action or toxins and this triggers an inflammatory response by attracting large numbers of white blood cells. Regional blood flow is increased causing erythema, and vascular permeability is increased under the influence of released cytokines resulting in tissue edema. Patients with systemic diseases such as diabetes, or who are immunocompromized are at greater risk for developing an abscess from relatively trivial trauma or from a surgical wound. Eyelid abscess can be associated with paranasal and sinus infections or with diseases such as tuberculosis. Obstruction of skin glands or lacrimal ducts can become infected leading to abscess formation.

CLINICAL PRESENTATION The cardinal features of an abscess are localized erythema, swelling, heat, and pain. An elevated soft, fluctuant mass is palpable with overlying injected skin that may be ulcerated and scaling. The abscess may rupture spontaneously and exude a purulent material sometimes mixed with blood. This site often seals over with dried blood and a mucoid crust. Any tissues of the eyelid can be involved. There is often a history of recent local infection, such as a chalazion, or trauma, surgery, or other treatment such as laser or cryosurgery. The infection can spread into the adjacent skin producing a spreading cellulitis. Organisms are often skin bacteria such as staphylococci, but occasionally can be parasites or fungi. Bacteremia can result with systemic manifestations.

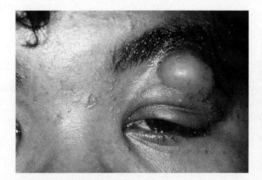 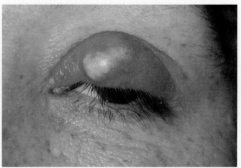

HISTOPATHOLOGY Abscesses are circumscribed areas of tissue necrosis containing a dense infiltrate of neutrophils along with necrotic debris. The edge of an abscess is usually edematous with dilated blood vessels. As abscesses age, they undergo progressive fibrosis beginning from their margins. Lymphocytes and macrophages predominate in chronic abscesses.

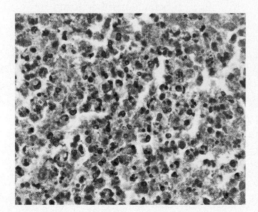 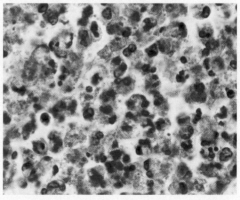

DIFFERENTIAL DIAGNOSIS   The differential diagnosis includes cellulitis, chalazion, and cutaneous malignancies. In the medial canthus one must include dacryocystitis.

TREATMENT   All abscesses should be carefully examined to make sure there is no foreign material present that must be removed. Local measures include warm compresses and topical antibiotics. Systemic antibiotics are administered for any abscess on the face because if the infection spreads to the angular or supraorbital vein it can spread to the cavernous sinus resulting in thrombosis. Medical therapy alone may not be effective and most cases will require surgical drainage. If the cavity is large a draining wick is placed to aid in continued drainage.

REFERENCES

Biswas J, Therese L, Kumarasamy N, Solomon S, Yesudian P. Lid abscess with extensive molluscum contagiosum in a patient with acquired immunodeficiency syndrome. Indian J Ophthalmol 1997; 45:234–236.

Cooper J, Notz R. Subcutaneous abscess following steroid injection of chalazia. Trans PA Acad Ophthalmol Otolaryngol 1986; 38:547–549.

Dispenza C, Saraniti S, Martines F, Caramanna C, Salzano FA. Frontal sinus osteomas and palpebral abscess: a case report. Rev Laryngol Otol Rhinol (Bord) 2005; 126:49–51.

Eifrig CW, Chaudhry NA, Tse DT, et al. Lacrimal gland ductal cyst abscess. Ophthal Plast Reconstr Surg 2001; 17:131–133.

Fayet B, Bernard JA. Eyelid and lacrimal abscesses. Rev Prat 1995; 45:461–464.

Kitagawa K. Blepharitis, hordeolum, abscess in the lids. Ryoikibetsu Shokogun Shirizu 1999; 25:329–332.

Laloyaux P, Vanpee D, Gillet JB. Orbital cellulitis with abscess formation caused by frontal sinusitis. J Emerg Med 2000; 18:253–254.

Raina UK, Jain S, Monga S, Arora R, Mehta DK. Tubercular preseptal cellulitis in children: a presenting feature of underlying systemic tuberculosis. Ophthalmology 2004; 111:291–296.

Acquired Melanosis

INTRODUCTION   Melanocytic lesions of the eyelids run the spectrum from benign nevi and acquired melanosis, to invasive malignant melanoma. Acquired melanosis is very common, with nearly one-third of individuals of European descent having at least one patch of conjunctival melanosis in one eye. It generally appears in middle age. Melanosis consists of abnormally prominent intra-epithelial melanocytes, in contrast to melanocytic nevi where nests of melanocytes occur at the dermal-epidermal junction or wholly within the dermis. Primary acquired melanosis (PAM) is often considered to be pre-malignant melanoma-in-situ. Benign melanosis is more common in young individuals less than 20 years of age, whereas PAM and malignant melanoma pre-dominate in older individuals. Risk factors for malignant change include white race, older age, history of intense sunlight exposure, and cellular atypia within PAM.

CLINICAL PRESENTATION   Acquired melanosis typically appears as one or more flat patches of superficial brown pigmentation involving the conjunctival epithelium. Faint melanotic stippling is often seen beyond the margins of the lesion. The perilimbal area is a common site of involvement, as is the bulbar conjunctiva within the palpebral fissure. The lesion may extend onto the cornea, into the fornices, or onto the palpebral conjunctiva. The eyelids, especially the upper lid, should be doubly everted to examine the entire conjunctival surface. The lesions are usually darkly pigmented, but may be amelanotic in rare cases. Darker focal thickenings or nodules, or involvement of the cornea or skin are suspicious for malignant transformation and must be biopsied.

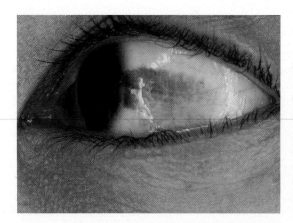 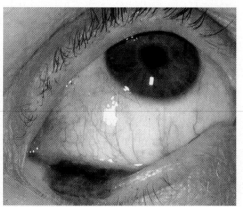

HISTOPATHOLOGY   Primary acquired melanosis (PAM) is classified as lacking atypia or having mild, moderate, or severe atypia based on cell morphology and the pattern of growth within the epithelium. Neoplastic melanocytes may be small polyhedral cells with round nuclei and scant cytoplasm; spindle cells; large melanocytes with complex arborizing dendrites; or round epithelioid cells with abundant eosinophilic cytoplasm. The degree of atypia is deemed more severe as the nucleus enlarges and the nucleolus becomes more prominent. Cells occur in five growth patterns: (*i*) basilar hyperplasia, with proliferated melanocytes along the basal layer of the epithelium; (*ii*) basilar nests of melanocytes that push upward but do not invade the overlying epithelium; (*iii*) intraepithelial nests; (*iv*) spread of individual atypical melanocytes into the epithelium (pagetoid spread); and (*v*) almost complete replacement of the epithelium by atypical melanocytes. PAM is highly variable histologically within different areas of the same lesion, and prognosis depends on the predominant growth pattern. The presence of epithelioid cells and the *lack* of dominant basal hyperplasia are histological features associated with progression to melanoma.

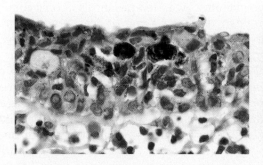 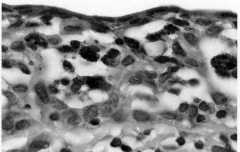

DIFFERENTIAL DIAGNOSIS   Melanosis can be confused with melanocytic nevi, and malignant melanoma. Oculodermal melanocytosis (Nevus of Ota) can look similar but usually also involves deeper tissues such as the sclera and surrounding eyelid skin. When amelanotic, the differential should also include squamous cell carcinoma. There are no clearly established criteria for distinguishing benign melanosis from pre-malignant PAM. However, suspicion should be raised and a biopsy performed for lesions that show progressive growth, are large or multifocal, or those that involve the caruncle, plica, fornices, or palpebral conjunctiva.

TREATMENT   Acquired melanosis can usually be followed with observation if it is limited in extent and growing slowly. For those that enlarge more rapidly or are extensive, excision or biopsy is warranted. If there is no atypia, then the lesion can continue to be observed safely. Repeat biopsies should be performed if worrisome changes occur later. If atypia is seen on the initial biopsy then complete excision should be performed since these carry a nearly 50% risk of transformation to melanoma. If the biopsy shows atypia and areas of invasive melanoma then aggressive excision of the remaining lesion is performed with double freeze-thaw cryotherapy and topical alcohol. Topical chemotherapy with mitomycin C has also been reported to produce regression.

REFERENCES

Baum TD, Adamis AP, Jakobiec FA. Primary acquired melanosis of the conjunctiva. Int Ophthalmol Clin 1997; 37:61–72.

Folberg R, McLean IW, Zimmerman LE. Primary acquired melanosis of the conjunctiva. Hum Pathol 1985; 16:129–135.

Folberg R, McLean IW. Primary acquired melanosis of the conjunctiva: terminology, classification, and biologic behavior. Hum Pathol 1986; 17:652–654.

Gloor P, Alexandrakis G. Clinical characteristics of primary acquired melanosis. Invest Ophthalmol 1995; 36:1721–1729.

Jakobiec FA, Folberg R, Iwamoto T. Clinicopathologic characteristics of premalignant and malignant melanocytic lesions of the conjunctiva. Ophthalmology 1989; 96:147–166.

Krohn J, Monge OR. Conjunctival primary acquired melanosis. Tidsskr Nor Laegeforen 2005; 125:2480–2482.

Ostergaard J, Prause JU, Heegaard S. Caruncular lesions in Denmark 1978–2002: a histopathological study with correlation to clinical referral diagnosis. Acta Ophthalmol Scand 2006; 84:130–136.

Pe'er J, Frucht-Pery J. The treatment of primary acquired melanosis (PAM) with atypia by topical Mitomycin C. Am J Ophthalmol 2005; 139:229–234.

Shields CL, Demirai H, Katatza E, Shields JA. Clinical survey of 1643 melanocytic and nonmelanocytic conjunctival tumors. Ophthalmology 2004; 111:1747–1754.

Shields CL, Demirai H, Shields JA, Spanich C. Dramatic regression of conjunctival and corneal acquired melanosis with topical mitomycin C. Br J Ophthalmol 2002; 86:244–245.

Shields JA, Shields CL. Tumors of the conjunctiva and cornea. In: Smolin G, Thoft RA, eds. The Cornea. 3rd ed. Boston: Little Brown & Co., 1993:588–589.

Actinic Keratosis

INTRODUCTION   Also known as *solar or senile keratoses*, these neoplasms are a common form of premalignant skin lesion seen on the face. Actinic keratoses are related to ultraviolet radiation damage of epidermal cells on sun-exposed areas of the face, hands, scalp, and eyelids. They occur more commonly in fair-skinned middle-aged or older individuals. The risk of malignant transformation is low, about 0.25% per year, but the ultimate development of squamous cell carcinoma in untreated lesions is as high as 20%. Up to 60% of squamous cell carcinomas are said to begin as actinic keratosis. Although some individual actinic keratoses will spontaneously resolve when sun-exposure is reduced, new lesions tend to develop. Squamous cell carcinomas arising from actinic keratoses are believed to be less aggressive than those developing de novo. Actinic keratosis may lie on a continuum toward squamous carcinoma, and recent chromosome aberration and gene mutation studies indicate an association between these two lesions. It has been suggested that actinic keratosis be referred to as "incipient intraepidermal squamous cell carcinoma."

CLINICAL PRESENTATION   Actinic keratoses usually appear as multiple, round, flat-topped erythematous papules with an adherent superficial white scale. Early lesions may be felt as gritty rough spots before they can be seen. On occasion they may develop hyperkeratosis and present as a cutaneous horn. Actinic keratosis can be pigmented which can confuse the diagnosis.

Actinic Keratosis *(Contd.)*

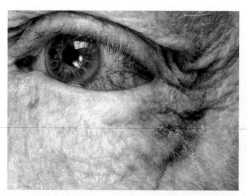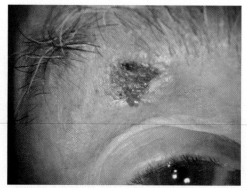

(Courtesy of Robert A. Goldberg, M.D.)

HISTOPATHOLOGY   The epidermis usually is slightly thickened with orthokeratosis, parakeratosis, hyper-granulosis, and cytologically atypical cells resulting in a variable loss of the normal orderly stratified arrangement of the epidermis. The atypical keratinocytes may form small buds or broad or elongated rete ridges. The dermis has actinic elastosis and may have a mild chronic inflammatory infiltrate. The hypertrophic (hyperplastic) form of actinic keratosis has prominent orthokeratosis and parakeratosis, which may result in formation of a cutaneous horn. The hyperplastic epidermis may exhibit conspicuous papillomatosis. Another example of actinic keratosis is shown in the terminology chapter under "parakeratosis."

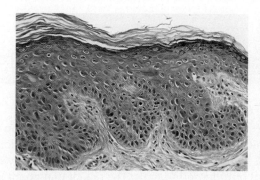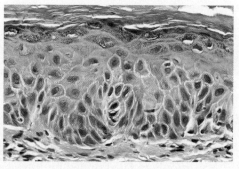

DIFFERENTIAL DIAGNOSIS   The differential diagnosis includes seborrheic keratosis, inverted follicular keratosis, basal cell carcinoma, and squamous cell carcinoma. When pigmented they can be confused with pigmented basal cell carcinoma, lentigo, or malignant melanoma.

TREATMENT   Simple surgical excision or less invasive destruction is recommended in most cases. Multiple lesions respond to topical 0.5% fluorouracil cream applied twice daily for two to three weeks, but this is associated with local skin irritation. Cryotherapy is associated with a 97% initial response rate, with a three year recurrence of 11%. Photodynamic therapy involving a combination of photosensitizing agents with intense pulsed light shows promise in the treatment of multiple or recurrent lesions. More recently topical 5% imiquimod cream has been shown to be effective in treating actinic keratosis. The mechanism of action may be related to its ability to stimulate a cutaneous immune response.

REFERENCES

Berner A. Actinic keratosis and development of cutaneous squamous cell carcinoma. Tidsskr Nor Laegeforen 2005; 125:1653–1654.

Cockerell CJ, Wharton JR. New histopathological classification of actinic keratosis (incipient intraepithelial squamous cell carcinoma). J Drugs Dermatol 2005; 4:462–467.

Jorizzo JL, Carney PS, Ko WT, et al. Treatment options in the management of actinic keratosis. Cutis 2004; 74:9–17.

Lee PK, Harwell WB, Loven KH, et al. Long-term clinical outcomes following treatment of actinic keratosis with imiquimod 5% cream. Dermatol Surg 2005; 31:659–664.

Ooi T, Barnetson RS, Zhuang L, et al. Imiquimod-induced regression of actinic keratosis is associated with infiltration by T lymphocytes and dendritic cells: a randomized controlled trial. Br J Dermatol 2006; 154:72–78.

Salama SD, Margo CE. Large pigmented actinic keratosis of the eyelid. Arch Ophthalmol 1995; 113:977–978.

Scott KR, Kronish JW. Premalignant lesions and squamous cell carcinoma. In: Albert DM, Jackobiec FA, eds. Principles and Practice of Ophthalmology: Clinical Practice. Vol. 3. Philadelphia: WB Saunders, 1994:1733–1744.

Spencer JM, Hazan C, Hsiung SH, Robins P. Therapeutic decision making in the therapy of actinic keratosis. J Drugs Dermatol 2005; 4:296–301.

Zouboulis CC, Rohrs H. Cryosurgical treatment of actinic keratoses and evidenced-based review. Hautarzt 2005; 56:353–358.

Amyloidosis

INTRODUCTION   Amyloidosis represents a variety of disorders that result in abnormal glycoprotein deposition. It can be associated with certain infections, inflammatory processes, and plasma cell dyscrasias. Primary amyloidosis occurs in the setting of no known predisposing disease. Secondary amyloidosis is typically superimposed on a chronic inflammatory disease such as leprosy, osteomyelitis, or rheumatoid arthritis. Amyloidosis occurring with multiple myeloma is considered a distinct entity. Skin deposits occur in up to 30% of patients with amyloidosis, predominantly on the lids, face, neck and extremities, and may be localized or generalized. The most common variety of amyloidosis to affect the eyelid skin is primary localized, representing 75% or more of all ophthalmic cases. In this variety the amyloid deposits consist of light chains secreted by bone marrow plasma cells. In contrast, generalized amyloidosis involving the eyelids may be associated with cardiac, renal, hepatic, or splenic involvement. The respiratory tract, bladder, adrenal glands and urethra may also be involved. Weakening of blood vessels by amyloid deposition can cause episodes of internal and intestinal bleeding. Involvement of the tongue causing macroglossia has been reported in about a third of systemic cases.

CLINICAL PRESENTATION   Ocular adnexal amyloidosis is characterized by amyloid deposition within the deep connective tissue layers of the eyelids, conjunctiva, and anterior orbit. It may not be associated with systemic amyloidosis. The eyelid deposits appear as small, yellowish or pink, waxy papules. Damage to associated vessels may lead to ecchymotic foci underlying the amyloid material, resulting in a very characteristic purple or magenta-colored lesion. Deposition within the upper eyelid tarsal plate and other tissues may present as ptosis with significant superior visual field loss. Yellowish papules or plaques can also occur on the conjunctiva and are associated with ocular discomfort. When the cornea is involved blurred vision is associated with a vascularized corneal mass. Presentation can be atypical including diffuse eyelid swelling, or recurrent eyelid bleeding without any other signs. Affected patients often present with weight loss and weakness.

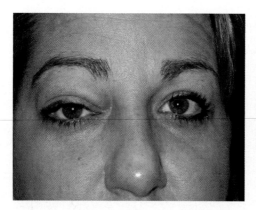
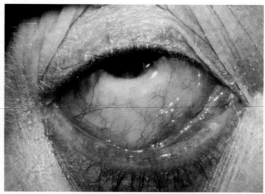

HISTOPATHOLOGY   Amyloid is an extracellular, amorphous, eosinophilic deposit that appears glassy and homogeneous ("hyaline") in H&E stained sections. Amyloidosis of the eyelid may be predominantly in the conjunctiva or skin, with deposits forming nodules replacing the connective tissue and surrounding blood vessels (shown on right below). The deposits contain few cells, usually fibroblasts or chronic inflammatory cells. Congo red causes the amyloid deposits to be orange to red under normal illumination; with polarized light the deposits have green to yellow birefringence (dichroism); an example of amyloid birefringence is illustrated in the terminology chapter under "birefringence." Collagen may stain weakly with Congo red, but it does not exhibit birefringence or dichroism when observed with polarization microscopy.

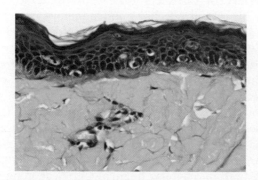
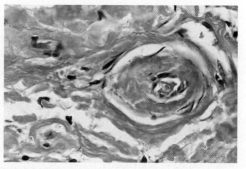

DIFFERENTIAL DIAGNOSIS   The differential diagnosis includes Darier's disease, lipoid proteinosis, xanthelasma, and acanthosis nigricans. Diagnosis can be established by punch, shave, or excisional biopsy and histopathologic evaluation.

TREATMENT   Treatment of the underlying condition is paramount. Although no proven effective treatment has yet been established to control localized involvement of the ocular adnexa, meticulous surgical debulking of the deposits has been reported to be effective. However, recurrences are common.

REFERENCES

Bernardini FP, Schneider S, de Conciliis C, Devoto MH. Advanced periocular, facial, and oral amyloidosis. Ophthal Plast Reconstr Surg 2005; 21:397–398.

Brownstein MH, Helwig EB. The cutaneous amyloidosis, I. Localized forms. Arch Dermatol 1970; 102:8–19.

Fett DR, Putterman AM. Primary localized amyloidosis presenting as an eyelid margin tumor. Arch Ophthalmol 1986; 104:584–585.

Hubbard AD, Brown A, Bonshek RE, Leatherbarrow B. Surgical management of primary localized conjunctival amyloidosis causing ptosis. Br J Ophthalmol 1995; 79:707.

Hill VE, Brownstein S, Jordon DR. Ptosis secondary to amylodosis of the tarsal conjunctiva and tarsus. Am J Ophthalmol 1997; 12:852–854.

Jacobiec FA, Jones IS. In: Duane T, ed. Clinical Ophthalmology. Vol. 2. Philadelphia: Harper & Row, 1983, Chap 35:42.

Kosch G, Meyer-Rusenberg HW. Primary localized amyloidosis of the eyelid and conjunctiva. Klin Monatsbl Augenheilkd 1993; 202:56–59.

Landa G, Aloni E, Milshtein A, et al. Eyelid bleeding and atypical amyloidosis. Am J Ophthalmol 2004; 138:495–496.

Natelson EA, Duncan WC, Macossay CR, Fred HL. Amyloidosis palpebrarum. Arch Intern Med 1970; 125:304–307.

Patrinely JR, Koch DD. Surgical management of advanced ocular adnexal amyloidosis. Arch Ophthalmol 1992; 110:882–885.

Pelton RW, Desmond BP, Mamalis N, et al. Nodular cutaneous amyloid tumors of the eyelids in the absence of systemic amyloidosis. Ophthalmic Surg Lasers 2001; 32:422–424.

Rubinow A, Cohen AS. Skin involvement in generalized amyloidosis. A study of clinically involved and uninvolved skin in 50 patients with primary and secondary amyloidosis. Ann Intern Med 1978; 88:781–785.

Smith M, Zimmerman LE. Amyloidosis of the eyelid and conjunctiva. Arch Ophthalmol 1996; 75:42–51.

Zuravleff JJ, Proia AD. Amyloid deposition in the eyelids. JAMA 1991; 266:2693.

Angioedema and Urticaria

INTRODUCTION   Angioedema and urticaria are common transient phenomena that result from mast cell degranulation with the release of mediators that promote vascular permeability, causing proteins and fluids to extravasate into the extracellular space. In urticaria fluid collects within the dermal tissue, whereas in angioedema fluid collects in the deeper subcutaneous space. The causes of mast cell degranulation are varied and include both immunologic and nonimmunologic mechanisms. Systemic involvement may include rhinitis, bronchospasm, or anaphylaxis. Severe reactions may lead to syncope, bronchial asthma, and hypotension. In rare cases both urticaria and angioedema may be triggered by exercise. Acute cases reach a peak in one to three days and usually fade in 7–21 days. In chronic cases the condition waxes and wanes for months or may even persist for years. There may be recurrent attacks separated by months to years. Inciting allergens are numerous and include foods, cosmetics, ophthalmic preparations, and environmental contactants. A hereditary form of angioedema is caused by a deficiency of the C1 esterase inhibitor, a component of complement.

CLINICAL PRESENTATION   Urticaria is characterized by edema and erythematous wheals which appear as pink edematous papules and plaques with normal overlying epidermis. They are accompanied by burning, stinging, and itching. Lesions may have blanched halos or may be so edematous as to be blanched themselves. They are rarely limited to the eyelids and may occur randomly scattered over the body. Associated edema of the lips, hands, and feet is common. The clinical finding of angioedema is an erythematous evanescent, eyelid swelling accompanied by severe pruritius. In both conditions the reaction usually occurs within 30 to 60 minutes after exposure to an allergen, though a delayed reaction of four to six hours can also occur. No one lesion lasts over 24 hours, but new ones may occur. Reactive conjunctival vascular dilation can also lead to boggy and sometimes massive conjunctival chemosis.

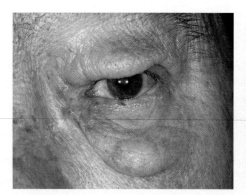 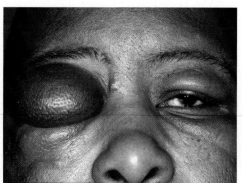

HISTOPATHOLOGY Angioedema is characterized by edema of the deep dermis and/or subcutis, which is recognized in histological sections as separation of the collagen bundles. Venules may appear dilated. There may be a sparse perivascular and interstitial infiltrate of lymphocytes, neutrophils, and eosinophils, though inflammatory cells are absent in hereditary angioedema.

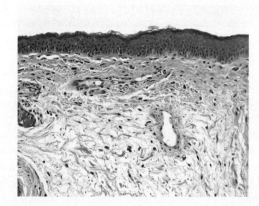 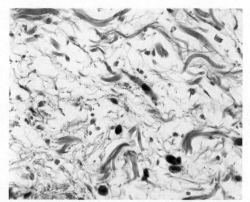

DIFFERENTIAL DIAGNOSIS The differential diagnosis includes contact dermatitis, atopic dermatitis, blepharochalasis, cellulitis, and conjunctivitis.

TREATMENT The key to treatment is to determine the underlying cause since urticaria is always present secondary to an underling immunologic process. Elimination of the inciting factor is curative. Allergy testing may be useful for recurrent cases. In acute urticaria, an etiology is found 20% to 30% of the time and most commonly includes drugs, food or food additives, intravenous radio-opaque contrast medium, hymenoptera stings, infections, or systemic inflammatory diseases. Marked emotional tension may precipitate or exacerbate the condition. Cold, pressure, and sunlight may trigger urticaria in rare familial or sporadic cases. Often, however, the cause cannot be determined. Cold compresses often give relief. Use of subcutaneous epinephrine injection may be necessary for hypotension or airway involvement. In chronic cases the etiology is found in less than 5% of cases.

REFERENCES

Braakenburg A, Nicolai JP. Bilateral eyelid edema: cutis laxa or blepharochalasis. Ann Plast Surg 2000; 45:538–540.

Daxecker F. Hereditary angioedema: pathogenesis, ophthalmological significance, diagnosis, and therapy. Klin Monatsbl Augenheilkd 1980; 177:390–393.

Kaplan AP, Greaves MV. Angioedema. J Am Acad Dermatol 2005; 53:373–388.

Kaplan AP. The pathogenic basis of urticaria and angioedema: recent advances. Am J Med 1981; 70:755–758.

Kato T, Komatsu H, Tagami H. Exercise-induced urticarial and angioedema: reports of two cases. J Dermatol 1997; 24:189–192.

Katz HI. In: Moschella SL, Hurley HJ, eds. Dermatology. Philadelphia: WB Saunders, 1985:269–279.

Margo CE, Stinson WG, Hamed LM. Ophthalmic manifestations of chronic angioedema with necrotizing vasculitis. Am J Ophthalmol 1992; 113:691–696.

Monroe EW, Jones HE. Urticaria. Arch Dermatol 1977; 113:80–90.

Soter NA, Wasserman SI. Urticaria/angioedema: a consideration of pathogenesis and clinical manifestations. Intl J Dermatol 1979; 18:517–532.

Angiosarcoma

INTRODUCTION   Angiosarcomas are aggressive malignant tumors of vascular endothelium that may originate anywhere in the body. They are relatively uncommon, with most occurring in the head and neck region of men over the age of 55 years. Only rarely does this tumor involve the eyelid. They show an aggressive course and have a high potential for metastasis. Metastases occur to the preauricular and cervical lymph nodes, lung, or liver and occur in approximately one third of cases. The prognosis is relatively poor, with a five-year survival rate of approximately 12% to 27%.

CLINICAL PRESENTATION   Angiosarcoma usually presents as innocuous single or multiple bruise-like macules, plaques, or nodules, in the skin or subcutaneously, and occasionally as chronic eyelid edema or cellulitis. On the eyelid they may take the appearance of a yellowish, reddish, or flesh-colored plaque that tends to bleed and ulcerate. Large advanced lesions are elevated, nodular, and occasionally ulcerated. Their variable appearance often leads to a delay in definitive diagnosis. The tumors often spread circumferentially and may extend deeply, eroding into the skull and orbit. They characteristically spread diffusely through the skin and soft tissue of the head and neck region before metastasizing.

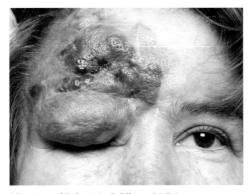

(Courtesy of Robert A. Goldberg, M.D.)

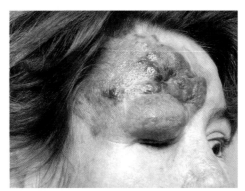

(Courtesy of Robert A. Goldberg, M.D.)

HISTOPATHOLOGY   These tumors vary widely in their degree of differentiation. Moderately differentiated angiosarcomas are most common and exhibit vascular spaces containing erythrocytes surrounded by dense clusters of irregular, moderately pleomorphic, spindle-shaped tumor cells. The endothelial nature of the tumor cells may be confirmed using antibodies to CD31 (shown on right below), CD34, or factor VIII-related antigen.

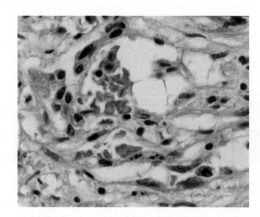 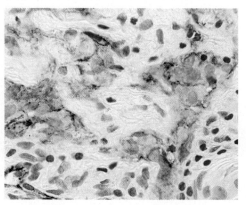

DIFFERENTIAL DIAGNOSIS   The differential diagnosis includes ecchymosis, hemangioma, rosacea, Kaposi's sarcoma, xanthelasma, contact dermatitis, lupus-related lesions, and focal bacterial or fungal infections.

TREATMENT   The preferred of treatment for angiosarcoma is wide-field electron-beam radiotherapy (5000–5600 cGy), often in combination wide local excision, including orbital exenteration when necessary. Chemotherapy is of no proven benefit. The prognosis is poor despite treatment.

REFERENCES

Bray LC, Sullivan TJ, Whitehead K. Angiosarcoma of the eyelid. Aust N Z J Ophthalmol 1995; 23:69–72.

Cernea P, Balan R, Brodicico G. Orbito-palpebral angiosarcoma. Klin Monatsbl Augenheilkd 1968; 153:52–56.

Conway RM, Hammer T, Viestenz A, Holbach LM, Conway RM. Cutaneous angiosarcoma of the eyelids. Br J Ophthalmol 2003; 87:514–515.

Gunduz K, Shields JA, Shields CL, Eagle RC, Nathan F. Cutaneous angiosarcoma with eyelid involvement. Am J Ophthalmol 1998; 125:870–872.

Lapidus, CS, Sutula FC, Stadecker MJ, Vine JE, Grande DJ. Angiosarcoma of the eyelid: yellow plaques causing ptosis. J Am Acad Dermatol 1996; 34:308–309.

Mehrens C, Anvari L, Grenzebach UH, Metze D. Unilateral eyelid swelling as an initial manifestation of angiosarcoma. Hautarzt 2000; 51:419–422.

Panizzon R, Schneider BV, Schnyder UW. Rosacea-like angiosarcoma of the face. Dermatologica 1990; 181:252–254.

Tay YK, Ong BH. Cutaneous angiosarcoma presenting as recurrent angio-oedema of the face. Br J Dermatol 2000; 143:1346–1348.

INTRODUCTION   Apocrine adenomas, also known as apocrine cystadenoma, are rare adnexal tumors that arise from apocrine Moll glands and ducts. The cystadenoma is derived from secretory epithelium, whereas the specific subtype tubular apocrine adenoma consists mainly of tubules with apocrine epithelium. More than 90% of such lesions occur on the face and scalp. Cystic spaces develop with lipid-rich decapitation material as found in apocrine cysts. Rarely, these lesions can undergo malignant change.

CLINICAL PRESENTATION   Apocrine adenomas are slow growing, single or multiple well-circumscribed dome-shaped or papillomatous dermal lesions. They can be solid or they may be cystic with a superior dome of yellowish or creamy material. These lesions occur more often on the eyelid margins where Moll glands are more abundant.

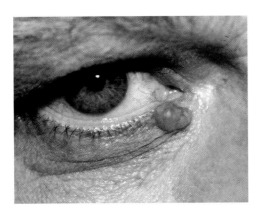

HISTOPATHOLOGY   The tubular variant of apocrine adenoma presents as a well-circumscribed intradermal nodule. The tumor is composed of variably-sized tubules usually composed of a double layer of cells with eosinophilic cytoplasm and round to oval nuclei. The inner lining of cells has prominent decapitation secretion characteristic of apocrine differentiation. Mitoses are rare and cellular pleomorphism is absent.

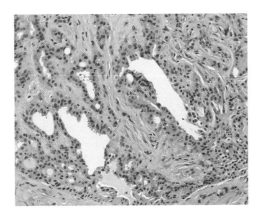 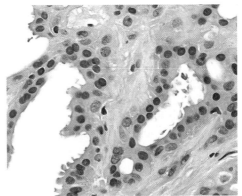

DIFFERENTIAL DIAGNOSIS   The differential diagnosis includes many dermal lesions such as syringoma, apocrine adenocarcinoma, nodular hidradenoma, fibroadenoma, sebaceous cell carcinoma, mucinous adenocarcinoma, myxoid chondrosarcoma, trichilemmal cyst, and trichoepithepthelioma.

TREATMENT   Treatment is usually not required unless the lesion is large and of cosmetic concern or functionally interferes with eyelid function. Surgical excision is easily accomplished. Trichloroacetic acid chemical ablation and electrocautery have also been reported to give good results. The diode laser has been advocated for facial lesions.

REFERENCES

Kruse TV, Khan MA, Hassan MO. Multiple apocrine cystadenomas. Br J Dermatol 1979; 100:675–681.

Matsumoto K, Inoue K, Fukamizu H, Moriguchi T. Apocrine cystadenoma in a child. Arch Dermatol 1983; 119:182–183.

Mehregan AH. Apocrine cystadenoma: a clinicopathologic study with special reference to the pigmented variety. Arch Dermatol 1964; 90:274–279.

Ni C, Dryja TP, Albert DM. Sweat gland tumors in the eyelids: a clinicopatholgical analysis of 55 cases. Intern Ophthalmol Clin 1982; 22:1–22.

Sacks E, Jakobiec FA, McMillan R, Frainfelder F, Iwamoto T. Multiple bilateral apocrine cystadenomas of the lower eyelids. Light and electron microscopic studies. Ophthalmology 1987; 94:65–71.

Seregard S. Apocrine adenocarcinoma arising in Moll gland cystadenoma. Ophthalmology 1993; 100:1716–1719.

Stokes J, Ironside J, Smith C, Dhillon B. Tubular apocrine adenoma—an unusual eyelid tumour. Eye 2005; 19:237–239.

Zumdick M, Milder P, Ruzicka T, Holzle E. Cutaneous apocrine mixed tumor with follicular differentiation. Hautarzt 1995; 46:481–484.

Apocrine Hidrocystoma

INTRODUCTION   Also known as a *cystadenoma*, *sudoriferous cyst*, or *cyst of the gland of Moll*, these lesions arise from apocrine glands of Moll and are true cystic adenomas of the secretory cells rather than retention cysts. These lesions are also associated with Schopf-Schulotz-Passarge syndrome, an ectodermal dysplasia in which patients display multiple periocular apocrine hydrocystomas, hypodontias, hypotrichosis, and palmoplantar hyperkeratosis.

CLINICAL PRESENTATION   Apocrine hidrocystoma lesions are small (less than 1 cm in diameter) solitary, translucent cysts on the eyelid, usually near the eyelid margin at the canthal angles. The overlying skin is shiny and smooth and the cyst is filled with clear or milky fluid. A layered precipitate of yellow or creamy material may be seen at the base of the cyst representing lipid-rich decapitation secretions. More rarely the cyst may display a bluish coloration. On occasion multiple lesions may occur and long standing lesions may reach several centimeters in size. They often occur bilaterally and symmetrically, and can become confluent and disfiguring.

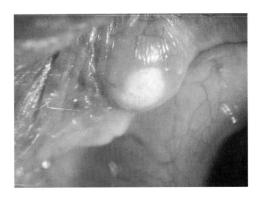 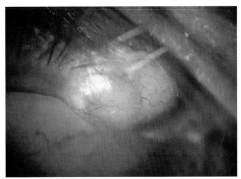

HISTOPATHOLOGY   Two layers of cells line these cysts, which may be unilocular or multilocular. The inner lining is composed of columnar cells with eosinophilic cytoplasm and decapitation secretion (buds of cytoplasm detaching from the luminal surface). Myoepithelial cells compose the outer layer; the cells are flat to low cuboidal. The epithelium may form papillary projections into the lumen. Cyst contents, when present, are lightly eosinophilic proteinaceous material.

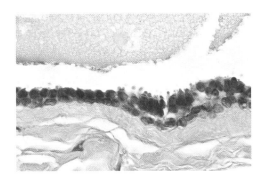

DIFFERENTIAL DIAGNOSIS   The differential diagnosis includes eccrine hidrocystoma, epidermoid cyst, and cystic basal cell carcinoma.

TREATMENT   In general, no treatment is necessary. But when removal of the lesion is desired for diagnosis, cosmesis, or to diminish irritation or obstruction of vision, complete surgical excision is appropriate with meticulous removal of the intact cyst wall. In cases of multiple or recurrent lesions adherent to the epithelium, en-bloc excision via a blepharoplasty type incision may be a useful approach. Chemical ablation of the cystic epithelium with trichloroacetic acid has been reported to yield excellent results without scarring. Carbon dioxide laser vaporization has also shown good results.

REFERENCES

Alessi E, Gianotti R, Coggi A. Multiple apocrine hidrocystomas of the eyelids. Br J Dermatol 1997; 137:642–645.

Dailey RA, Saulny SM, Tower RN. Treatment of multiple apocrine hidrocystomas with trichloroacetic acid. Ophthal Plast Reconstr Surg 2005; 21:148–150.

del Pozo J, Garcia-Silva J, Pena-Penabad C, Fonseca E. Multiple apocrine hidrocystomas: treatment with carbon dioxide laser evaporation. J Dermatolog Treat 2001; 12:97–100.

Hampton PJ, Angus B, Carmichael AJ. A case of Schopf-Schultz-Passarge syndrome. Clin Exp Dermatol 2005; 30:528–530.

Hassan MO, Khan MA, Kurse TV. Apocrine cystadenoma. An ultrastructural study. Arch Dermatol 1979; 115:194–200.

Henderer JD, Tanenbaum M. Excision of multiple eyelid apocrine hidrocystomas via an en-bloc blepharoplasty incision. Ophthalmic Surg Lasers 2000; 31:157–161.

Lahav M, Albert DM, Bahr R, Craft J. Eyelid tumors of sweat gland origin. Albtecht Von Graefes Arch Klin Exp Ophthalmol 1981; 216:301–311.

Shields JA, Eagle RC, Shields CL, de Potter P, Markowitz G. Apocrine hydrocystoma of the eyelid. Arch Ophthalmol 1993; 111:866–867.

Smith JD, Chernosky ME. Apocrine hydrocystoma (cystadenoma). Arch Dermatol 1974; 109:700–702.

Arteriovenous Hemangioma/Malformation

INTRODUCTION   The nomenclature of vascular lesions of the skin remains very unclear and there are no clear-cut guidelines for clinicians. Despite attempts at better classifications hemangiomas and malformations are still often confused. Most authorities classify vascular lesions as hemangiomas (hamartomas) or malformations (developmental anomalies). This is further refined based on endothelial characteristics and flow type. When arteriovenous lesions occur in the skin they are often referred to as hemangiomas, but are synonymous with what are referred to as arteriovenous malformations (AVM) elsewhere. These fast-flow lesions can occur either as congenital defects or less commonly they can develop following trauma, surgery or even as a sequel to inflammation. They are uncommon on the face and particularly rare on the eyelids. Unlike capillary hemangiomas, AVM's do not involute, and often become progressively worse.

CLINICAL PRESENTATION   The lesion appears as a pulsating single vessel or mass, or a tangle of blood vessels, red to purple in coloration. It is compressible and spongy, but refills quickly after compression. There is often a palpable thrill and sometimes an auditory bruit in this pulsatile lesion. Bleeding often occurs either into the surrounding tissue or onto the surface. The Valsalva maneuver or bending forward often increases the size of the lesion and gives the subjective perception of throbbing. Orbital involvement may result in proptosis and can affect vision. Diagnosis is often aided with Doppler ultrasonography, CT scan and carotid arteriography, or digital subtraction angiography.

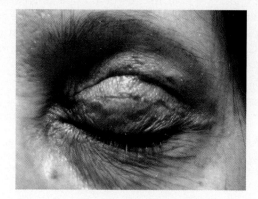 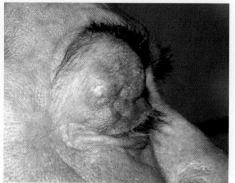

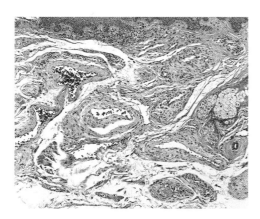 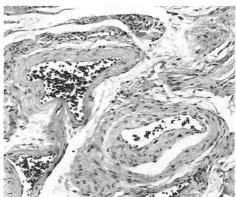

HISTOPATHOLOGY   This form of hemangioma is composed of numerous mostly thick walled vessels resembling both arteries and veins. The muscular walls have variable elastic lamina, and arteriovenous anastomoses and/or thrombi may be present. Eyelid arteriovenous hemangiomas are usually well-circumscribed intradermal masses.

DIFFERENTIAL DIAGNOSIS   The differential diagnosis includes lymphangioma, hemangioma, venous lake, plexiform neurofibroma, varicose veins, and carotid-cavernous fistula.

TREATMENT   Treatment is not indicated during infancy or childhood unless visual symptoms or amblyopia threatens. When treatment is required surgical resection with prior occlusion of feeder vessels is best, but is usually very difficult and can be mutilating. Identification and ligation of feeder vessels will give only temporary relief since rapid recruitment of flow from nearby arteries will reestablish blood supply in most cases. Embolization can be considered, but it carries a risk of undesirable intracranial or retinal vessel obstruction when employed in periorbital lesions. Sclerotherapy can be useful if the feeder vessels are first ligated. While laser therapy is useful for slow flow venous malformations they are less useful for the AVM.

REFERENCES

Buckmiller LM. Update on hemangiomas and vascular malformations. Curr Opin Otolaryngol Head Neck Surg 2004; 12:476–487.

Fishman SJ, Mulliken JB. Hemangiomas and vascular malformations of infancy and childhood. Pediatr Clin North Am 1993; 40:1177–1200.

Forman AR, Lussenhop AJ, Limaye SR. Ocular findings in patients with AVM of the head and neck. Am J Ophthalmol 1975; 79:626–633.

Holt JE, Holt GR, Thornton WR. Traumatic arteriovenous malformation of the eyelid. Ophthalmic Surg 1980; 11:771–777.

Hundeiler M. What is a hemangioma, what is a malformation? On the differential diagnosis of vascular tumors. Kongressbd Dtsch Ges Chir Kongr 2001; 118:439–442.

Marler JJ, Mulliken JB. Current management of hemangiomas and vascular malformations. Clin Plast Surg 2005; 32:99–116.

Mulliken JB, Glowacki J. Hemangiomas and vascular malformations in infants and children. A classification based on endothelial characteristics. Plast Reconstr Surg 1982; 69:412–422.

Rootman J. Vascular malformations of the orbit: hemodynamic concepts. Orbit 2003; 22:103–120.

Rusin LJ, Harrell ER. Arteriovenous fistula: Cutaneous manifestations. Arch Dermatol 1976; 112:1135–1138.

Spring MA, Bentz ML. Cutaneous vascular lesions. Clin Plast Surg 2005; 32:171–186.

Very M, Nagy M, Carr M, Collins S, Brodsky L. Hemangiomas and vascular malformations: Analysis of diagnostic accuracy. Laryngoscope 2002; 112:612–615.

Zweep HP, Rieu PN, van Die CE, Boll AP, Steijlen PM, Spauwen PH. Haemangiomas and congenital vascular malformations: their classification and diagnosis. Ned Tijdschr Geneeskd 2002; 146:1072–1077.

Atopic Dermatitis

INTRODUCTION   The eyelids can be affected by various types of dermatitis that can be difficult to diagnose. Of these types 70% result from allergic contact dermatitis, and about 9% to 10% each from irritant contact dermatitis, atopic dermatitis, and seborrheic dermatitis. Atopic dermatitis is a chronically relapsing inflammatory skin disease. It is a genetically fixed disease that remains with the patient all their lives, whether they show symptoms or not. It occurs in approximately 2% of the population. In several large series 80% to 90% of patients with eyelid dermatitis were female. Distinct infantile, juvenile, and adult stages of the disease have been reported. Associated diffuse eczematous skin changes vary with the age of the patient and often disappear during puberty or adolescence. In the infantile stages associated manifestations include facial erythema and crusting. After age two to three years erosions, lichenification, and hyper or hypopigmentaton develop particularly on the face and flexural surface of the extremities. In adults the rash may be bright red, edematous and oozing or more chronic appearing with lichenified and hyperpigmented patches, or it may present as a mixture of both. Infectious complications are common and it has been shown that 87% of patients with atopic dermatitis harbor bacterial colonization in the conjunctival sac and eyelid margins compared to 25% in nonaffected controls. A family history of atopy manifested by atopic dermatitis, asthma, or hay fever exists in 70% of affected individuals. Eyelash length has been shown to be longer in children and adolescents with allergic diseases, including atopic dermatitis.

CLINICAL PRESENTATION   Eyelid changes consist of edematous, indurated, or weeping eczematous lesions. Pruritis aggravated by heat, sweat, or wool often leads to chronic rubbing and as a result, the eyelid skin becomes violaceous early on and hyperpigmented with time. Coalescent papules, fissures, and fine scaling may occur. If the condition becomes chronic, thickening and accentuation of normal skin lines (lichenification) can occur on the periocular skin, and scaling plaques occur predominantly on the upper eyelids. With time eversion or stenosis of the lacrimal puncta may occur and frank ectropion may be seen in severe cases. Loss of eyelashes can occur. Darkening of periorbital skin suggests the diagnosis of atopy and is frequently of cosmetic concern to patients. Secondary staphylococcal infection or colonization of the eczematous skin is common leading to chronic anterior blepharitis. Associated ocular changes include keratoconjunctivitis, chemosis, symblepharon, corneal pannus, Tranta's dots, anterior and posterior subcapsular cataracts, and keratoconus.

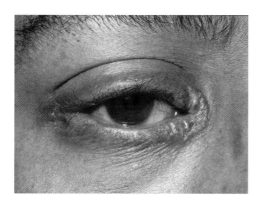 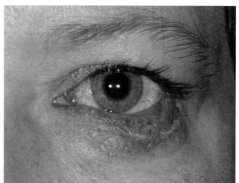

HISTOPATHOLOGY   The histological appearance is dependent on the phase of the process. Acute lesions show spongiosis, lymphocytes, and macrophages around blood vessels of the superficial dermis, and extension of inflammatory cells into the epidermis (exocytosis). Subacute lesions exhibit irregular acanthosis, mild spongiosis, hyperkeratosis, small foci of parakeratosis, and mild exocytosis. Chronic lesions have further thickening of the epidermis, diminished spongiosis, focal parakeratosis, and dermal fibrosis from persistent rubbing. A sparse infiltrate of eosinophils is common in the dermis.

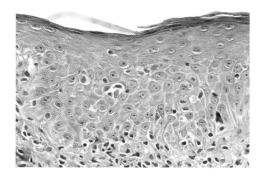

DIFFERENTIAL DIAGNOSIS   The differential diagnosis includes seborrheic dermatitis, lichen simplex chronics, allergic contact dermatitis, irritant contact dermatitis, urticaria, angioedema, and rosacea.

TREATMENT   The "itch-scratch" cycle must be broken in order to control the dermatitis. Treatment generally relates to intensive patient education, avoidance of known exacerbating factors such as irritant exposure, emotional stress, and infection. Topical corticosteroid preparations, oral antihistamines, and use of bland emollients (Aquaphor®, white petrolatum, and absorbase) that decrease dryness (*xerosis*) are important. Avoidance of hot humid climates and harsh skin detergents together with frequent skin hydration with oils or creams is important to minimize flare-ups. Cool, damp compresses often aid in relieving pruritis. Periodic flare-ups are treated aggressively with low potency nonfluorinated topical corticosteroids such as hydrocortisone or dexamethasone. Secondary staphylococcal infection is treated with oral antibiotics or bland topical antibiotic ointments. Topical corticosteroids and mast cell stabilizers are often needed to control acute keratoconjunctivitis. Surgical intervention for the eyelid changes may be necessary, but is associated with an increased incidence of peri-operative complications.

Atopic Dermatitis (Contd.)

REFERENCES

Ayala F, Fabbrocini G, Bacchilega R, et al. Eyelid dermatitis: an evaluation of 447 patients. Am J Contact Dermat 2003; 14:69–74.

Dogru M, Nakagawa N, Tetsumotot K, Katakami C, Yamamoto M. Ocular surface disease in atopic dermatitis. Jpn J Ophthalmol 1999; 43:53–57.

Garrity JA, Liesegang TJ. Ocular complications of atopic dermatitis. Can J Ophthalmol 1984; 19:21–24.

Guin JD. Eyelid dermatitis: a report of 215 patients. Contact Dermatitis 2004; 50:87–90.

Guin JD. Eyelid dermatitis: experience in 203 cases. J Am Acad Dermatol 2002; 47:755–765.

Hanifin JM. Atopic dermatitis. J Allergy Clin Immunol 1984; 73:211–226.

Hanifin JM. Atopic dermatitis. Special clinical complications. Postgrad Med 1983; 74:188–193, 196–199.

Inoue Y. Ocular infections in patients with atopic dermatitis. Int Ophthalmol Clin 2002; 42:55–69.

Levy Y, Segal N, Ben-Amitai D, Danon YL. Eyelash length in children and adolescents with allergic diseases. Pediatr Dermatol 2004; 21:534–537.

Nakata K, Inoue Y, Harada J, et al. A high incidence of Staphylococcus aureus colonization in the external eyes of patients with atopic dermatitis. Ophthalmology 2000; 107:2167–2171.

Valsecchi R, Imerti G, Martino D, Cainelli T. Eyelid dermatitis: an evaluation of 150 patients. Contact Dermatitis 1992; 27:143–147.

Zug KA, Palay DA, Rock A. Dermatologic diagnosis and treatment of itchy red eyelids. Surve Ophthalmol 1996; 40:293–305.

Basal Cell Carcinoma

INTRODUCTION   Basal cell carcinoma is a malignant tumor derived from cells of the basal layer of the epidermis. It represents the most common malignant tumor of the eyelids, comprising 85–90% of all malignant epithelial eyelid tumors. The etiology of basal cell carcinomas is linked to excessive ultraviolet light exposure in fair-skinned individuals. Several types of basal cell carcinoma can occur on the eyelids. The nodular-type is the most common, followed by the morphea variety. Over 99% of basal cell carcinomas occur in Caucasians. They are seen typically in middle aged and elderly adults, but are more frequently being seen in younger adults, and several cases have been reported in children without pre-existing genetic syndrome or a history of radiotherapy. Predisposing factors include ionizing radiation, arsenic exposure, and pre-existing scars. Having had one basal cell carcinoma is risk for the development of additional lesions. While metastases are rare (0.028–0.55%), local invasion is common and can be very destructive. Basal cell nevus syndrome, also known as *Gorlin-Goltz syndrome* or *nevoid basal cell carcinoma syndrome*, is an autosomal dominantly inherited disorder associated with multiple basal cell carcinomas affecting the face, trunk, and extremities with a high rate of recurrence.

CLINICAL PRESENTATION   Basal cell carcinomas are often located on the lower eyelid (50–60%) and near the medial canthus (25–30%). Uncommonly they may occur on the upper eyelid (15%), and lateral

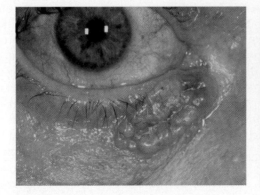
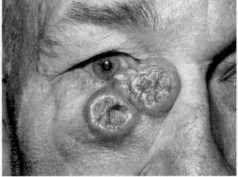

canthus (5%). The nodular-type is the most common form to affect the eyelid and has the classic appearance of a pink or pearly papule or nodule with overlying telangiectatic vessels. As the tumor grows in size a central ulceration may occur surrounded by a rolled border (also known as a "rodent ulcer"). Cystic varieties may occur. The pigmented basal cell carcinoma is similar, but with brown or black pigmentation. These lesions represent the most common pigmented malignancy on the eyelids, and may resemble malignant melanoma. The morphea or sclerosing type appears as a flat, indurated yellow to pink plaque with ill-defined borders. It may simulate blepharitis or dermatitis. This form of basal cell carcinoma is aggressive and can invade the dermis deeply. It characteristically occurs in the medial canthal region and can invade into the paranasal sinuses, lacrimal system, and orbit. Superficial basal cell carcinomas appear as an erythematous, scaling patch with raised pearly borders. Recurrent tumors tend to be more aggressive and infiltrative and show a lower rate of cure than with primary lesions.

HISTOPATHOLOGY   Basophilic tumor cells with hyperchromatic nuclei form irregular lobules. Along the periphery of the tumor lobules, the cells often are arranged radially with their long axes parallel to each other, creating so-called "peripheral palisading". Stroma surrounding the tumor is often mucinous and artifactually shrinks away from the tumor islands during histological processing, creating thin clefts. Clefts and mucinous matrix help to distinguish poorly differentiated basal cell carcinoma from poorly differentiated squamous cell carcinoma. Tumor lobules may have central necrosis, a prominent adenoid pattern, or strands of basaloid cells in a dense fibrous stroma (morphea or sclerosing pattern).

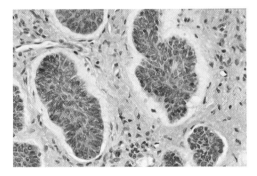 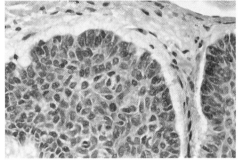

DIFFERENTIAL DIAGNOSIS   The differential diagnosis includes malignant melanoma, sebaceous cell carcinoma, squamous cell carcinoma, actinic keratosis, radiation dermatitis, keratoacanthoma, cutaneous horns, dermoid and sebaceous cysts, eccrine and apocrine cysts, papillomatous lesions, seborrheic kertosis, blepharitis, chalazion, eczema, psoriasis, and seborrheic dermatitis.

TREATMENT   The goal of therapy is the complete removal of tumor cells with preservation of uninvolved eyelid and periorbital tissues. If excision is done without histologic control, a 4 mm margin will give adequate results in most cases. It has been shown that even with residual tumor at the cut margin the recurrence rate is only 38%. Mohs' micrographic surgery with frozen section control has proven to yield the highest cure rate with the most effective preservation of normal tissue. Recurrence rates with this technique are reported at 0.5–1%. Radiation therapy in doses of 4,000–6,500 cGy has been reported to yield a 5-year tumor free control rate of 91%. While some have advocated its use for small nodular lesions, it may be more appropriate for the treatment of advanced invasive or recurrent tumors. Cryotherapy is often used to treat non-periorbital lesions but when used on the eyelid, notching of the lid margin, malpositions of the eyelid, symblepharon formation with fornix foreshortening, and pigmentary changes of the eyelid skin may be seen as complications. It is also associated with a higher recurrence rate. Tumor regression has been reported with topical 5% neomycin cream.

REFERENCES

Al-Bouloushi A, Filho JP, Cassie A, Arthurs B, Burnier MN Jr. Basal cell carcinoma of the eyelid in children: a report of three cases. Eye 2005; 19:1313–1314.

Arlette JP, Carruthers A, Threlfall WJ, Warshawski LM. Basal cell carcinoma of the periocular region. J Cutan Med Surg 1998; 2:205–208.

Buschmann W. A reappraisal of cryosurgery for eyelid basal cell carcinomas. Br J Ophthalmol 2002; 86:453–457.

D'Hermies F, Morel X, Meyer A, et al. Pigmented basal cell carcinoma of the eyelid. Apropos of a clinical case. J Fr Ophtalmol 1998; 21:462–463.

Hamada S, Kersey T, Thaller VT. Eyelid basal cell carcinoma: non-Mohs excision, repair, and outcome. Br J Ophthalmol 2005; 89:992–994.

Karcioglu ZA, al-Hussain H, Svedberg AH. Cystic basal cell carcinoma of the orbit and eyelids. Ophthal Plast Reconstr Surg 1998; 14:134–140.

Leibovitch I, McNab A, Sullivan T, Davis G, Selva D. Orbital invasion by periocular basal cell carcinoma. Ophthalmology 2005; 112:717–723.

Leshin B, Yeatts P, Anscher M, Montano G, Dutton JJ. Management of basal cell carcinoma: Mohs' micrographic surgery versus radiotherapy. Surv Ophthalmol 1993; 38:193–212.

Lindgren G, Lindholm B, Bratel AT, Molne L, Larko O. Mohs' micrographic surgery for basal cell carcinomas on the eyelids and medial canthal area. I. Characteristics of the tumours and details of the procedure. Acta Ophthalmol Scand 2000; 78:425–429.

Nerad JA. Periocular basal cell carcinoma in adults 35 years of age and younger. Am J Ophthalmol 1988; 106:723–729.

Pieh S, Kuchar A, Novak P, et al. Long-term results after surgical basal cell carcinoma excision in the eyelid region. Br J Ophthalmol 1999; 83:85–88.

Shields CL. Basal cell carcinoma of the eyelids. Int Ophthalmol Clin 1993; 33:1–4.

Torre D. Cryosurgery of basal cell carcinoma. J Am Acad Dermatol 1986; 15:917–929.

Blepharitis

INTRODUCTION Blepharitis is a general term referring to eyelid margin inflammation. The two most prevalent factors appear to be a dysfunction of the sebaceous glands (meibomian glands), and colonization by pathogenic staphylococci. Additional common features include a diminished or abnormal tear production, chronic conjunctivitis, and structural changes in the lid margin due to chronic inflammation. Several organisms have at times been implicated in the etiology of blepharitis, including *Moraxalla*, *Demodex folliculorum*, and *Malassezia furfur* (*Pityrosporum ovale*), however, it now appears the most likely organism is *Staphylococcus*. Once the bacteria colonize the lid margin and meibomian glands they are virtually impossible to eradicate. Through their production of aggravating exotoxins and enzymes that convert lipids to fee fatty acids, they are responsible for many of the ongoing tissue changes and chronic inflammation seen in blepharitis. They remain sequestered deep in the meibomian glands and can also survive within phagocytizing cells where they remain isolated from antibodies or host defense systems. Once in the tear film free fatty acids can contribute to corneal epithelial breakdown and subsequent punctate keratitis. Although the majority of symptomatic patients are adults, most cases of chronic blepharitis begin in childhood as a localized form of seborrhea.

CLINICAL PRESENTATION   Blepharitis is characterized by small brittle scales and collarettes at the base of the lashes, and moderate erythema along the eyelid margin. A more severe ulcerative form has larger mottled crusts surrounding the base of the lashes, which upon removal result in small ulcers and even bleeding. With time the lid margins develop telangiectasias and become permanently thickened, roughened, and keratinized on the inner surface. The orifices of the meibomian glands may be dilated and inflamed, and become capped by a dome of inspissated oil or it may take on a "pouting" appearance. The tear film may appear foamy with suspended particulate debris over the surface of the cornea. Recurrent hordeola and loss of lashes are often seen. Angular blepharitis represents a distinct form of blepharitis characterized by a subacute or chronic inflammation of the skin of the lateral canthal region associated with a low-grade conjunctivitis. Symptoms of blepharitis include burning, itching, tearing, blurred vision, and discharge. Due to a disruption in the lipid layer of the corneal tear film, the cornea may lose its lubricant ability, eventuating in chronic keratitis sicca. Marginal corneal infiltrates representing antigen-antibody precipitates are also intermittently seen.

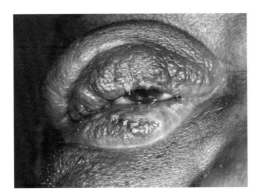 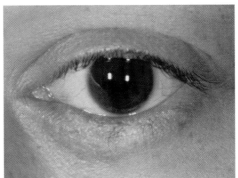

HISTOPATHOLOGY   Seborrheic dermatitis is a chronic dermatosis that characteristically involves the scalp, ears, eyebrows, eyelid margins, and nasolabial areas. In common with other chronic forms of blepharitis, there is mild, superficial perivascular chronic inflammation in the dermis, along with acanthosis of the epidermis. Orthokeratosis, parakeratosis, and spongiosis may be present.

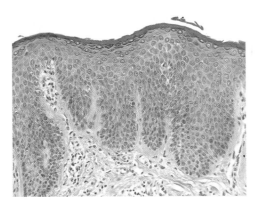 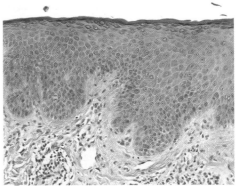

Blepharitis *(Contd.)*

DIFFERENTIAL DIAGNOSIS   The differential diagnosis includes acne rosacea, mucous membrane pemphigoid, pagetoid meibomian cell or basal cell carcinoma, discoid lupus erythematous, psoriasis, and atopic dermatitis.

TREATMENT   Patients should understand that this condition will likely be a life-long problem that can be controlled, but seldom eliminated. The main goals of treatment are to reduce meibomian gland inflammation and to reduce increased tear osmolality. Eyelid cosmetics may be an aggravating factor and should be avoided for a time. Scalp seborrhea must be controlled with 1% selenium sulfide shampoo, and a "baby" or "no tears" shampoo can be used for lid scrubs. Scales and crusts should be soaked and removed daily with cotton-tipped applicators or a moist washcloth wrapped around a finger. Cultures of the lid margins and of material expressed from the meibomian glands should be obtained for antibiotic sensitivities prior to starting topical antibiotics to suppress the bacterial growth. Preferred anti-infective agents in topical ointment form are bacitracin, sulfacetamide, and erythromycin. In the most severe cases a short course of systemic antibiotic, preferably a semisynthetic penicillin, may be needed. For more symptomatic patients mild topical steroids will give earlier relief, but should be promptly discontinued to avoid their adverse effects. Topical cyclosporine 0.05% may be useful in reducing lid margin telangiectasias and meibomian gland inclusions. Milking the meibomian glands on a weekly or bimonthly schedule will reduce the amount of inspisated glandular debris in which the bacteria thrive. In older patients, particularly those with established blepharitis, tear function abnormalities are treated with topical lubrication. Severe cases may benefit from oral tetracycline, 250 mg daily to alter the character of the meibomian secretions.

REFERENCES

Bron, AJ, Benjamin L, Snibson GR. Meibomian gland disease. Classification and grading of lid changes. Eye 1991; 5:395–411.

Driver PJ, Lemp MA. Meibomian gland dysfunction. Surv Ophthalmol 1996; 40:343–367.

Gilbard JP. Dry eye, blepharitis, and chronic eye irritation: divide and conquer. J Ophthalmic Nurs Technol 1999; 18:109–115.

Kaercher T, Brewitt H. Blepharitis. Ophthalmologie 2004; 101:1135–1147.

McCulley JP, Dougherty JM, Deneau DG. Classification of chronic blepharitis. Ophthalmology 1982; 89:1173–1180.

McCulley JP, Sciallis GF. Meibomian keratoconjunctivitis. Am J Ophthalmol 1977; 84:788–793.

Perry HD, Doshi-Carnevale S, Donnenfeld ED, Solomon R, Biser SA. Efficacy of commercially available topical cyclosporine A 0.05% in the treatment of meibomian gland dysfunction. Cornea 2006; 25:171–175.

Raskin EM, Speaker MG, Laibson PR. Blepharitis. Infect Dis Clin North Am 1992; 6:777–787.

Smith RE, Flowers CW Jr. Chronic blepharitis: a review. CLAO J 1995; 21:200–207.

Smolin G, Okumoto M. Staphylococcal blepharitis. Arch Ophthalmol 1977; 95:812–816.

Thygeson P. Complications of staphylococci blepharitis. Am J Ophthalmol 1969; 68:446–449.

Van Bijsterveld OP. New Moraxella strain isolated from angular conjunctivitis. Appl Microbiol 1970; 20:405–408.

Blue Nevus

INTRODUCTION   The blue nevus was first described by Tièche in 1906. It gets its name from its blue color that results from the concentration of melanin in its location in the deep dermis and the Tyndall effect of differential absorption of long wavelengths of light. It is believed to represent dermal arrest in embryonal migration of neural crest melanocytes that fail to reach the epidermis. The blue nevus is composed of pigmented dermal melanocytes and is represented by two histologic types: the common blue nevus and the cellular blue nevus. These two variants can sometimes be differentiated on clinical appearance. LAMB syndrome is the association of blue nevi with lentigines and skin papules and underlying atrial cardiac myxomas.

CLINICAL PRESENTATION   The common blue nevus appears as a solitary, smooth surfaced, well-circumscribed oval lesion that is flat to slightly elevated. It is usually less than 1 cm in diameter. Blue nevi vary in color from blue to blue-black and may have a grey or whitish center. They occur most often on the back of the hands, face, and on the buttocks. While they usually occur in the skin, blue nevi can also be seen in the sclera, conjunctiva, and orbit. When present from birth the nevus typically remains unchanged throughout life, but most develop later in life and can show very slow growth.

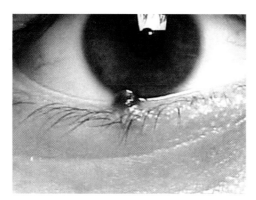
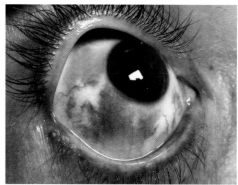

(Courtesy of Robert A. Goldberg, M.D.)

HISTOPATHOLOGY   The common blue nevus is characterized by elongated melanocytes present between collagen bundles of the mid and upper dermis. Melanophages contain much of the pigment present in these lesions.

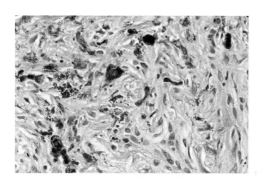
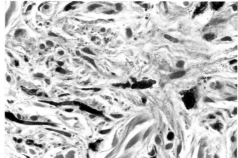

DIFFERENTIAL DIAGNOSIS   The differential diagnosis includes cellular blue nevus, dermatofibroma, oculodermal melanocytosis, malignant melanoma, pigmented basal cell carcinoma, Kaposi's sarcoma, and vascular lesions.

TREATMENT   Treatment is not necessary as long as the diagnosis is assured. If there is any change in pigmentation a biopsy should be performed. When removal is desired for diagnosis or cosmesis, simple surgical excision is recommended. It is important to include deep subcutaneous tissue because these nevi often extend into the subcutis.

REFERENCES

Dorsey CS, Montgomery H. Blue nevus and its distinction from Mongolian spot and the nevus of Ota. J Invest Dermatol 1954; 22:225–236.

Haye C, Dhermy P. Blue nevus of the eyelid. J Fr Ophtalmol 1978; 1:73.

Mishima Y. Cellular blue nevus: melanogenic activity and malignant transformation. Arch Dermatol 1970; 101:104–110.

Rodriguez HA, Ackerman LV. Cellular blue nevus: clinicopathologic study of forty-five cases. Cancer 1968; 21:393–405.

Silverberg GD, Kadin ME, Dorfman RF, Handberry JW, Prolo DJ. Invasion of the brain by a cellular blue nevus of the scalp: a case report with light and electron microscopic studies. Cancer 1971; 27:349–355.

Capillary Hemangioma

INTRODUCTION   Also known as a benign *hemangioendothelioma* or *strawberry nevus*, this common vascular lesion occurs in 1% to 2% of infants and is the most common orbital tumor found in children. It is felt to represent a vascular hamartoma derived from endothelial rests. Periorbital hemangiomas may present as a superficial cutaneous lesion (strawberry hemangioma), subcutaneous lesion, deep orbital tumor, or can occur in a combination of these different locations. Approximately one-third of lesions are clinically noticed at birth, with virtually all-remaining lesions becoming apparent by six months of age. Typically an initial phase of rapid growth of the lesion occurs within 6 to 12 months of diagnosis. This is usually followed by a period of dormancy and then subsequent spontaneous involution over the course of several years. It is estimated that approximately 74% to 90% will regress to some extent by seven to nine years of age. Girls are more commonly affected than boys, with a ratio of 3:2. The most significant ocular complication is amblyopia, which may result from occlusion of the visual axis or from anisometropia due to pressure-induced astigmatism.

CLINICAL PRESENTATION   Superficial capillary hemangiomas initially present as a flat red lesion with telangiectatic surface vessels. As they enlarge they typically become a red, elevated, domed mass with a soft consistency. The lesion is compressible and blanches easily with gentle pressure. Subcutaneous lesions present as a bluish-purple mass seen through the skin. Like its superficial counterpart it has a soft, spongy consistency. With the Valsalva maneuver or

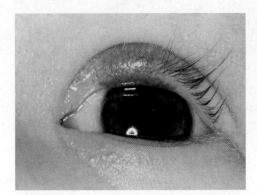
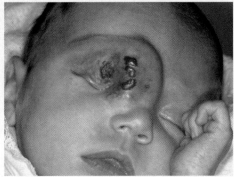

when the child is crying, capillary hemangiomas will show a transient enlargement and darkening in color as they fill with blood. Involuted lesions develop a pale pink or white mottled appearance with fibrosis and inability to blanch. Ultrasound, computed tomography, and magnetic resonance imaging may aid in diagnosis and in determining the extent of orbital involvement.

HISTOPATHOLOGY   Capillary hemangiomas are composed of closely packed, thin-walled capillaries. Lobules are separated by thin fibrous septa. The capillaries may be lined by flattened endothelium and contain erythrocytes, or they may have plump endothelial cells making the vascular lumen inconspicuous. The tumors are usually well circumscribed by fibrous connective tissue.

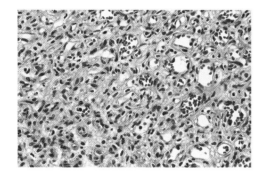 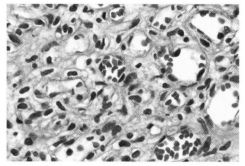

DIFFERENTIAL DIAGNOSIS   The differential diagnosis includes other vascular lesions such as nevus flammeus, cavernous hemangioma, and lymphangioma, as well as other lesions including dermoid cyst, encephalocele, rhabdomyosarcoma, neuroblastoma, and inflammatory masses.

TREATMENT   Since most capillary hemangiomas will undergo some degree of spontaneous regression conservative observation is appropriate. Intervention should be reserved for those patients who develop functional limitations of the eyelid, amblyopia, or astigmatism. Intralesional corticosteroid injection or systemic corticosteroids typically result in dramatic reduction in the size of the lesion, but treatment may have to be repeated. However, prolonged adrenal suppression and failure to thrive has been documented following such treatment, and steroid injection has been associated with visual loss form embolization of ocular arterial flow by retrograde pressure. A topical fluorinated corticosteroid, clobetasol propionate, may produce a measurable reduction in the size of these lesions with no obvious systemic manifestations. Limited experience with injections of interferon-alpha has shown arrest in lesion progression and a possible accelerated rate of regression. Radiotherapy has also been advocated, but carries a risk of secondary orbital tumors. Laser treatment and surgery should be considered for selected localized lesions, or for those that fail to respond to corticosteroids. In some cases residual tumor may have to be left behind to avoid injury to important eyelid structures.

REFERENCES

Aldave AJ, Shields CL, Shields JA. Surgical excision of selected amblyogenic periorbital capillary hemangiomas. Ophthalmic Surg Lasers 1999; 30:754–757.

Brown BZ, Huffaker G. Local injection of steroids for juvenile hemangiomas which disturb the visual axis. Ophthalmic Surg 1982; 13:630–633.

Cruz OA, Zarnegar SR, Myers SE. Treatment of periocular capillary hemangioma with topical clobetasol propionate. Ophthalmology 1995; 102:2012–2015.

Deans RM, Harris GJ, Kivlin JD. Surgical dissection of capillary hemangiomas. An alternative to intralesional corticosteroids. Arch Ophthalmol 1992; 110:1743–1747.

Egbert JE, Paul S, Engle WK, Summers CG. High injection pressure during intralesional injection of corticosteroids into capillary hemangiomas. Ach Ophthalmol 2001; 119:677–683.

Fledelius HC, Illum N, Jensen H, Prause JU. Interferon-alfa treatment of facial infantile haemangiomas: with emphasis on the sight-threatening varieties. A clinical series. Acta Ophthalmol Scand 2001; 79:370–373.

Glatt HJ, Putterman AM, Van Aalst JJ, Levine MR. Adrenal suppression and growth retardation after injection of periocular capillary hemangioma with steroids. Ophthalmic Surgery 1991; 22:95–97.

Goyal R, Watts P, Lane CM, Beck L, Gregory JW. Adrenal suppression and failure to thrive after steroid injection for periocular hemangioma. Ophthalmology 2004; 111:389–395.

Haik BG, Karcioglu ZA, Gordon RA, Pechous BP. Capillary hemangioma (infantile periocular hemangioma). Surv Ophthalmol 1994; 38:399–426.

Hidano A, Nakajima S. Earliest features of the strawberry mark in the newborn. Br J Dermatol 1972; 87:138–144.

Hiles DA, Pilchard WA. Corticosteroid control of neonatal hemangiomas of the orbit and ocular adnexa. Am J Ophthalmol 1971; 71:1003–1008.

Kushner B. Intralesional corticosteroid injection for infantile adnexal hemangioma. Am J Ophthalmol 1982; 93:496–506.

Momtchilova M, Pelosse B, Diner PA, Vazques MP, Laroche L. Amblyopia and peri-ocular capillary hemangioma of infancy: screening and clinical course before and after surgery. J Fr Ophtalmol 2004; 27:1135–1140.

O'Keefe M, Lanigan B, Byrne SA. Capillary haemangioma of the eyelids and orbit: a clinical review of the safety and efficacy of intralesional steroid. Acta Ophthalmol Scand 2003; 81:294–298.

Shorr N, Goldberg RA, David LM. Laser treatment of juvenile hemangioma. Ophthal Plast Reconstr Surg 1988; 4:131–134.

Slaughter K, Sullivan T, Boulton J, O'Reagan P, Gole G. Early surgical intervention as definitive treatment for ocular adnexal capillary haemangioma. Clin Experimental Ophthalmol 2003; 31:418–423.

Walker RS, Custer PL, Nerad JA. Surgical excision of periorbital capillary hemangiomas. Ophthalmology 1994; 101:1333–1340.

Cavernous Hemangioma

INTRODUCTION   Cavernous hemangioma represents a hamartoma that seldom appears prior to middle childhood, with the majority arising after the second decade. Although this lesion is the most common benign orbital tumor in adults, it only occasionally occurs as an isolated eyelid lesion. A rare syndrome termed the blue rubber bleb nevus syndrome, exists which is characterized by multiple cutaneous cavernous hemangiomas associated with gastrointestinal hemangiomas that often bleed. A subtype of cavernous hemangioma, termed sinusoidal hemangioma, has been described to involve the eyelid with a more aggressive growth pattern invading adjacent areas of the brow and cheek.

CLINICAL PRESENTATION   Superficial skin lesions are slow growing, dark blue, lobulated, compressible lesions. When large they can cause amblyopia from ptosis with obstruction of the visual axis, and from astigmatism from ocular compression. Unlike their orbital counterpart, isolated superficial hemangiomas are not encapsulated.

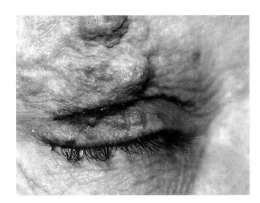 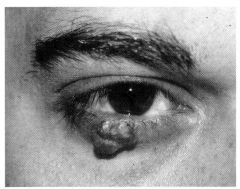

HISTOPATHOLOGY   Cavernous hemangiomas are composed of large, dilated, endothelium-lined, blood-filled spaces. Fibrous stroma separates the vascular spaces and may have focal chronic inflammation. Cavernous hemangiomas of the eyelid are usually well circumscribed but not encapsulated. Cavernous hemangiomas of the eyelid are not as common, in our experience, as arteriovenous hemangiomas, which are well-circumscribed masses of vessels with varying wall thickness comprising both arteries and veins.

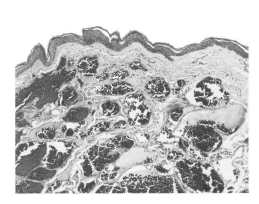 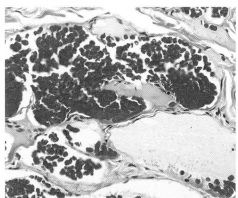

DIFFERENTIAL DIAGNOSIS   The differential diagnosis includes capillary hemangioma, varix, arteriovenous malformation, and lymphangioma.

TREATMENT   Spontaneous regression of cavernous hemangiomas has been reported, but it is not as typical as for capillary hemangiomas. Treatment of eyelid lesions may be necessary for threatening amblyopia or for cosmetic purposes. Definitive treatment is usually with local surgical excision. Intralesional sclerosing agents and cryotherapy have been used with some success, as has brachytherapy in doses of 800 to 1500cGy in fractionated doses.

REFERENCES

Basta LL, Anderson LS, Acers TE. Regression of orbital hemangioma detected by echography. Arch Ophthalmol 1977; 95:1383–1386.

Beare MJ, Rogers S. Giant cavernous hemangiomata. Mod Probl Pediatr 1976; 20:58–68.

Enjolras O, Wassef M, Brocheriou-Spelle I, et al. Sinusoidal hemangioma. Ann Dermatol Venereol 1998; 125:575–580.

Jakobiec F, Jones I. In: Tasman W, Jeager EA (eds). Duane's Clinical Ophthalmology. Vol. 2. Philadelphia: Harper & Row, 1983; 37:6–8.

McCannel CA, Hoenig J, Umlas J, et al. Orbital lesions in the blue rubber bleb nevus syndrome. Ophthalmology 1996; 103:933–936.

Cellular Blue Nevus

INTRODUCTION   Cellular blue nevus is a variant of the common blue nevus, but was first described as a variant of melanoma. Although these can be similar clinically to the common blue nevus, they tend to be larger, elevated, and have more pronounced celluarity composed of nonpigmented spindle-shaped melanocytes. They are most common in Asian populations, and rare in blacks. The cellular blue nevus is believed to represent a dermal arrest of embryonal migration of neural crest melanocytes that fail to reach the epidermis. They tend to remain unchanged throughout life, but there have been rare reports of malignant transformation to melanoma.

CLINICAL PRESENTATION   Cellular blue nevus can appear at any age but generally develops in the second decade of life or later. They start out as singular smooth surfaced flat macules that slowly develop into dome-shaped papules. Color varies from gray-blue to bluish black. The dark color results from their deep location in the dermis and the Tyndall effect where differential absorption of long wavelengths of light and scattering of short wavelengths by melanin favors the blue end of the spectrum. Malignant change is heralded by a sudden increase in size and occasional ulceration.

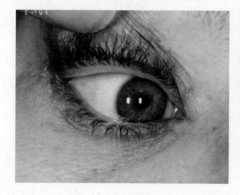 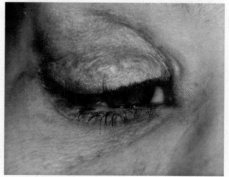

HISTOPATHOLOGY   Lesions are usually well circumscribed and composed of nests and interweaving fascicles of mostly non-pigmented spindle-shaped melanocytes having pale cytoplasm. Melanophages may be found between the cellular islands. The presence of melanin-containing dermal

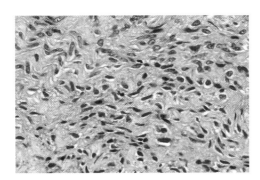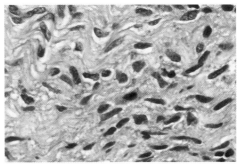

melanocytes interspersed with the non-pigmented cells aids in differentiating the lesion from other spindle-cell tumors such as dermatofibroma or leiomyoma. The melanocytic nature of the process may be confirmed immunohistochemically since the cells express S-100 protein and HMB-45.

DIFFERENTIAL DIAGNOSIS   The differential diagnosis includes melanocytic nevus, oculodermal melanocytosis, malignant melanoma, and dermatofibroma.

TREATMENT   A biopsy is indicated for any change in size or pigmentation. Malignant degeneration can occur in part of the lesion so that it can be missed on routine biopsy. When therapy is indicated for cosmesis or for malignant change, surgery is necessary. For small lesions simple excision is curative. Larger lesions can be infiltrative into eyelid tissues and the orbit making complete excision difficult.

REFERENCES

Barnhill RL, Barnhill MA, Berwick M, Mihm MC Jr. The histologic spectrum of pigmented spindle cell nevus: a review of 120 cases with emphasis on atypical variants. Hum Pathol 1991; 22:52–58.

Gunduz K, Shields JA, Shields CL, Eagle RC Jr. Periorbital cellular blue nevus leading to orbitopalpebral and intracranial melanoma. Ophthalmology 1998; 105:2046–2050.

Rodriguez HA, Ackerman LV. Cellular blue nevus. Clinicopathologic study of forty-five cases. Cancer 1968; 21:393–405.

Temple-Camp CR, Saxe N, King H. Benign and malignant cellular blue nevus. A clinicopathological study of 30 cases. Am J Dermatopathol 1988; 10:289–296.

Tran TA, Carlson JA, Basaca PC, Mihm MC. Cellular blue nevus with atypia (atypical blue nevus): a clinicopathologic study of nine cases. J Cutan Pathol 1998; 25:252–258.

Zembowicz A, Granter SR, McKee PH, Mihm MC. Amelanotic cellular blue nevus: a hypopigmented variant of the cellular blue nevus; clinicopathologic analysis of 20 cases. Am J Surg Pathol 2002; 26:1493–1500.

Cellulitis

INTRODUCTION   Preseptal cellulitis is defined as inflammation and infection confined to the eyelids and periorbital structures anterior to the orbital septum. The orbital structures posterior to the septum are not involved, but may be secondarily inflamed. In children, the most common cause of preseptal cellulitis is underlying sinusitis. Preseptal cellulitis in children under age 5 was often associated with bacteremia, septicemia, and meningitis caused by *Haemophilus influenzae*, however, this cause of preseptal and orbital cellulitis has virtually been eliminated by the introduction of the HIB vaccine. Currently, most cases of preseptal and orbital cellulitis in children are due to gram-positive cocci. In teenagers and adults preseptal cellulitis usually arises from a superficial source such as traumatic inoculation, or a chalazion. The site of the infected focus is often difficult to find because the eyelid tissues become markedly swollen.

CLINICAL PRESENTATION   The initial skin lesion is often a small, erythematous focus, suggesting an early furuncle, but instead of localizing, it rapidly spreads through the adjacent subcutaneous tissues after 5 to 10 days. Eyelid edema, erythema, and inflammation may be severe. Unless the infection spreads to the post-septal orbit, the globe is uninvolved; pupillary reaction, visual acuity, and ocular motility are not disturbed; pain on eye movement and chemosis are absent. Complications can result in lagophthalmos, ectropion, and lid necrosis.

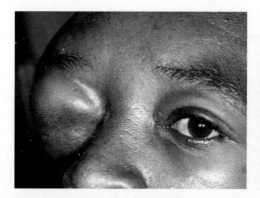 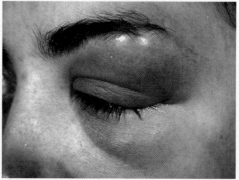

HISTOPATHOLOGY   Cellulitis, or diffuse inflammation of the connective tissue of the skin or deeper soft tissues, may be acute or chronic. Acute cellulitis is characterized histopathologically by an infiltrate of neutrophils throughout the dermis and/or subcutaneous tissue. There may be subepidermal edema and vascular ectasia. In chronic cellulitis the inflammatory infiltrate consists mostly of lymphocytes and macrophages and is accompanied by fibrosis and angiogenesis.

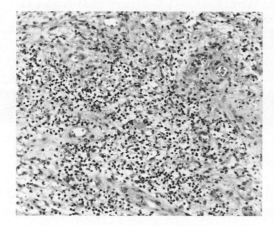 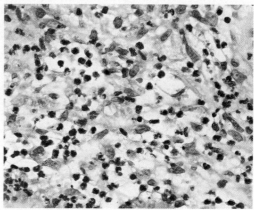

DIFFERENTIAL DIAGNOSIS   The differential diagnosis includes orbital cellulitis, erysipelas, Mucormycosis, and ruptured dermoid or epidermoid cyst.

TREATMENT   Initial antibiotic selection is based on the history, clinical findings, and initial laboratory studies. With positive culture, prompt sensitivity studies are indicated so that the antibiotic selection can be revised, if necessary. *Staphylococcus aureus* is the most common pathogen in patients with preseptal cellulitis from trauma. The infection usually responds quickly to penicllinase-resistant penicillin. Imaging studies should be performed to rule out underlying sinusitis if no direct inoculation site is identified. If the patient does not respond quickly to oral antibiotics or if orbital involvement becomes evident, prompt hospital admission, CT scanning and intravenous antibiotics are usually indicated. Surgical drainage may be necessary if the preseptal cellulitis progresses to a localized abscess. Incision and drainage can usually be performed directly over the abscess. The orbital septum should not be opened to avoid contaminating the orbital soft tissue. Affected children should be treated in consultation with a pediatrician, and hospitalization and intravenous antibiotics may be indicated.

REFERENCES

Baker C. Group B streptococcal cellulitis-adenitis in infants. Am J Dis Child 1982; 136:631.

Casady DR, Zobal-Ratner JL, Meyer DR. Eyelid abscess as a presenting sign of occult sinusitis. Ophthal Plast Reconstr Surg 2005; 21:368–370.

Donahue SP, Schwartz G. Preseptal and orbital cellulitis in childhood. A changing microbiologic spectrum. Ophthalmology 1998; 105:1902–1905.

Feingold D. Gangrenous and crepitant cellulitis. J Am Acad Dermatol 1982; 6:289–299.

Harris GJ. Subperiosteal abscess of the orbit: age as a factor in the bacteriology and response to treatment. Ophthalmology 1994; 101:585–595.

Harris GJ. Subperiosteal abscess of the orbit: computed topography and the clinical course. Ophthal Plast Reconstruct Surg. 1996; 12:1–8.

Parunovic A. Proteus mirabilis causing necrotic inflammation of the eyelid. Am J Ophthalmol 1973; 76:543–544.

Rao VA, Hans R, Mehra AK. Pre-septal cellulitis—varied clinical presentations. Indian J Ophthalmol 1996; 44:225–227.

Chalazion and Hordeolum

INTRODUCTION   A chalazion and hordeolum are focal inflammatory lesions of the eyelid that results from the obstruction of secretory glands. In a chalazion there is no acute bacterial infection, but rather a chronic inflammatory lesion with circumferential fibrosis. When this involves the meibomian glands they form a deep chalazion, whereas when there is involvement of the more superficial glands of Zeis in the dermis or glands of Moll associated with the pilosebaceous unit a more superficial chalazion results. A hordeolum is an acute bacterial abscess filled with pus and associated with pain and inflammatory signs. They can involve the meibomian glands (deep hordeolum) or the Zeis and Moll glands (superficial hordeolum). Superficial hordeola are usually found near the eyelid margin where the Zeis glands are concentrated. Two-thirds of chalazia show mixed-cell cytology, and one-third are suppurating granulomas. The latter tend to occur in older patients with a longer duration of symptoms and larger lesions. When the impacted gland ruptures, extravasated lipid material produces a surrounding chronic lipogranulomatous inflammation. Both chalazia and hordeola often occur in patients with blepharitis and rosacea.

CLINICAL PRESENTATION   A hordeolum presents acutely with pain, eyelid edema, and erythema, and it evolves into a subcutaneous nodule which may point anteriorly to the skin surface or through the posterior surface of the lid where the tarsus is closer to the conjunctival surface. Exuberant lesions will sometimes erode through the conjunctiva presenting as a type of pyogenic granuloma. They may drain spontaneously or under medical therapy. In contrast, chalazia usually present insidiously as a firm, painless mass. Multiple lesions of both types are not uncommon and very large lesions on the upper lid may even induce astigmatism and amblyopia in children.

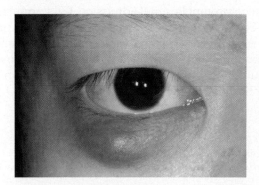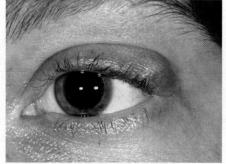

HISTOPATHOLOGY   A chalazion is a localized lipogranulomatous reaction to the sebaceous glands of the eyelids (either the meibomian glands or the glands of Zeiss). Obstruction of sebaceous gland ducts results in a granulomatous response surrounding vacuoles that remain when lipid is dissolved during histological processing. Epithelioid cells predominate in the granulomas, and the number of multinucleated giant cells is highly variable. Neutrophils may be prominent in early lesions, while lymphocytes and varying degrees of fibrosis are seen in more chronic chalazia. Chalazia arising from the meibomian glands may rupture into the conjunctival substantia propria or involve the dermis of the eyelid. Chalazia developing from a gland of Zeiss usually remain localized to the eyelid margin.

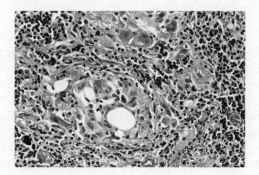

DIFFERENTIAL DIAGNOSIS   About 6 % to 7% of chalazia and hordeola are misdiagnosed at presentation, with about 1 to 2% actually being malignant. The differential diagnosis includes chronic inflammation, abscess, sebaceous cell carcinoma, and basal cell carcinoma.

TREATMENT   Small hordeola may resolve spontaneously. Acute lesions are initially treated with hot compresses to encourage localization and drainage, combined with a topical steroid-antibiotic preparation. When further treatment is required the technique varies according to the stage and nature of a lesion. Chronic chalazia may be treated using intralesional corticosteroid injection or surgical drainage. Injection of soluble steroids such as tiramcinolone acetonide, can be effective but carries a very small risk of central retinal artery obstruction, the result of retrograde arterial infusion. It can also induce focal depigmentation in darker skinned patients. Inadvertent ocular penetration has been reported. If a viral etiology is suspected, steroids should be used only cautiously. Suppurating granulomas in long-standing chalazia respond better to surgery than to steroid injections so that larger, long-standing lesions (>8 months duration) are best treated surgically. When medical therapy or steroids fail to resolve the lesion surgical drainage is performed. This is best accomplished with vertical transconjunctival incisions that allow adequate curettage of the lesion while limiting damage to surrounding meibomian glands. Thermal cautery of the cyst wall has no demonstrable effect on recurrence rate. In recurrent lesions, biopsy is necessary to exclude sebaceous gland carcinoma.

REFERENCES

Ben Simon GJ, Huang L, Nakra T, et al. Intralesional tiramcinolone acetonide injection for primary and recurrent chalazia: is it really effective? Ophthalmology 2005; 112:913–917.

Dhaliwal U, Bhatia A. A rationale for therapeutic decision-making in chalazia. Orbit 2005; 24:227–230.

Donaldson MJ, Gole GA. Amblyopia due to inflamed chalazion in a 13-month old infant. Clin Experiment Ophthalmol 2005; 33:332–333.

Goldberg RA, Shorr N. 'Vertical slat' chalazion excision. Ophthalmic Surg 1992; 23:120–122.

Hosal BM, Zilelioglu G. Ocular complications of intralesional corticosteroid injection of a chalazion. Eur J Ophthalmol 2003; 13:798–799.

Lempert SL, Jenkins MS, Brown SI. Chalazia and rosacea. Arch Ophthalmol 1979; 97:1652–1653.

Ozdal PC, Codere F, Callejo S, Caissie AL, Burbier MN. Accuracy of the clinical diagnosis of chalazion. Eye 2004; 18:135–138.

Sendrowski DP, Maher JF. Thermal cautery after chalazion surgery and its effect on recurrence rates. Optom Vis Sci 2000; 77:605–607.

Chondroid Syringoma

INTRODUCTION   Chondroid syringoma is also known as *pleomorphic adenoma* or *mixed tumor of the skin*. These benign lesions are of possible eccrine gland or hair follicle origin, although several reports showed apocrine differentiation. They usually occur on the head and neck. They only occasionally involve the eyelid. Rarely, malignant variants have been reported.

CLINICAL PRESENTATION   These lesions present as an asymptomatic solitary nodule 0.5 to 2.0 cm in diameter. They generally show slow growth over 2 to 10 years or longer before coming to medical attention. When they occur on the eyelid they tend to be fixed to the underlying tarsus, but they do not cause changes in the overlying epidermis except occasionally for some pigmentation.

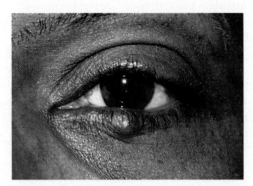

(Courtesy of J. Justin Older, M.D.)

HISTOPATHOLOGY   Epithelial cells are distributed singly or form tubules or ducts that are usually lined by two or more rows of epithelial cells. The outer layer of epithelial cells lining the tubules tends to be more flattened than the inner layer of cells. The epithelial cells are within a stroma that varies in appearance from chondroid to myxoid to fibrous. The chondroid stroma is bubbly and blue in H&E stained sections and contains abundant glycosaminoglycans (mucopolysaccharides) that stain positively using alcian blue, colloidal iron, and mucicarmine techniques.

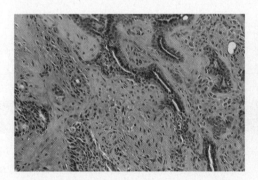
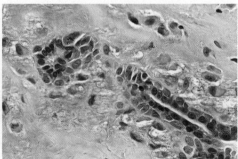

DIFFERENTIAL DIAGNOSIS   The differential diagnosis includes epidermoid cyst, neurofibroma, and pilomatrixoma.

TREATMENT   Treatment is not indicated except for cases of cosmesis or when the lesion interferes with vision. Surgical excision within its capsule is curative.

REFERENCES

D'Hermies F, Mourier L, Wastl JP, et al. Palpebral form of mixed tumor of the lacrimal gland. Apropos of a case. J Fr Ophtalmol 1992; 15:220–223.

Jordan DR, Nerad JA, Patrinely JR. Chondroid syringoma of the eyelid. Can J Ophthalmol 1989; 24:24–27.

Mandeville JT, Roh JH, Woog JJ, et al. Cutaneous benign mixed tumor (chondroid syringoma) of the eyelid: clinical presentation and management. Ophthal Plast Reconstr Surg 2004; 20:110–116.

Martorina M, Capoferri C, Dessanti P. Chondroid syringoma of the eyelid. Int Ophthalmol 1993; 17:285–288.

Mencia-Gutierrez E, Bonales-Daimiel JA, Gutierrez-Diaz E, et al. Chondroid syringomas of the eyelid: two cases. Eur J Ophthalmol 2001; 11:80–82.

Meythaler H, Koniszewski G. Pleomorphic adenoma of Moll's glands. Klin Monatsbl Augenheilkd 1979; 175:825–828.

Saini JS, Mukherjee AK, Naik P. Pleomorphic adenoma of Krause's gland in the lower lid. Indian J Ophthalmol 1985; 33:181–182.

Tong JT, Flanagan JC, Eagle RC Jr, Mazzoli RA. Benign mixed tumor arising from an accessory lacrimal gland. Ophthal Plast Reconstr Surg 1995; 11:136–138.

Tyagi N, Abdi U, Tyagi SP, Maheshwari V, Gogi R. Pleomorphic adenoma of skin (chondroid syringoma) involving the eyelid. J Postgrad Med 1996; 42:125–126.

Cicatricial Pemphigoid

INTRODUCTION   Cicatricial pemphigoid, also known as *benign mucous membrane pemphigoid, essential conjunctival shrinkage*, or *ocular pemphigus* is a progressive inflammatory disease of presumed autoimmune etiology. It variously involves mucous membranes of the mouth, conjunctiva, pharynx, nose, esophagus, vagina, urethra, and anus. Oral bullae and erosions occur in 90% of cases. Strictures of the esophagus, urethra, or anus sometimes occur late in the disease. Skin involvement is seen in less than 25% of cases and takes one of two forms: a recurrent nonscarring vesiculobullous eruption, mainly involving the extremities and inguinal region, or in the form of localized erythematous plaques with associated vesicles and bullae on the face and scalp. The latter variant heals with small atrophic scars. Another variant of localized pemphigoid known as *Brunsting-Perry type* has skin lesions limited to the face and neck but with no mucosal involvement. Significant scarring of affected areas often occurs, sometimes involving the eyelids. The average age of onset of cicatricial pemphigoid is in the seventh decade, but it can occur at any age, including childhood. The incidence is approximately 1:30,000 and there is a slight female predominance.

CLINICAL PRESENTATION   In ocular cicatricial pemphigoid the conjunctival bullae are evanescent and therefore are seldom visualized. The initial symptoms usually include irritation and tearing due to ruptured conjunctival bullae. Subepithelial scarring with gradual obliteration of tear gland openings and loss of mucous glands ultimately results in keratoconjunctivitis sicca. In addition, surfaces on the bulbar and palpebral conunctiva fuse together, resulting in symblepharon. Eventually these symblephara obliterate the conjunctival fornices impairing lid closure. A band of symblepharon extending across the medial part of the lower cu-de-sac is typical of early ocular pemphigoid. The resulting entropion, tear deficiency, and lagophthalmos conspire to cause corneal opacification and loss of vision. Although a few unilateral cases have been seen, cicatricial pemphigoid almost always eventually becomes bilateral. However, involvement of the second eye may be delayed for up to two years.

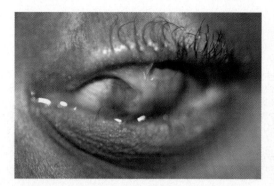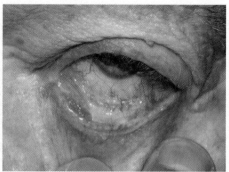

(Courtesy of Charles S. Soparkar, M.D.)

HISTOPATHOLOGY   By routine light microscopy, cicatricial pemphigoid has subepidermal vesicles containing fibrin, edema fluid, and inflammatory cells. The dermis has a perivascular infiltrate of mainly lymphocytes and plasma cells, along with lesser numbers of neutrophils and eosinophils. Scarring may be prominent. Subepithelial bullae are not commonly seen in conjunctival lesions. Light microscopic features are nonspecific; diagnosis rests on demonstrating by direct immuno-fluorescence the linear deposition of immunoglobulin (usually IgG) and often of complement component C3 along the basement membrane zone.

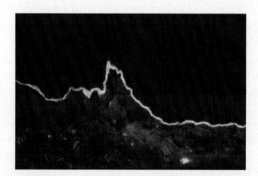

DIFFERENTIAL DIAGNOSIS   The differential diagnosis includes porphyria, bullous pemphigoid, sebaceous gland carcinoma, dermatitis herpetiformis, pemphigus vulgaris, Sjogren's disease, beta-hemolytic strep-tococcal infections, diphtheria, adenoviral and herpes simplex infections, trachoma, prolonged use of oral practolol, and reactions to epinephrine, pilocarpine, and/or phospholidine iodide eye drops.

TREATMENT   Diagnosis can sometimes be established with a biopsy of an oral mucosal bulla, with histopatho-logic examination showing a sub-epidermal locus. Immunofluorescent antibodies fixed to conjunctiva basement membrane can be demonstrated in up to 80% of cases. Assays for circulating auto-antibodies also exist, but are positive in only about 10% of affected patients. During exacerbations, topical steroids will reduce the severity and perhaps diminish scarring. Because up to half of patients will harbor staphylococci, the lids and conjunctivae should be periodically cultured, and a course of appropriate antibiotics started if necessary. Artificial tears often help the signs and symptoms of aqueous tear deficiency. In severe cases combined therapy using systemic steroids and immunosuppressive agents is usually of benefit. Dapsone (diaminodiphenylsulfone) in doses of 25–50 mg daily can show early benefit, but its effect appears to diminish after one to two years. Conjunctival surgery, including cryosurgery, should be avoided because it often precipitates exacerbations, ultimately leaving the patient worse off. Marked loss of conjunctiva can be repaired with mucous membrane or amniotic membrane grafts. Eyelid surgery for trichitic lashes should avoid insults to the conjunctiva if possible, and eyelid margin rotation through an anterior approach is preferred for entropion. No matter the intervention, some patients will inexorably progress despite all therapeutic measures.

REFERENCES

Bartley GB. Surgical reconstruction of the ocular surface in advanced ocular cicatricial pemphigoid and Stevens-Johnson syndrome. Am J Ophthalmol 1996; 122:752–753.

Bean S, Furey N, West C, Andrews T, Esterly NB. Ocular cicatricial pemphigoid (immunologic studies). Trans Sect Ophthalmol Am Acad Ophthal Otoloaryngol 1976; 81:806–812.

Dutton JJ, Tawfik HA, DeBacker CM, Lipham WJ. Anterior tarsal V-wedge resection for cicatricial entropion. Ophthal Plast Reconstr Surg 2000; 16:126–130.

Elder MJ, Collin R. Anterior lamellar repositioning and grey line split for upper lid entropion in ocular cicatricial pemphigoid. Eye 1996; 10:439–442.

Elder MJ, Collin R. Lid surgery: the management of cicatricial entropion and trichasis. Dev Ophthalmol 1997; 28:207–218.

Elder MJ, Collin R. The eyelid sequelae of chronic progressive conjunctival cicatrisation. Dev Ophthalmol 1997; 28:176–181.

Griffith MR, Fukuyama K, Tuffanelli D, Silverman S Jr. Immunofluorescent studies in mucous membrane pemphigoid. Arch Dermatol 1974; 109:195–199.

Holsclaw DS. Ocular cicatricial pemphigoid. Int Ophthalmol Clin 1998; 38:89–106.

Mondino BJ, Brown SI, Lempert S, Jenkins MS. The acute manifestations of ocular cicatricial pemphigoid: Diagnosis and treatment. Ophthalmology 1979; 85:543–555.

Mondino BJ, Brown SI. Ocular cicatricial pemphigoid. Ophthalmology 1981; 88:95–100.

Mondino BJ, Brown SI. Immunosuppressive therapy in ocular cicatricial pemphigoid. Am J ophthalmol 1983; 96:453–459.

Mondino BJ, Ross AN, Rabin BS, Brown SI. Autoimmune phenomena in ocular cicatricial pemphigoid. Am J Ophthalmol 1977; 83:443–450.

Rogers RS, Perry HO, Bean SF, Jordan RE. Immunopathology of cicatricial pemphigoid: studies of complement deposition. J Invest Dermatol 1977; 58:39–43.

Shore JW, Foster CS, Westfall CT, Rubin PA. Results of buccal mucosal grafting for patients with medically controlled ocular cicatricial pemphigoid. Ophthalmology 1992; 383–385.

Cutaneous Horn

INTRODUCTION

The term cutaneous horn, also known as *cornu cutaneum*, is a descriptive designation for a protuberant projection of packed keratin that resembles an animal horn. It is more common in elderly individuals, but can be seen in young adults as well. It is associated with a large variety of benign, premalignant, and malignant lesions at the base, thus masking the true diagnosis. About 60% to 75% of such inciting lesions are benign and 8% to 10% malignant. Malignant diagnoses tend to occur more commonly in males and in patients 8 to 10 years older than those with benign diagnoses. The most common inciting diagnoses are seborrheic keratosis, actinic keratosis, and squamous cell carcinoma.

Cutaneous Horn *(Contd.)*

CLINICAL PRESENTATION   Cutaneous horns are usually seen on areas of exposed skin. They may attain a very large size causing mechanical ptosis or other eyelid malpositions, and may completely occlude vision. Lesions present as a dry, white to yellowish, firm, hornlike projection of keratin that extends upward from the skin surface. It may have several distinct projections that coalesced at the base.

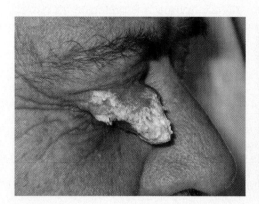 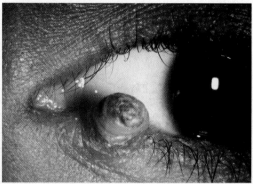

HISTOPATHOLOGY   Cutaneous horn is a clinical diagnosis that corresponds histologically to a protuberant mass of keratin. To be designated a "horn", the height should exceed at least one-half of the greatest diameter of the lesion from which it arises. Cutaneous horns are most commonly associated with actinic (solar) keratosis, verruca vulgaris, seborrheic keratosis, squamous cell carcinoma, inverted follicular keratosis, or tricholemmoma.

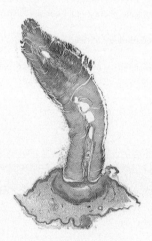

DIFFERENTIAL DIAGNOSIS   The cutaneous horn is easy to diagnose, but its significance is determining the underlying lesion. They can develop from a variety of underlying lesions, including seborrheic keratosis, actinic keratosis, inverted follicular keratosis, verruca vulgaris, tricholemmoma, subepidermal calcified nodules, basal cell carcinoma, squamous cell carcinoma, metastatic tumors, and other epidermal tumors.

TREATMENT   Treatment is dependent on the underlying cause. For benign lesions simple excision or shave biopsy may be adequate. However, when the basal lesion is malignant, surgical excision with adequate clear margins will be necessary to affect a cure. In most cases, however, the diagnosis is not apparent until the specimen has been submitted for histologic examination. Because of the possibility of an underlying malignant lesion, complete surgical excision should be performed.

REFERENCES

Brauninger GE, Hood CI, Worthen DM. Sebaceous carcinoma of lid margin masquerading as cutaneous horn. Arch Ophthalmol 1973; 90:380–381.

Copcu E, Sivrioglu N, Culhaci N. Cutaneous horns: are these lesions as innocent as they seem to be? World J Surg Oncol 2004; 2:18.

D'Hermies F, Gerolami-Favreul I, Meyer A, et al. A cutaneous horn of the free margin of the eyelid: an anatomical and clinical observation. J Fr Ophtalmol 2003; 26:534–537.

Ferry AP. Subepidermal calcified nodules of the eyelid. Am J Ophthalmol 1990; 109:85–88.

Mencia-Gutierrez E, Gutierrez-Diaz E, Redondon-Marcos I, Ricoy JR, Garcia-Torre JP. Cutaneous horns of the eyelid: a clinicopathological study of 48 cases. J Cutan Pathol 2004; 31:539–543.

Thappa DM, Laxmisha C. Cutaneous horn of eyelid. Indian Pediatr 2004; 41:195.

Yu RC, Pryce DW, Macfarlane AW, Stewart TW. A histopathologic study of 643 cutaneous horns. Br J Dermatol 1991; 124:449–452.

Cylindroma

INTRODUCTION

Cylindromas are rare tumors of primitive sweat gland origin. They occur in two settings: either as nonfamilial solitary lesions or as dominantly inherited multiple tumors. There is a well-established association of multiple cylindromas in association with trichoepitheliomas in some familial cases. Rarely, cylindromas (usually of the multiple type) undergo malignant degeneration capable of lymph node and visceral metastases. Brooke-Spiegler syndrome is an autosomal dominantly inherited disease characterized by cutaneous adnexal neoplasms, most commonly cylindromas and tirchoepitheliomas. Lesions may show histologic hybrid features of apocrine, follicular, and sebaceous differentiation. The occurrence of combined sebaceous and trichoblastic features suggests that cylindromas are not eccrine tumors but neoplasms of the folliculosebaceousapocrine unit.

CLINICAL PRESENTATION

Solitary lesions usually appear as dome-shaped, smooth, firm dermal nodules of varying size on the eyelid or brow. The color ranges from flesh toned to pinkish-blue with white specks. The multiple, inherited variety shows numerous nodules of varying size, mainly on the scalp, but some may be found on the forehead and face. Such extensive involvement is known as a "turban tumor." A case of dermal cylindroma has been reportred in the superomedial orbit.

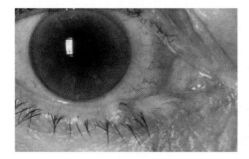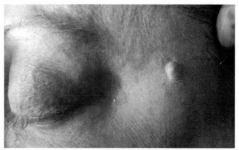

Rarely, they can be extensive enough to cover the scalp and forehead, and even can erode through the skull into the cranial vault.

HISTOPATHOLOGY   These poorly circumscribed dermal tumors are formed of irregularly shaped cords and islands of basaloid cells. Prominent eosinophilic hyaline bands of basement membrane material surround the islands and cords of cells. The nests of cells may contain droplets of this eosinophilic basement membrane material. The islands have peripheral cells with dark nuclei and a tendency for palisading and more centrally located larger cells with vesicular nuclei. The stroma is loose collagenous tissue with an increased number of fibroblasts. Loss of the sheath of basement membrane material and larger islands composed predominantly of larger cells without peripheral palisading are features associated with aggressive or malignant behavior.

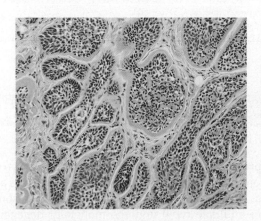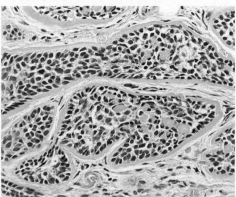

DIFFERENTIAL DIAGNOSIS   The differential diagnosis includes neurofibroma, pilar cyst, or epidermal inclusion cyst. When multiple the differential also includes basal cell nevoid syndrome, neurofibromatosis, and metastatic disease.

TREATMENT   Surgical excision is effective management for symptomatic lesions or for cosmetic concerns. Lesions on the face and scalp can be treated with Nd:Yag laser ablation leaving limited superficial scars.

REFERENCES

Bondeson L. Malignant dermal eccrine cylindroma. Acta Dermatol Venereol 1979; 59:92–94.

Chaer RA, Lipnick S. Images in clinical medicine. Cylindroma. N Engl J Med 2004; 351:2530.

Cucurell M, Diaz C, Barranco C, Gimenez-Arnau A, Camarasa JG. Multiple facial cylindromas in twins. Acta Derm Venereol 1996; 76:333–334.

Given K, Pickrell K, Smith D. Dermal cylindroma (turban tumor). Case report. Plast Reconstr Surg 1977; 59:582–587.

Goette DK, McConnell MA, Fowler VR. Cylindroma and eccrine spiradenoma coexistent in the same lesion. Arch Dermatol 1982; 118:272–274.

Gupta R, Jain R, Sood S, Mohan H. Dermal cylindroma presenting as a mass lesion in superomedial orbit. Indian J Ophthalmol 2003; 51:257–259.

Rubin MG, Mitchell AJ. Generalized cutaneous cylindromatosis. Cutis 1983; 33:568.

Stoll C, Alembik Y, Wilk A, Grosshans E. Familial cylindromatosis. Genet Couns 2004; 15:175–182.

Welch JP, Wells RS, Kerr CB. Anell-Spiegler cylindromas (turban tumors) and Brooke-Fordyce trichoepitheliomas: Evidence for a single genetic entity. J Med Genet 1968; 5:29–35.

Wyld L, Bullen S, Browning FS. Transcranial erosion of a benign dermal cylindroma. Ann Plast Surg 1996; 36:194–196.

INTRODUCTION   Dermatofibroma is also known as a *fibrous histiocytoma*. It is a common benign cutaneous tumor of unknown etiology that is more common in females. Although these tumors occur most commonly on the extremities, they have also been described on the eyelids. These lesions represent multiple variants of tumors derived from fibroblast precursors and are frequently referred to as fibrous histiocytoma, nodular subepidermal fibrosis, and sclerosing hemangioma.

CLINICAL PRESENTATION   These lesions are usually asymptomatic, but can be associated with tenderness and pruritus. They most often present as slowly growing 2 to 10 mm, hard, singular, skin colored to yellowish dome-shaped nodules attached to the overlying skin. This attachment results in a central dimple when compressed laterally. They may be present and static for years or even decades. In immunocompromized hosts, lesions may be multiple. Occasionally the color can be reddish due to hemosiderin deposits. If near the surface the mass may have a yellow or pearly white appearance.

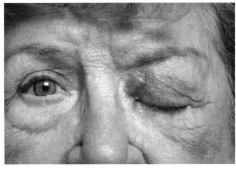

(Courtesy of Robert A. Goldberg, M.D.)

Prominent vascularity may result in a picture simulating a regressing capillary hemangioma. Such tumors are often referred to sclerosing hemangiomas. Spontaneous regression has been reported leaving a depressed hypopigmented postinflammatory scar.

HISTOPATHOLOGY   These are poorly demarcated lesions composed of varying numbers of fibroblast-like cells, histiocytes, and blood vessels. Numerous histological variants occur in the skin. These are uncommon tumors of the eyelid, and they usually have interlacing spindle cells in a vague cartwheel (storiform) pattern. There may be scattered multinucleated giant cells of the foreign body or Touton giant cell types or large histiocytic cells mixed in with the spindle cells. The overlying epidermis may be acanthotic and papillomatous. Immunostains for factor XIIIa and CD34 may assist in differentiating a dermatofibroma (factor XIIIa positive and CD34 negative) from an early dermatofibrosarcoma protuberans (CD34 positive and factor XIIIa negative).

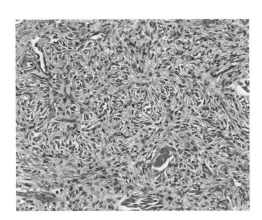
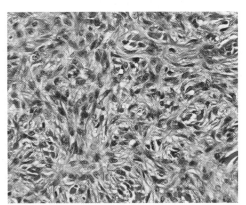

DIFFERENTIAL DIAGNOSIS The differential diagnosis includes keloid, blue nevus, xanthogranuloma, keratoacanthoma, pilomatrixomas, melanocytic nevus, trichomatrixoma, basal cell carcinoma, squamous cell carcinoma, and malignant melanoma.

TREATMENT Treatment is generally not necessary as long as the diagnosis has been established. For lesions that are of cosmetic concern simple surgical excision is recommended.

REFERENCES

Baraf CS, Shapiro L. Multiple histiocytomas: Report of a case. Arch Dermatol 1970; 101:588–590.

Betharia SM, Ramakrishna K, Sen S, Kashyap S, Thanikachalam S. Dermatofibroma of the eyelid: a case report. Orbit 2000; 10:161–164.

Henkind P, Schultz D. Dermatofibroma of the eyelid. Am J Ophthalmol 1968; 65:420–425.

Jakobiec FA, DeVoe AG, Boyd J. Fibrous histiocytoma of the tarsus. Am J Ophthalmol 1977; 84:794–797.

John T, Yanoff M, Scheie HG. Eyelid fibrous histiocytoma. Ophthalmology 1981; 88:1193–1195.

Jordan DR, Addison DJ, Anderson RL. Fibrous histiocytoma. An uncommon eyelid lesion. Arch Ophthalmol 1989; 107:1530–1531.

Kargi E, Kargi S, Gun B, Hosnuter M, Altinyazar C, Aktune E. Benign fibrous histiocytoma of the eyelid with an unusual clinical presentation. J Dermatol 2004; 31:27–31.

Singh Gomez C, Calonje E, Fletcher CD. Epithelioid benign fibrous histiocytoma of skin: clinico-pathological analysis of 20 cases of a poorly known variant. Histopathology 1994; 24:123–129.

Ulloa TK, Anderson SF. Orbital fibrous histiocytoma: case report and literature review. Am Optom Assoc 1999; 70:253–260.

Dermoid Cyst

INTRODUCTION Dermoid cysts are congenital choristomas containing components of both the epidermis and skin appendages. They account for 15–20% of all eyelid lesions in childhood. These cysts can occur as superficial, subcutaneous, or deep eyelid and orbital lesions. They presumably result from entrapment of skin along embryonic closure lines. Attachment to underlying bony sutures often is present and most commonly involves the frontozygomatic suture. Lesions may extend posteriorly into the orbit and into soft tissues such as the lacrimal gland. Erosion or remodeling of bone can occur. Dermoid cysts of conjunctival origin are usually located in the medial conjunctiva, caruncle, or orbit and appear to represent sequestration of epithelium destined to become caruncle.

CLINICAL PRESENTATION Superficial lesions usually are recognized in early childhood and present as somewhat fluctuant round, slowly enlarging, non-tender masses beneath the skin of the upper eyelid. Most commonly they are seen in the lateral upper eyelid and brow region, but can be seen medially as well. Very rarely, they may be bilateral. Deeper orbital dermoids may not become clinically evident until adulthood. Eyelid dermoid cysts are usually freely movable, but can be more firmly adherent to the underlying periosteum. They may become irritated and inflamed with repeated manipulation causing eyelid edema. They range in size from less than one, to several centimeters and rarely can be sufficiently large to partially close the lid or press on the globe resulting in amblyopia. Less commonly, the clinical presentation may be orbital inflammation, incited by leakage of oil and keratin from the cyst.

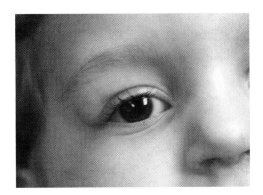 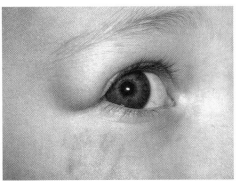

HISTOPATHOLOGY   These cysts are lined by keratinized, stratified squamous epithelium, identical to that of the epidermis, with adnexal structures including sebaceous and eccrine glands and hair follicles. The cyst cavity contains keratin, hair shafts, and sebaceous secretions. If the cyst ruptures, it incites an intense granulomatous inflammatory response. Occasional specimens submitted for histopathological analysis will show only keratin debris, hair fragments, and a granulomatous reaction.

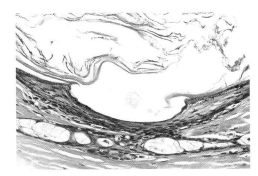 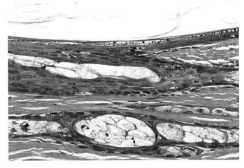

DIFFERENTIAL DIAGNOSIS   The differential diagnosis includes epidermoid cyst, ectopic lacrimal gland, lacrimal gland tumors, neurofibromas, fibromas, hemangiopericytomas, mucoceles, and rarely meningoceles.

TREATMENT   These lesions are benign and when small can safely be observed. In most cases, however, cosmetic issues warrant treatment. Management is with complete surgical excision which can usually be accomplished through an upper eyelid crease incision, even for lesions under and above the brow. Preoperative orbital imaging is indicated if the entire cyst cannot be palpated or if they are fixed to periosteum and orbital extension is suspected. The surgeon must be prepared to manage an occult extension into the orbit or into the intracranial cavity. Recurrences are rare, but can occur if the lesion is rupture during removal.

REFERENCES

Brownstein MH, Helwig EB. Subcutaneous dermoid cysts. Arch Dermatol 1973; 107:237–239.

Ditmar S, Daus W, Volcher HE. Covered rupture of periocular dermoid cysts. Clinicohistologic study. Klin Monatbl Augenheilkd 1993; 203:403–407.

Eibl KH, Kampik A, Hintschich C. Upper eyelid oedema from a dumbbell-shaped dermoid cyst. Acta Ophthalmol Scand 2005; 83:126–127.

Dermoid Cyst *(Contd.)*

Elahi MM, Glat PM. Bilateral frontozygomatic dermoid cysts. Ann Plast Surg 2003; 51:509–512.

Ghafouri A, Rodgers IR, Perry HD. A caruncular dermoid with contiguous eyelid involvement: embryologic implications. Ophthal Plast Reconstr Surg 1998; 14:375–377.

Hsu HC, Lin HF. Eyelid tumors in children: a clinicopathologic study of a 10-year review in southern Taiwan. Ophthalmologica 2004; 218:274–277.

Jakobiec FA, Bonanno PA, Sigelman J. Conjunctival adnexal cysts and dermoids. Arch Ophthalmol 1978; 96:1404–1409.

Kersten RC. The eyelid crease approach to superficial lateral dermoid cyst. J Pediatr Ophthalmol Strabismus. 1998; 25:48–51.

Kiratli H, Bilgic S, Sahin A, Tezel GG. Dermoid cyst of the lacrimal gland. Orbit 2005; 24:145–148.

Kronish JW, Dortzbach RK. Upper eyelid crease surgical approach to dermoid and epidermoid cysts in children. Arch Ophthalmol 1988; 106:1625–1627.

Shields JA, Shields CL. Orbital cysts of childhood—classification, clinical features, and management. Surv Ophthalmol 2004; 49:281–299.

Dermolipoma

INTRODUCTION   The dermolipomas are congenital choristomas that typically occur on the superotemporal conjunctiva. They contain more adipose tissue that the solid dermoid, and are more common in patients with Goldenhar syndrome (oculoauriculovertebral dysplasia). When they contain variable combinations of ectopic tissues such as cartilage, smooth muscle, and acinar glands, they are referred to as complex choristomas. Dermolipomas account for about 5% of all conjunctival tumors in childhood.

CLINICAL PRESENTATION   Dermolipomas usually present in childhood and occur in the superotemporal conjunctiva. They can extend onto the corneal surface or posteriorly into the fornix or even into the orbit. They are well-defined, elevated pink to yellowish, fatty lesions that may contain fine telangiectasias. Hair can grow from these lesions resulting in corneal abrasion. When large they can irritate the palpebral conjunctiva inciting a papillary conjunctivitis.

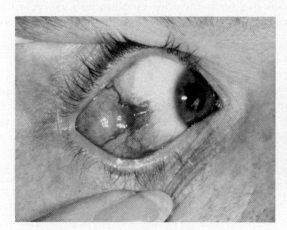 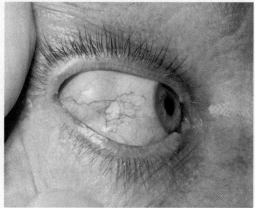

HISTOPATHOLOGY   Dermolipomas are composed of mature adipose tissue and bundles of dense collagenous tissue. Hair follicles and adnexal glands are usually absent. The conjunctival epithelium may be irregularly thickened, or it may be thin and smooth.

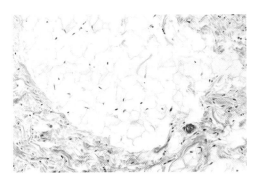 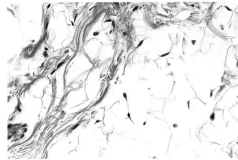

DIFFERENTIAL DIAGNOSIS   The differential diagnosis includes prolapsed orbital fat, dermoid cysts, and conjunctival tumor.

TREATMENT   Treatment is indicated for cosmesis or for symptoms related to corneal exposure from eyelid displacement away from the globe. When removal is desired a simple lamellar dissection is appropriate for the corneal portion. For the remainder of the lesion conjunctival resection should be kept to a minimum and only that portion of the tumor anterior to the orbital rim should be removed. Care must be taken to avoid injury to the lateral rectus muscle insertion and the ductules of lacrimal secretion. Complications include damage to the lacrimal secretory system, restrictive strabismus, diplopia, and symblepharon formation.

REFERENCES

Beard C. Dermolipoma surgery, or, "an ounce of prevention is worth a pound of cure." Ophthal Plast Reconstr Surg 1990; 6:153–157.

Beby F, Kodjikian L, Roche O, et al. Conjunctival tumors in children. A histopathologic study of 42 cases. J Fr Ophtalmol 2005; 28:817–823.

D'Hermies F, Saragoussi JJ, et al. Limbal dermoid and Goldenhar syndrome. Report of an anatomical study. J Fr Ophthalmol 2001; 24:893–896.

Francoise P, Lekieffre M, Woillez M, Ryckewaert M. Complications of dermolipoma ablation. Bull Soc Ophtalmol Fr 1989; 89:289–290.

Fry CL, Leone CR Jr. Safe management of dermolipomas. Arch Ophthalmol 1994; 112:1114–1116.

Kamali K, El-Rifai. Dermolipoma adherent to the lacrimal gland. Bull Ophthalmol Egypt 1975; 68:633–636.

Kim YD, Goldberg RA. Orbital fat prolapse and dermolipoma: two distinct entities. Korean J Ophthalmol 1994; 8:42–43.

Manners RM, Vardy SJ, Rose GE. Localized giant papillary conjunctivitis secondary to a dermolipoma. Eye 1995; 9:376–378.

McNab AA, Wright JE, Caswell AG. Clinical features and surgical management of dermolipomas. Aust N Z J Ophthalmol 1990; 18:159–162.

Touzri RA, Beltaief O, Romdhane BB, Kriaa L, Ouertani AM. Complications of dermolipoma surgery. Two observations. J Fr Ophtalmol 2004; 27:1156–1158.

Eccrine Hidrocystoma

INTRODUCTION   Eccrine hidrocystoma represents a common cystic lesion with a lining that resembles that of eccrine sweat glands. Thought to represent ductal retention cysts, they occur commonly on the face with a predilection for the canthal angles. Immunohistochemical studies suggest that these lesions are of eccrine origin.

CLINICAL PRESENTATION   Such lesions present as solitary or multiple, small translucent 1 to 5 mm fluid filled cysts. The lesions are typically flesh-colored to bluish, tense shiny vesicles usually near the eyelid margins. They are located in the dermis and the overlying epidermis is uninvolved. They tend to increase in size in hot, humid weather associated with increased perspiration. When the cyst wall is punctured the cyst collapses and exudes a clear thin fluid and there is no evidence of layered debris from cellular decapitation as with apocrine cysts.

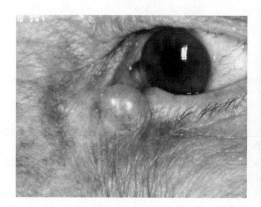 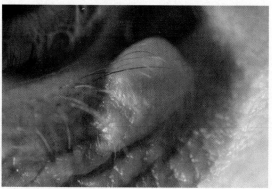

HISTOPATHOLOGY   Two layers of epithelium line these unilocular cysts, commonly termed *sudoriferous cysts* by ophthalmologists. The inner layer is cuboidal and the outer layer is usually low cuboidal to flat. The cyst contents are often absent from histological sections; when present, there is lightly eosinophilic proteinaceous material.

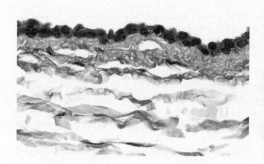 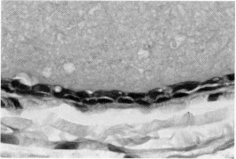

DIFFERENTIAL DIAGNOSIS   The differential diagnosis includes apocrine hidrocystoma, milia, pilar cyst, epidermal inclusion cyst, and syringoma.

TREATMENT   When removal is desired, complete surgical excision including the cyst wall is the treatment of choice. Pulsed dye laser ablation has been reported to give good results after multiple treatment sessions. Botulinum toxin has been suggested as an alternative therapeutic option because of its effect on reducing sweat production.

REFERENCES

Alfadley A, Al Aboud KA, Tulba A, Mourad MM. Multiple eccrine hidrocystomas of the face. Int J Dermatol 2002; 40:125–129.
Blugerman G, Schavelzon D, D'Angelo S. Multiple eccrine hidrocystomas: a new therapeutic option with botulinum toxin. Dermatol Surg 2003; 29:557–559.

Cordero AA, Montes LF. Eccrine hidrocystoma. J Cutan Pathol 1976; 3:292–293.

DeViragh PA, Szeimes RM, Eckert F. Apocrine cystadenoma, apocrine hidrocystoma, and eccrine hidrocystoma: three distinct tumors defined by expression of keratins and milk fat globulin 1. J Cutan Pathol 1997; 24:249–255.

Kaur C, Sarkar R, Kanwar AJ, Mohan H. Multiple eccrine hidrocystomas. J Eur Acad Dermatol Venereol 2002; 16:288–290.

Smith JD, Chernosky ME. Hidrocystomas. Arch Dermatol 1974; 109:700–702.

Sperling LC, Sakas EL. Eccrine hidrocystomas. J Am Acad Dermatol 1992; 7:763–770.

Tanzi E, Alster TS. Pulsed dye laser treatment of multiple eccrine hidrocystomas: a novel approach. Dermatol Surg 2001; 27:898–900.

Yasaka N, Iozumi K, Nashiro K, Tasuchida T, et al. Bilateral periorbital eccrine hidrocystoma. J Dermatol 1994; 21:490–493.

Eccrine Nodular Hidradenoma

INTRODUCTION   Eccrine hidradenoma is also referred to as *nodular hidradenoma, eccrine spiradenoma, or clear cell hidradenoma*. These lesions are uncommon on the eyelids. They presumably arise from eccrine sweat glands and do not show any apocrine differentiation. These tumors occur primarily in middle-aged females and have a predilection for the head region. Very rarely they may undergo malignant change.

CLINICAL PRESENTATION   The eccrine hidradenoma presents as a solitary slowly progressive nodular intradermal swelling. Occasionally it may be exophytic in growth with a translucent appearance and fine telangiectatic vessels. Some lesions have been known to undergo spontaneous regression. Malignant change is suggested by ulceration and infiltration around the borders and these have a high potential for metastatic spread.

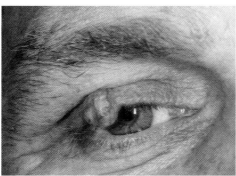 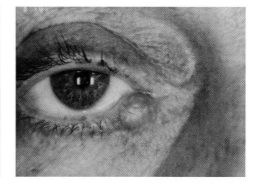

(Courtesy of Bettina Meekins, M.D.)

HISTOPATHOLOGY   These tumors, usually located in the dermis, are well circumscribed and composed of lobules of cells forming tubules and solid sheets. The tubules vary widely in luminal diameter and number, and cuboidal or columnar cells line them. Solid areas of the tumor have a mixture of polyhedral cells with rounded nuclei and slightly basophilic cytoplasm and other cells that are round with clear cytoplasm due to glycogen dissolution during histological processing. The proportion of the two cell types varies considerably between tumors, and there may be cells that have features between the two extremes.

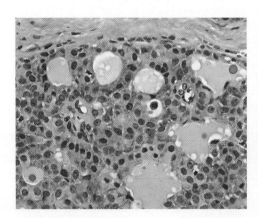 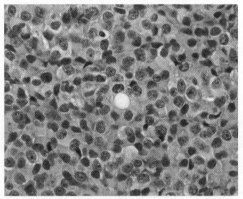

DIFFERENTIAL DIAGNOSIS   These can be confused with many skin lesions. The differential diagnosis includes basal cell carcinoma, apocrine hidradenoma, seborrheic keratosis, leiomyosarcoma, and syringoma.

TREATMENT   Treatment is usually with complete surgical excision. Recurrences are common, reported in up to 50% of cases. Malignant tumors are managed with wide surgical excision and regional lymph node dissection, with ancillary radiotherapy or chemotherapy.

REFERENCES

Agarwala NS, Rane TM, Bhaduri AS. Clear cell hidradenoma of the eyelids: a case report. Indian J Pathol Microbiol 1999; 42:361–363.

Amann J, Spraul CW, Mattfeld T, Lang GK. Eccrine spiradenoma of the eyelid. Klin Monatsbl Augenheilkd 1999; 214:53–54.

Greer CH. Clear cell hidradenoma of the eyelid. Arch Ophthalmol 1968; 80:220–222.

Grosniklaus HE, Knight SH. Eccrine Acrospiroma (clear cell hidradenoma) of the eyelid. Immunohistochemical and ultrastructural features. Ophthalmology 1991; 98:347–352.

Jagannath C, Sandhya CS, Venugopalachari K. Eccrine Acrospiroma of the eye lid—a case report. Indian J Ophthalmol 1990; 38:182.

Stratigos AJ, Olbricht S, Kwan TH, Bowers KE. Nodular hidradenoma. A report of three cases and review of the literature. Dermatol Surg 1998; 24:387–391.

Tsuda Y, Kitaoka T, Amemiya T, Tsuda K. Nodular hidradenoma of the eyelid. Arch Ophthalmol 1996; 114:1287–1288.

Epibulbar Osseous Choristoma

INTRODUCTION   Epibulbar osseous choristoma is a choristomatous lesion of the conjunctiva containing bone in an otherwise normal eye. It is usually a congenital lesion arising as an abnormal development of embryonic pleuripotential mesenchyme, presenting in childhood. However, some lesions may be associated with trauma, presenting in adulthood, and possibly related to inflammation. 70% of cases are in females and 80% occur in the superotemporal quadrant. Lesions can sometimes be associated with other choristomatous lesions such as cartilage, dermoid cyst, and ectopic lacrimal tissue.

CLINICAL PRESENTATION   This lesion most commonly presents as an isolated epibulbar lesion in the super-otemporal conjunctival quadrant, but it can be seen in other areas as well. It is typically present at birth and shows slow growth. It appears as a fatty yellowish subconjunctival mass without hair, and resembles a dermolipoma. A central hard core of bone is present surrounded by a more fibrous mass. The lesion may have a firm attachment to the underlying sclera or to the insertion of an extraocular muscle.

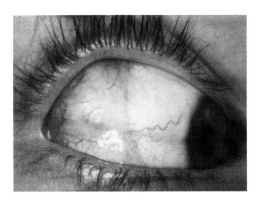

HISTOPATHOLOGY   This choristomatous lesion of the conjunctiva is composed of mature, compact bone surrounded by fibrous connective tissue. Haversian canals are present and are surrounded by concentric lamellae of bone. Other choristomatous tissues including fibroadipose tissue, nerves, and lacrimal acini have been seen occasionally in these rare lesions of the conjunctiva.

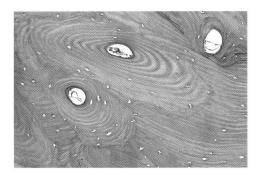

DIFFERENTIAL DIAGNOSIS   The differential diagnosis includes limbal dermoid, epithelial inclusion cyst, prolapsed orbital fat, papilloma, dermolipoma, and complex choristoma.

TREATMENT   Since these are benign lesions that are usually asymptomatic, they can be safely observed without treatment. Indications for treatment include cosmetic improvement, ocular inflammation, or chronic epiphora. Surgical excision can be achieved with care taken to preserve the insertion of extraocular muscles.

REFERENCES

Dreizen NG, Schacat AP, Shields JA, Augsburger JJ. Epibulbar osseous choristoma. J Pediatr Ophthalmol Strabismus 1983; 20:247–249.

Gayre GS, Proia AD, Dutton JJ. Epibulbar osseous choristoma: case report and review of the literature. Ophthal Surg Lasers 2002; 33:410–415.

Gonnering RS, Fuerste FH, Lemke BN, Sonneland PR. Epibulbar osseous choristomas with scleral involvement. Ophthal Plast Reconstr Surg 1988; 4:63–66.

Melki TS, Zimmerman LE, Chavis RM, Ellsworth R, O'Neill JF. A unique epibulbar osseous choristoma. J Pediatr Ophthalmol Strabismus 1990; 27:252–254.

Oritz JM, Yanoff M. Epipalpebral conjunctival osseous choristoma. Br J Ophthalmol 1979; 63:173–176.

Shields JA, Eagle RC, Sheilds CL, DePotter P, Schnall BM. Epibulbar osseous choristoma: computed tomography and clinicopathologic correlation. Ophthalmic Practice 1997; 15:110–112.

Trojet S, Kamoun H, El Afrit MA, et al. Epibulbar osseous choristoma: two case reports. J Fr Ophtalmol 2003; 26:481–483.

Epidermoid Cyst

INTRODUCTION   The epidermoid cyst is also referred to as *infundibular cyst, epidermal inclusion cyst, keratinous cyst,* or frequently and erroneously *sebaceous cyst.* The sebaceous cyst is similar clinically but arises from obstruction in the hair follicle and is referred to as a pilar or trichilemmal cyst. The epidermoid cyst is a very common skin lesion that arises from traumatic entrapment of surface epithelium or from aberrant healing of the infundibular epithelium of the hair follicle following episodes of follicular inflammation. They can also be seen following any injury to the skin, including surgery. When congenital, they likely arise from sequestration of epidermal rests along embryonic fusion planes. Epidermoid cysts are not of sebaceous origin, but rather produce normal keratin rather than sebum. These cysts may present anytime from adolescence through adulthood, but commonly in the third and fourth decades.

CLINICAL PRESENTATION   On the eyelid epidermoid cysts present as a slow-growing round, firm flesh-colored to yellow or white lesion within the dermis or subcutaneous tissue. On the face they may be associated and causally related to the obstructing effects of acne vulgaris and seborrhea. Epidermoid cysts are usually solitary, fluctuant, and freely movable, and are generally less than 1 to 2 cm in diameter. Sometimes a central pore or depression is seen, but this is an inconsistent finding. The cyst can be pigmented in darker skinned individuals. A foul-smelling cheese-like material may discharge from the lesion. Rupture of the cyst wall may cause an inflammatory foreign body reaction, with associated tenderness or pain. Less frequently the cyst can become infected. Rarely carcinomas, such as basal cell carcinoma, may arise within an epidermoid cyst.

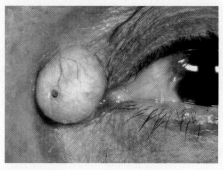
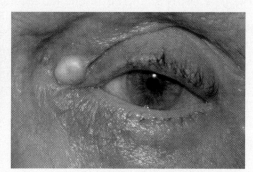
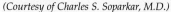

(Courtesy of Charles S. Soparkar, M.D.)

HISTOPATHOLOGY   Epidermoid cysts are lined by keratinized, stratified squamous epithelium nearly identical to the epidermis. Keratohyaline granules are often prominent in the epithelial cells nearer the cyst lumen. Adnexal structures are absent from the cyst wall. Laminated keratin fills the cyst lumen.

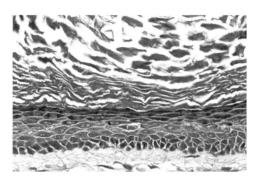 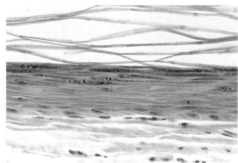

DIFFERENTIAL DIAGNOSIS   The differential diagnosis includes dermoid cyst, pilar cyst, milia, lipoma, and neurofibroma.

TREATMENT   Asymptomatic epidermoid cysts may respond to injections of intralesional tiramcinolone, particularly when they are inflamed. Incision and drainage is a fast and easy method, but the keratin-producing lining remains and recurrence is common. Dissection of the overlying epithelium and shelling out of the cyst is very effective. However, after inflammation the cyst may be more firmly adherent to surrounding tissues so that a full-thickness elliptical excision including the entire cyst wall may be required.

REFERENCES

Folberg R. Eyelids: Study of specific conditions. In: Folberg R, ed. Pathology of the Eye. [CD-ROM]. St Louis: Mosby-Year Book, 1996.

Ikeda I, Ono T. Basal cell carcinoma originating from an epidermoid cyst. J Dermatol 1990; 17:643–646.

Jordan DR. Multiple epidermal inclusion cysts of the eyelid: a simple technique for removal. Can J Ophthalmol 2002; 37:39–40.

Kligman AM. The myth of the sebaceous cyst. Arch Dermatol 1964; 89:253–256.

Kronish JW, Sneed SR, Tse DT. Epidermoid cyst of the eyelid. Arch Ophthalmol 1988; 106:270.

Mao WS, Yue KK. Epidermoid cyst of the eyelid. Chin Med J 1951; 69:248–450.

McGavran MH, Binnington B. Keratinous cysts of the skin. Identification and differentiation of pilar cysts from epidermal cysts. Arch Dermatol 1966; 94:499–508.

Erysipelas

INTRODUCTION   Erysipelas is an acute cellulitis-lymphangiitis usually caused by a group A hemolytic *Streptococcus*. The organism usually gains access through a break in the skin, or occasionally through a surgical incision, and proceeds along the superficial lymphatics. The disease affects mainly older adults. The most common sites of occurrence are the lower legs and face. If the infection extends into the deep subcutaneous and fascial tissues it may spread remarkably rapidly, and is known as necrotizing fasciitis.

CLINICAL PRESENTATION   In 40% of cases the portal of entry may not be obvious. After an incubation period of several days the disease commences abruptly with fever, malaise, and sometimes mental confusion. A small erythematous patch at the infected site rapidly spreads. The erythema is irregular with extensions or tongues along lymphatic vessels. The clinical appearance of an elevated, erythematous, indurated area with a sharp border is very characteristic. The area is hot to the touch, and tiny vesicles may be seen at the advancing margin. The tense edema gives the skin a shiny glazed appearance and is sufficient to greatly distort the facial features. Local complications include hemorrhagic infarction, ulceration, and necrosis. Regional lymphadenopathy accompanies the infection. Chronic lymphedema is a possible sequel resulting from occlusion of lymph vessels. As with many streptococcal infections acute glomerulonephritis may develop later in the convalescent period.

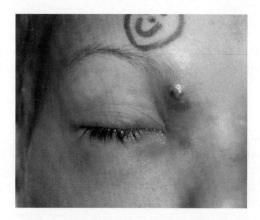

HISTOPATHOLOGY   This distinctive form of cellulitis has marked subepidermal edema, which may result in formation of vesiculobullous lesions. Beneath the zone of marked edema, there is a diffuse and heavy infiltrate of neutrophils without abscess formation. The neutrophils may be accentuated around blood vessels. Blood vessels and lymphatics may be dilated. As the lesions heal, granulation tissue may form subjacent to the zone of subepidermal edema.

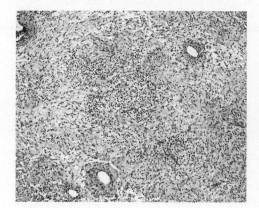
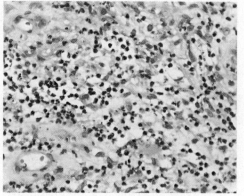

DIFFERENTIAL DIAGNOSIS   The differential diagnosis includes mucormycosis, preseptal cellulitis, dermatitis, necrotizing fasciitis, orbital cellulitis, and Herpes zoster.

TREATMENT With the early institution of systemic antibiotic therapy most patients will begin to show improvement in 24 to 48 hours. While oral antibiotics may be acceptable intravenous antibiotic therapy is generally needed with penicillin as the drug of choice. General supportive measures are important including bed rest, elevation of the head to reduce edema, and topical antibiotics. The infection does not impart immunity and, in fact, victims seem to harbor an increased susceptibility to recurrence.

REFERENCES
Abbott RL, Shekter WB. Necrotizing erysipelas of the eyelids. Ann Ophthalmol 1979; 11:381–384.

Aichmair H. Erysipelas of the lids. Klin Monatsbl Augenheilkd 1977; 171:614–615.

Bonnetblanc JM, Bedane C. Erysipelas: recognition and management. Am J Dermatol 2003; 4:157–163.

Brennecke S, Hartmann M, Schofer H, Rasokat H, Tschachler E, Brockmeyer NH. Treatment of erysipelas in Germany and Austria—results of a survey in German and Austrian dermatological clinics. J Dtsch Dermatol Gees 2005; 3:263–270.

Jegou J, Hansmann Y, Chalot F, et al. Hospitalization criteria for erysipelas: prospective study in 145 cases. Ann Dermatol Venereol 2002; 129:375–379.

Krasagakis K, Saminis G, Maniatakis P, Georgala S, Tosca A. Bullous erysipelas: clinical presentation, staphylococcal involvement, and methicillin resistance. Dermatology 2006; 212:31–35.

McHugh D, Fison PN. Ocular erysipelas. Ach Ophthalmol 1992; 110:1315.

Erythema Multiforme/Stevens-Johnson Syndrome/Toxic Epidermal Necrolysis Disease Spectrum

INTRODUCTION Erythema multiforme is an acute mucocutaneous hypersensitivity reaction. Although once believed to be distinct diseases, many observers currently consider erythema multiforme, Stevens-Johnson syndrome, and toxic epidermal necrolysis (TENS) to represent a mild to severe continuum of the same process. Erythema multiforme minor represents the mildest form. These three entities share certain clinical, histologic, and etiologic characteristics in common. Although ocular involvement in erythema multiforme minor is rare, it is seen frequently in both Stevens-Johnson syndrome and TENS. The majority of cases occur in children and young adults. Most cases follow exposure to a drug or infectious agent. The most frequently implicated organisms have been herpes simplex, *Mycoplasma pneumoniae*, and *Streptococcus*. Drugs include antibiotics and seizure medications. Recurrences can occur and the disease is fatal in 10% of cases.

CLINICAL PRESENTATION Erythema multiforme minor is characterized by round erythematous rapidly progressive mucocutaneous macules or papules. The borders are bright red with central petichiae, vesicles, or purpura. Conjunctivitis with blisters and ulcerations can be seen, and secondary infection is common. Lesions may coalesce and become generalized. Burning may be significant, but pruritis is generally absent. These lesions usually resolve over one to several weeks, but postinflammatory hyper- or hypopigmentation may occur. In EM major (Stevens-Johnson syndrome) prodromal symptoms occur in 50% of cases and include fever, malaise, sore throat, arthralgia, vomiting, and diarrhea. Mucocutaneous involvement shows bullous lesions which become hemorrhagic and necrotic, leading to extensive denuded areas of skin and mucous membrane including the mouth and conjunctiva. Scarring results in lagophthalmos, trichiasis, symblepharon, and eyelid malpositions such as entropion and ectropion. Loss of mucin producing goblet cells contributes to a severe dry eye syndrome. TENS produces even more severe disease characterized by large flaccid bullae that quickly progress to peeling off of epithelium in great sheets exposing the raw, weeping dermis. This is a medical emergency and may be life-threatening.

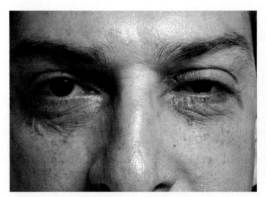

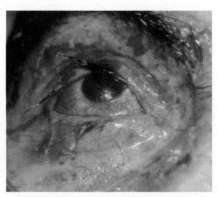

(Courtesy of Robert A. Goldberg, M.D.)   *(Courtesy of Charles S. Soparkar, M.D.)*

HISTOPATHOLOGY   In early lesions, there are vacuolated basal epidermal cells, mild spongiosis, lymphocytes along the epidermal-dermal junction and migrating into the epidermis ("exocytosis"), and a mild perivascular lymphohistiocytic infiltrate in the superficial dermis. Apoptosis of individual basal cells results in eosinophilic, rounded keratinocytes that may be anucleate or have pyknotic nuclei; these are the hallmark of erythema multiforme. Lymphocytes may surround dying keratinocytes ("satellite cell necrosis"). More edematous lesions have greater spongiosis and papillary edema, and a more intense inflammatory infiltrate.

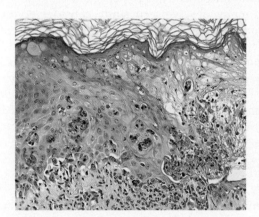

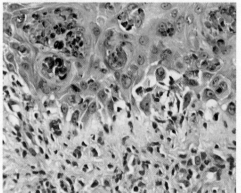

DIFFERENTIAL DIAGNOSIS   The differential diagnosis includes cicatricial ocular pemphigoid, IgA linear dystrophy, rosacea, and pityriasis rosea.

TREATMENT   Clinical diagnosis may be difficult; therefore a skin biopsy can be extremely helpful. Withdrawal of the causative agent is essential. For EM minor symptomatic treatment is offered. Acute episodes should be managed with topical corticosteroids and ocular lubrication. For recurrent disease, prophylactic oral acyclovir may be effective in reducing episodes. For EM major hospitalization is required. Systemic immunosuppressive agents such as cyclophosphamide or azathioprine, either alone or in combination with systemic steroids are indicated. Local measures such as tear replacement, and topical steroids and antibiotics are used for ocular involvement. Debridement of the fornices with lysis of symblephara using a glass rod may be helpful. Surveillance cultures should be taken every few days, and secondary infections should be treated aggressively. Once the acute phase has resolved surgical therapy including skin grafts to treat lagophthalmos, lysis of symblephara with or without conjunctival or amniotic membrane grafting, and tarsorraphy may be necessary. Trichiasis may require treatment with epilation, electrocautery, or cryosurgery.

REFERENCES

Amon RB, Dimond RL. Toxic epidermal necrolysis: Rapid differentiation between staphylococcal and drug induced disease. Arch Dermatol 1975; 111:1433–1437.

Arstikaitis MJ. Ocular aftermath of Stevens-Johnson syndrome. Arch Ophthalmol 1973; 90:376–379.

Bennett TO, Sugar J, Sahgal S. Ocular manifestations of toxic epidermal necrolysis associated with allopurinol use. Arch Ophthalmol 1977; 95:1362–1364.

Beyer CK. The management of special problems associated with Stevens-Johnson syndrome and ocular pemphigoid. Trans Am Acad Ophthalmol Otolaryngol 1977; 83:701–707.

Bushkell LL, Mackel SE, Jordan RE. Erythema multiforme: direct immunofluorescence studies and detection of circulating immune complexes. J Invest Dermatol 1980; 74:372–374.

Kazmierowski JA, Wuepper KD. Erythema multiforme immune complex vasculitis of the superficial cutaneous microvasculature. J Invest Dermatol 1978; 71:366–369.

Manzella JP, Hull CB, Green JL, McMeekin TO. Toxic epidermal necrolysis in childhood: differentiation from staphylococcal scalded skin syndrome. Pediatrics 1980; 66:291–294.

Powers WJ, Ghoraishi M, Merayo-Lloves J, Neves RA, Foster CS. Analysis of the acute ophthalmic manifestations of the erythema multiforme/Stevens-Johnson Syndrome/toxic epidermal necrolysis disease spectrum. Ophthalmology 1995; 102:1669–1676.

Rasmussen JE. Erythema multiforme in children: response to treatment with systemic steroids. Br J Dermatol 1976; 95:181–186.

Tonneson MG, Soter NA. Erythema multiforme. J Am Acad Dermatol 1979; 1:357–364.

Watts MT, Nelson ME. External Eye Disease: A Color Atlas. Edinburgh: Churchill Livingstone, 1992.

Whitmore PV. In: Duane TD ed Clinical Ophthalmology. Vol. 5. Philadelphia: Harper & Row, 1983, Chap. 27.

Wilkins J, Morrison L, White CR Jr. Oculocutaneous manifestations of the erythema multiforme/Stevens-Johnson syndrome/toxic epidermal necrolysis spectrum. Dermatol Clin 1992; 10:571–582.

Granuloma Annulare

INTRODUCTION

Granuloma annulare, also known as *pseudorheumatoid nodule*, is a benign self-limited lesion of uncertain etiology with characteristic clinical and histopathologic appearance. It has been suggested that lesions are triggered by trauma, insect bites, sun exposure, viral infection, and tuberculin skin tests, but there is no convincing evidence to support these claims. Lesions most often occur on the dorsum of the hands, legs, and trunk, and less frequently on the face and eyelids. Several varieties have been recognized including subcutaneous, generalized, and perforating types. The subcutaneous form occurs most often in children and young adults and is most likely to involve the face. Deep granuloma annulare is a subtype of the subcutaneous form and can involve periosteum and be fixed to bone.

CLINICAL PRESENTATION   Lesions present as one or more skin colored erythematous or violaceous dermal plaques, nodules or papules arranged in rings. They are seen most frequently on the lateral upper eyelid and lateral canthus. Lesions appear as nontender mobile cutaneous masses generally less than 1 to 1.5 cm in diameter. Eyelid edema may be moderate, and there may be ptosis of the upper eyelid. With deep lesions they may involve fascia and tendons, and are rubbery in consistency, immobile and often fixed to the orbital rim.

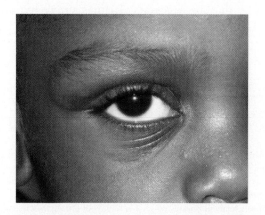

HISTOPATHOLOGY   In "classical" granuloma annulare, a palisade of histiocytes surrounds a zone of degenerated collagen containing prominent mucin. The mucin is light blue in sections stained with hematoxylin and eosin, and its presence can be confirmed using alcian blue or colloidal iron stains. In other cases of granuloma annulare, the histiocytes may be interstitial without organization or they may be aggregated but without palisading. Often, there is a mixture of histiocytes that are not palisaded, slightly palisaded, and well palisaded. Multinucleated giant cells are usually scant. Usually, all layers of the dermis contain the histiocytic infiltrate. A lower magnification image of granuloma annulare is shown in the terminology chapter under "necrobiosis."

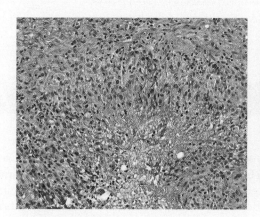 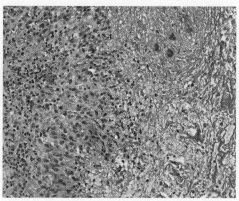

DIFFERENTIAL DIAGNOSIS   The differential diagnosis includes insect bites, erythema multiforme, syphilis, rheumatoid nodules, tuberculous granulomas, metastatic lesions, fibrosarcoma, and amyloidosis.

TREATMENT Granuloma annulare lesions tend to be self-limited, resolving over several months without scarring. Therefore, treatment is generally not needed and surgical intervention should be avoided. However, in 20% of cases lesions will recur in the same location and in 26% they will appear at other sites. When treatment is required because of persistence, varying degrees of success have been reported with surgical excision, cryotherapy, radiotherapy, and intralesional steroids.

REFERENCES

Burnstein MA, Headington JT, Reifler DM, et al. Periocular granuloma annulare, nodular type. Arch Ophthalmol 1994; 112:1590–1593.

Cronquist SD, Stashower ME, Benson PM. Deep dermal granuloma annulare presenting as an eyelid tumor in a child, with review of pediatric eyelid lesions. Ped Dermatol 1999; 16:377–380.

Dutton JJ, Escaravage GK. Periocular subperiosteal deep granuloma annulare in a child. Ophthal Plast Reconstr Surg 2006; 22:141–143.

Ferry AP. Subcutaneous granuloma annulare ("pseudorheumatoid nodule") of the eyebrow. J Ped Ophthalmol 1977; 14:154–157.

Floyd BB, Brown B, Isaacs H, Minckler DS. Pseudorheumatoid nodule involving the orbit. Arch Ophthalmol 1982; 100:1478–1480.

Goldstein SM, Douglas RS, Binenbaum G, Katowitz JA. Paediatric periocular granuloma annulare. Acta Ophthalmol Scand 2003; 81:90–91.

Grogg KL, Nasimento MD. Subcutaneous granuloma annulare in childhood: clinicopathologic features in 34 cases. Pediatrics 2001; 107:E42.

Rao NA, Font RL. Pseudorheumatoid nodules of the ocular adnexa. Am J Ophthalmol 1975; 79:471–478.

Ross MJ, Cohen KL, Peiffer RL Jr, Grimson BS. Episcleral and orbital pseudorheumatoid nodules. Arch Ophthalmol 1983; 101:418–421.

Hemangiopericytoma

INTRODUCTION This vascular neoplasm arises from the primitive pericytes, which are cells that normally reside in the outer capillary wall. They may occur at any age, and are rare in the eyelids and orbit. Hemangiopericytomas have a great propensity for local spread, especially when recurrent. Although more common in the orbit, localized eyelid hemangiopericytomas have been reported. About 20% of these lesions are malignant, and these may progress rapidly with a poor prognosis.

CLINICAL PRESENTATION Hemangiopericytomas of the eyelid or periorbital region grow slowly over several years and as a well-circumscribed, painless subcutaneous mass. It may be beneath the skin or even in the lacrimal sac. The lesion is firm and often bluish in color. When the conjunctiva is involved the lesion appears as a red nodule. Orbital involvement is more common and presents with proptosis with or without decreased vision. Hemangiopericytoma can also involve the choroid or ciliary body.

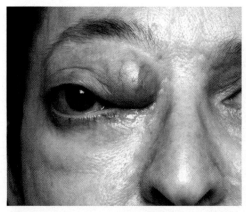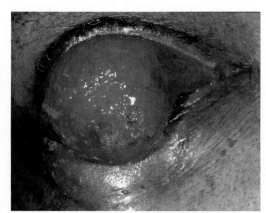

(Courtesy of Robert A. Goldberg, M.D.)

HISTOPATHOLOGY   Hemangiopericytomas are formed of closely packed tumor cells surrounding thin-walled, endothelium-lined, branching vascular spaces that vary widely in caliber. Large branching vessels have been referred to as having "antler" or "staghorn" configurations. Tumor cells are arranged haphazardly around the vessels and have round to oval nuclei, moderate amounts of cytoplasm, and indistinct cell borders. The tumor cells react with antibodies to factor XIIIa and CD34, but these are not markers specific for this tumor. The cells do not express factor VIII-related antigen, nor do they react with *Ulex europaeus* I lectin, which distinguishes them from the endothelial cells lining the vascular channels. Predicting biological behavior from the histological appearance is fraught with difficulty, but frequent mitotic figures, necrosis, hemorrhage, and increased cellularity are features associated with a poor prognosis.

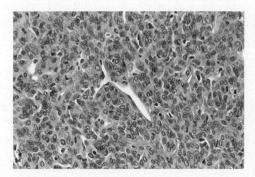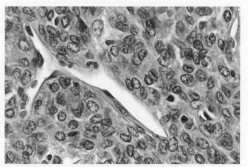

DIFFERENTIAL DIAGNOSIS   The differential diagnosis of hemangiopericytomas includes cavernous hemangioma, arteriovenous malformations, fibrous histiocytoma, and leiomyoma.

TREATMENT   Early complete excision is recommended because of the tendency toward relentless growth. Surgical violation of the capsule without total removal of the neoplasm can result in a rapid infiltration of surrounding tissues and possible malignant transformation. Intra-arterial chemotherapy may be useful for diffuse recurrent lesions. Radiotherapy is of little benefit and may precipitate sarcomatous change.

REFERENCES

Battifora H. Hemangioperictoma: Ultrastructural study of five cases. Cancer 1973; 31:1418–1432.

Brown HH, Brodsky MC, Hembree K, Mrak RE. Supraciliary hemangiopericytoma. Ophthalmology 1991; 98:378–382.

Charels NC, Palu RN, Jagirdar JS. Hemangiopericytoma of the lacrimal sac. Arch Ophthalmol 1998; 116:1677–1680.

Enzinger FM, Smith BH. Hemangiopericytoma: an analysis of 106 cases. Hum Pathol 1976; 7:61–82.

Henderson JW, Farrow GM. Primary orbital hemangiopericytoma: an aggressive and potentially malignant neoplasm. Arch Ophthalmol 1978; 96:666–673.

Lee JT, Pettit TH, Glasgow BJ. Epibulbar hemangiopericytoma. Am J Ophthalmol 1997; 124:547–549.

Lee YC, Wang JS, Shyu JS. Orbital hemangiopericytoma—a case report. Kaohsiung J Med Sci 2003; 19:33–37.

Lim KH, Kim YD, Kim YI. Hemangiopericytoma of the lacrimal sac. Korean J Ophthalmol 1991; 5:88–91.

Macoul KL. Hemangiopericytoma of the lid and orbit. Am J Ophthalmol 1968; 66:731–733.

McMaster MJ, Soule EG, Ivins JC. Hemangioperictoma. A clinicopathologic study and long-term follow-up of 60 patients. Cancer 1975; 36:2232–2244.

Oshida N, Hisatomi U, Takemura M, Kobayashi Y. A hemangiopericytoma of the eyelid. Nippon Ganka Kiyo 1970; 21:269–272.

Sekundo W, Roggenkanper P, Tschubel K, Fischer HP. Hemangiopericytoma of the inner canthus. Am J Ophthalmol 1996; 121:445–447.

Shimura M, Suzuki K, Fuse N, et al. Intraocular hemangiopericytoms. A case report. Ophthalmologica 2001; 215:378–382.

Herpes Simplex

INTRODUCTION   Herpes simplex is caused by a DNA virus that is estimated to infect 60% to 90% of individuals at sometime during their life. Clinically evident infections however are much less common. Involvement of the facial region is predominantly due to type I herpes virus, with the exception of newborns, in whom overwhelming exposure to the type II variety during birth can result in development of typical skin lesions during the first few days of life, often associated with devastating CNS and systemic involvement. Primary herpes occurs in previously uninfected individuals. The chief mode of transmission is by kissing or other forms of intimate contact with an individual who has an active, usually recurrent, herpetic lesion.

CLINICAL PRESENTATION   Following a 2 to 14 day incubation period there develops a mild fever with moderately painful, usually unilateral, edema and erythema of the eyelid region. This is soon followed by the development of multiple discrete 2 to 3 mm vesicles that generally have a central umblilication. These break, crust over, and most often resolve without bacterial infection or scarring over the ensuing few weeks. There is a mildly tender preauricular lymphadenopathy, and often vesicular lesions are found elsewhere on the face or mucous membranes. Atypical dermal manifestations include the development of a black eschar early on, or edema without obvious vesicles. A careful search often reveals a few minute vesicles sometimes hidden at the base of the lashes. Following resolution the herpes virus retreats to the trigeminal ganglion where it can later reactivate and incite recurrent infections. Recurrent herpetic infections frequently follow a fever, head cold, sun exposure, or some other trivial physical or emotional insult. Onset is often preceded by a 24-hour prodrome with focal dysethesia, numbness, and tingling. The recurrent eruption is usually less severe than the primary and is more limited. Associated ocular involvement may include a follicular conjunctivitis, dendritic keratitis, disciform keratitis, acute anterior uveitis, and rarely a necrotizing retinitis or optic neuritis.

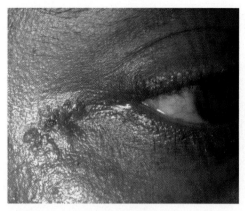

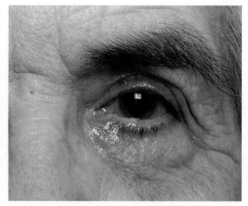

(Courtesy of Kenneth Cohen, M.D.)   *(Courtesy of Robert A. Goldberg, M.D.)*

HISTOPATHOLOGY   The histological features of herpes simplex virus (HSV), varicella, and herpes zoster virus skin infections are similar. In HSV, the earliest changes are seen in the epidermal cell nuclei, which enlarge, develop a homogenous "ground glass" appearance, and have peripherally clumped chromatin. Changes begin along the basal epidermal layer and progress to involve all layers. Intraepidermal vesicles soon form secondary to ballooning and acantholysis of keratinocytes. Subepidermal vesicles may result from destruction of the basal layer of epidermis. Multinucleated keratinocytes are more conspicuous in lesions that have been present for several days. The histopathological clue to diagnosis is eosinophilic nuclear inclusions, which are more common in the multinucleated cells. Diagnosis is confirmed using immunohistochemistry.

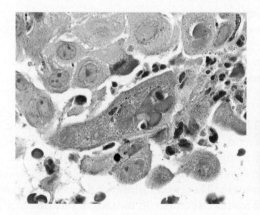

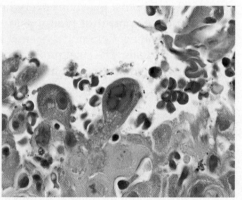

DIFFERENTIAL DIAGNOSIS   The differential diagnosis includes acute stye, insect bite, chickenpox, herpes zoster, contact dermatitis, and ulcerative blepharitis.

TREATMENT   The diagnosis can usually be made clinically; however, confirmation can be accomplished by finding multinucleated giant cells on a Giemsa-stained smear. Viral cultures can be obtained and would be needed to exclude herpes zoster, which will look the same on smear. An enzyme-linked immunosorbent assay (ELISA) is also available. Because of the high risk of secondary corneal involvement in cases involving the eyelids, prophylactic treatment with idoxuridine or vidarabine ointment to the eye four times a day until the skin lesions have dried and crusted, and then twice a day for an additional two weeks, reduces the incidence and severity of ocular infection. Use of antiviral medications on the skin lesions is also recommended in the hope of suppressing the shed of viral particles. For recurrent attacks prophylactic use of topical antiviral agents in the prodromal phase will often abort the attack. Bacterial infection occurs only occasionally, so antibiotics are not generally employed until or unless secondary infection becomes manifest. Steroids should not be used because they exacerbate ocular infections. In younger children without corneal involvement the disease can be self-limited with spontaneous resolution.

REFERENCES

Besada E. Clinical diagnosis of recurrent herpes simplex blepharitis in an adult: a case report. J Am Optom Assoc 1994; 65:235–238.

Campanella PC, Rosenwasser GO, Sassani JW, Goldberg SH. Herpes simplex blepharoconjunctivitis presenting as complete acquired ankyloblepharon. Cornea 1997; 16:360–361.

Honig P, Holzwanger J, Leyden J. Congenital herpes simplex virus infections. Report of three cases and review of the literature. Arch Dermatol 1979; 115:1329–1333.

Long J, Wheeler C, Briggaman R. Varicella-like infection due to herpes simplex. Arch Dermatol 1978; 114:406–409.

Nauheim J, Sussman W. Herpes simplex of the lids and adjacent areas. Trans Am Acad Ophthalmol Otolaryngol 1971; 75:1236–1241.

Overall JC Jr. Persistent problems with resistant herpes viruses. N Engl J Med 1981; 305:95–97.

Pavan-Langston D. Diagnosis and management of herpes simplex ocular infection. Int Ophthalmol Clin 1975; 15:19–35.

Parisi ML. A case of recurrent, isolated, simultaneous, bilateral herpes simplex lid infection. J Am Optom Assoc 1998; 69:49–56.

Pazin G, Ho M, Jannetta P. Reactivation of herpes simplex virus after decompression of the trigeminal nerve root. J Infect Dis 1978; 138:405–409.

Schneidman DW, Barr, RJ, Graham JH. Chronic cutaneous herpes simplex. JAMA 1980; 241:592–594.

Simon JW, Longo F, Smith RS. Spontaneous resolution of herpes simplex blepharoconjunctivitis in children. Am J Ophthalmol 1986; 102:598–600.

Stumpf TH, Case R, Shimeld C, Easty DL, Hill TJ. Primary herpes simplex virus type I infection of the eye triggers similar immune responses in the cornea and the skin of the eyelids. J Gen Virol 2002; 83:1579–1590.

Whallett EJ, Pahor AL. Herpes and the head and neck: the difficulties in diagnosis. J Laryngol Otol 1999; 113:573–577.

Herpes and Varicella Zoster

INTRODUCTION

Herpes zoster (*shingles*) and varicella zoster (*chickenpox*) are both systemic infections with manifestations caused by herpes virus varicellae. The virus is an obligate human parasite requiring person-to-person transmission for its survival. Varicella most commonly occurs in children and is almost always a mild, self-limited disease; however, when the disease occurs in adults it is often a much more severe process. Zoster, meaning belt or girdle in Greek, is felt to be a reactivation of a previous varicella infection within a single dermatome. Herpes zoster is most prevalent in middle to late adulthood; however, it can occur in children and rarely even in infants, in whom it is usually a mild disease. Eyelid symptoms result from involvement of the first or ophthalmic division of the trigeminal (5th cranial) nerve and are seen in up to 10% of cases of zoster infections. Adults with herpes zoster are contagious during the early stages and often transmit the virus to susceptible youngsters who then develop chickenpox. The incidence of post herpetic neuralgia increases with age; it is seldom seen under age 50 years but occurs in up to 50% of victims over 70 years old. Most cases subside after several months, but those that persist can be sever enough to lead to incapacitation and may even result in suicide.

CLINICAL PRESENTATION   Following an incubation period of approximately two weeks and a prodrome of fever and malaise, the cutaneous lesions begin as a mild maculo-papular eruption. The papules evolve into clear vesicles that show an umbilicated center. Characteristic vesicles overlie a larger patch of erythema and develop in several successive crops. The vesicles become cloudy, rupture, and form crusts. Healing occurs over the ensuing few weeks with little or no scarring unless they become infected. In contrast to varicella, the lesions in herpes zoster are limited to a single dermatome; however, hematologic dissemination of the virus can result in a few distant skin lesions as well. Pain in the region supplied by the involved nerve is not common but can precede the skin changes by several days. Preauricular adenopathy is often seen. The nasociliary branch of the ophthalmic nerve supplies sensation to the eye, with terminal branches going to the tip of the nose. Lesions on the tip of the nose, therefore, are usually accompanied by ocular manifestations (Hutchinson's sign). Associated ocular involvement may include a follicular conjunctivitis, nummular keratitis, dendritic keratitis, disciform keratitis, acute anterior uveitis, or rarely a necrotizing retinitis. Less often, optic nerve involvement or selective palsies of the oculomotor, trochlear, or abducens nerves may be seen. Late ocular sequelae may include glaucoma, neuroparalytic keratopathy, and Addie's tonic pupil due to ciliary ganglion damage may occur.

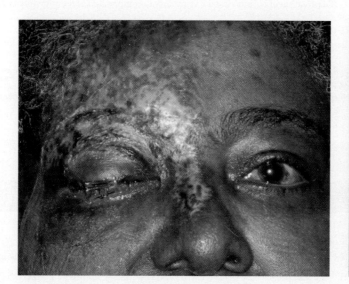
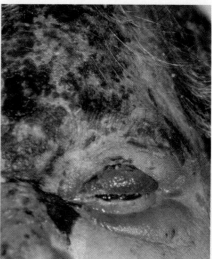

HISTOPATHOLOGY   The characteristic lesion of herpes zoster infection is an intraepidermal vesicle (blister) with swollen and multinucleated epidermal cells. Swollen epidermal cells lose their attachment to adjacent cells and separate from them; a subepidermal vesicle may result if this process involves the basal epidermal cells. Eosinophilic nuclear inclusions are found in some of the multinucleated keratinocytes. Neutrophils are present within vesicles and within the subjacent dermis. The lesions of herpes zoster resemble those of herpes simplex, but they can be distinguished using immunohistochemical stains.

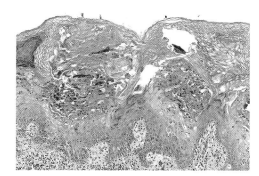
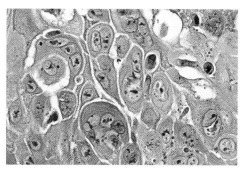

DIFFERENTIAL DIAGNOSIS The differential diagnosis includes Herpes simplex, impetigo, and Coxsackie virus infections.

TREATMENT A vaccine against varicella is now available and may limit its occurrence in future generations. For active disease oral antihistamines may be useful in decreasing pruritis and scratching which may lead to scarring. Systemic antivirals including acyclovir and valcyclovir may limit the duration of the disease in adults. Systemic steroids should be avoided owing to the risk of inducing encephalitis. Herpes zoster also runs a limited course, however the incidence of post herpetic neuralgia is much higher. Antiviral agents such as valcyclovir and famcyclovir may limit the course, and in the case of famcyclovir may actually reduce the instance of post herpetic neuralgia. High-dose systemic steroids during the acute disease, in the range of 60 mg of prednisone daily, also appear to reduce the incidence and severity of post herpetic neuralgia. In debilitated or immunosuppressed individuals systemic steroids carry a considerable risk of inducing disseminated zoster. In patients with immunologic defects, varicella can be devastating and even fatal, therefore, when known exposure has occurred or is suspected, gamma globulin or zoster immune globulin can abort or reduce the severity of the disease.

REFERENCES

Eaglestein WH, Katz R, Brown JA. The effects of early corticosteroid therapy on the skin eruption and pain of herpes zoster. JAMA 1970; 211:1681–1683.

Grimson BS, Glaser JS. Isolated trochlear nerve palsies in herpes zoster ophthalmicus. Arch Ophthalmol 1978; 96:1233–1235.

Liesegang TJ. Corneal complications from herpes zoster ophthalmicus. Ophthalmology 1985; 92:316–324.

Marsh RJ. Current management of ophthalmic zoster. Aust N Z J Ophthalmol 1990; 18:273–279.

Mok CH. Zoster-like disease in infants and young children. N Engl J Med 1971; 285:294.

Naumann G, Gass JD, Font RL. Histopathology of herpes zoster ophthalmicus. Am J Ophthalmol 1968; 65:533–541.

Pavan-Langston D, McCully JP. Herpes zoster dendritic keratitis. Arch Ophthalmol 1973; 89:25–29.

Pavan-Langston D. Varicella-zoster ophthalmicus. Int Ophthal Clin 1975; 15:171–185.

Piebenga LW, Laibson PR. Dendritic lesions in herpes zoster ophthalmicus. Arch Ophthalmol 1973; 90:268–270.

Severson EA, Baratz KH, Hodge DO, Burke JP. Herpes zoster ophthalmicus in Olmsted County, Minnesota: have systemic anitvirals made a difference? Arch Ophthalmol 2003; 121:386–390.

Yoshida M, Hayasaka S, Yamada T, et al. Ocular findings in Japanese patients with varicella-zoster virus infection. Ophthalmologica 2005; 219:272–275.

Ichthyosis

INTRODUCTION   Ichthyosis represents a heterogeneous group of disorders of skin keratinization. Four major classes of ichthyosis are recognized. The most common type is *ichthyosis vulgaris*, an autosomal dominant disease with onset prior to age five years. Fine, light scales with flexural sparing is present. The eyelids and eyelashes are often involved. In *X-linked ichthyosis* affected males manifest large, dark scales with flexural involvement during the first year of life due to a deficiency of microsomal enzyme cholesterol sulfatase. *Lamellar ichthyosis* is an autosomal recessive condition present at birth. The infant is invested in a thick collodion membrane that is usually shed in 10 to 12 days. Large, thick uniform scales with generalized involvement is characteristic. *Epidermolytic hyperkeratosis*, a rare autosomal dominant disorder, presents at birth with red, moist skin and blisters. Thick scales form within several days. Facial involvement is usually mild. Associated corneal changes include gray stromal opacities, punctate epithelial erosions, gray elevated nodules, and band keratopathy.

CLINICAL PRESENTATION   In lamellar ichthyosis the skin shows, course, yellow scales with raised corners which range is size from fine to large and plate-like. These scales are arranged in a mosaic pattern resembling fish skin and are easily shed. Fine, light to dark thick scales are present on the eyelid skin and at the base of the eyelashes. Alopecia of the scalp and loss of eyelashes is common. Often there is keratinization of the lid margin and palpebral conjunctiva, accompanied by a papillary reaction. With time the skin tightens resulting in ectropion which may be very severe. Corneal exposure with secondary scarring and vascularization is a constant threat.

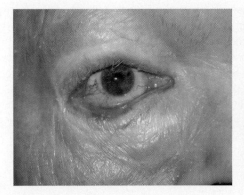 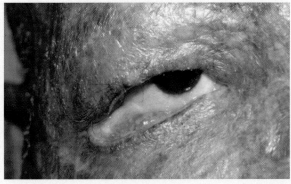

HISTOPATHOLOGY   A moderate degree of hyperkeratosis and a thin or absent granular cell layer are the usual findings in ichthyosis vulgaris. Keratotic follicular plugs may result from extension of hyperkeratosis into hair follicles.

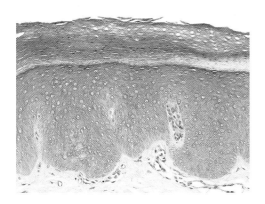

DIFFERENTIAL DIAGNOSIS   Few other disorders give the clinical picture of ichthyosis. Most notably the differential includes psoriasis, exfoliative dermatitis, collodion baby syndrome, harlequin fetus, Refsum's disease, Sjogren-Larsson syndrome, Conradi's disease, KID syndrome, and Trichothiodystrophy.

TREATMENT   When seen in newborn infants care in a neonatal intensive care unit is essential for placement in a high humidity incubator and general hydration, and to monitor for infection. Systemic steroids may be lifesaving in the bullous forms of infantile ichthyosis. In adults steroids and antimetabolites have not been of value. Topical hydration techniques, keratolytic agents, and retinoids are applied to help soften the scales. Newer therapies include alpha hydroxyl acids to reduce itching and treat mild eczemas, topical retinoids to inhibit microcomodo formation and to reduce cohesiveness of follicular epithelial cells, and topical tazarotene (Tazorac) 0.05% gel which is a retinoid prodrug that moduolates epithelial tissue differentiation and proliferation and may also have anti-inflammatory and immunomodulatory properties. Ectropion repair will usually require skin grafts, but it may be difficult to find an adequate donor site. However, the grafts tend to scale and contract often making any surgical gains short-lived. Foreskin may not be involved and may make an acceptable donor site.

REFERENCES

Cruz AA, Menezes FA, Chaves R, et al. Eyelid abnormalities in lamellar ichthyosis. Ophthalmology 2000; 107:1895–1898.

Hosal BM, Abbasogglu OE, Gursel E. Surgical treatment of cicatricial ectropion in lamellar Ichthyosis. Orbit 1999; 19:37–40.

Jay B, Blach R, Wells RS. Ocular manifestations of ichthyosis. Br J Ophthalmol 1968; 52:217–226.

Messmer EM, Kenyon KR, Rittinger O, Janecke AR, Kampik A. Ocular manifestations of keratitis-ichthyosis-deafness (KID) syndrome. Ophthalmology 2005; 112:1–6.

Peled I, Bar-Lev A, Wexler MR. Surgical correction of ectropion in lamellar Ichthyosis. Ann Plast Surg 1982; 8:429–431.

Rose HM. Lid changes in non-bullous ichthyosiform erythemoderma. Br J Ophthalmol 1971; 55:750–752.

Sever R, Frost P, Weinstein G. Eye findings in ichthyosis. JAMA 1968; 206:2283–2286.

Singh AJ, Atkinson PL. Ocular manifestations of congenital Ichthyosis. Eur J Ophthalmol 2005; 15:118–122.

Uthoff D, Gorney M, Teichmann C. Cicatricial ectropion in ichthyosis: a novel approach to treatment. Ophthal Plast Reconstr Surg 1994; 10:92–95.

Impetigo

INTRODUCTION   Impetigo represents a superficial invasion of the skin by pathogenic streptococci, staphylococci, or sometimes a mixture of both. Infections tend to occur in areas of previously compromised or diseased skin, such as skin affected by dermatitis, especially eczema, or in a recently lasered resurfaced skin. Owing to the superficial location there is rarely any systemic reaction of consequence. However, in rare instances the bacterial infection may result in the formation of antigen-antibody complexes that can lead to a life-threatening nephritis.

CLINICAL PRESENTATION   Impetigo can begin in either a bullous or vesicular form, with both types eventuating in pustule formation and then in ulceration. Invasion of the superficial regions of the skin by pathogenic streptococci or staphylococci produces small erythematous macules followed by dissolution of the basal epithelial layers and the formation of superficial vesicles or bullae ranging from 2 to 20 mm in diameter and surrounded by a narrow halo of erythema. These soon become pustules that, upon rupturing, spread the infection to new areas. A tan crust made of dried blood and cellular debris forms over the lesion. Most lesions will heal without scarring; however, when

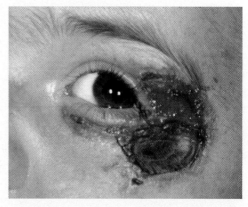

deeper involvement occurs (ecthyma), it can result in cicatrix formation and lid deformity. Conjunctivitis or keratitis may occur which may lead to ankyloblepharon or corneal scarring.

HISTOPATHOLOGY   Common impetigo has subcorneal accumulation of neutrophils and gram-positive cocci, and a few acantholytic cells may be present. Neutrophils often extend through the epidermis into the underlying dermis. As the lesions age, there is a surface crust of serum, neutrophils undergoing degeneration, and parakeratosis (shown on right). In bullous impetigo, the subcorneal bullae contain neutrophils, gram-positive cocci, and a few acantholytic cells, and the papillary dermis has a mild to moderate mixed acute and chronic inflammatory infiltrate.

DIFFERENTIAL DIAGNOSIS   Fungal infections as well as viral eruptions such as herpes zoster and varicella zoster may be mistaken for impetigo.

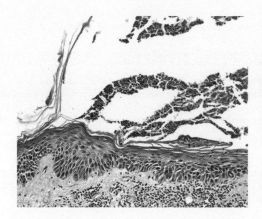
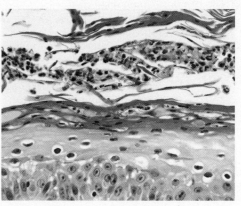

TREATMENT   The diagnosis, suspected from the clinical appearance, can be confirmed on culture, which will virtually always show a combination of streptococci and staphylococci. On rare occasions other organisms, including gram-negative varieties, will be recovered. Mild cases can sometimes be managed with local skin hygiene alone. Antibiotic therapy is governed by culture and sensitivity results. Topical therapy is helpful but of limited value owing to pharyngeal colonization and wide dissemination of organisms. For deeper lesions, systemic antibiotics are indicated in the form of a semisynthetic penicillin or erythromycin. In severe cases dicloxacillin or a cephalosporin may be needed.

REFERENCES

Albert S, Baldwin R, Czeckajewski S, et al. Bullous impetigo due to group II Staphylococcus aureus. An epidemic in a normal newborn nursery. Am J Dis Child 1970; 120:10–13.

Dajani AS, Ferrieri P, Wannamaker L. Endemic superficial pyoderma in children. Arc Dermatol 1973; 108:517–522.

Duke-Elder S. System of Ophthalmology. Vol. 13. St. Louis: Mosby, 1974:91.

Esterly NB, Markowitz M. The treatment of pyoderma in children. JAMA 1970; 212:1667–1670.

Elias PM, Levy SW. Bullous impetigo. Occurrence of localized scalded skin syndrome in an adult. Arch Dermatol 1976; 112:856–858.

Ferrieri P, Dajani AS, Wannamaker LW, Chapman SS. Natural history of impetigo. J Clin Invest 1972; 51:2851–2852.

Hughes WT, Wan RT. Impetigo contagiosa: Etiology, complications and comparison on erythromycin and antibiotic ointment. Am J Dis Child 1967; 113:449–453.

Lissauer TJ, Sanderson PJ, Valman HB. The re-emergence of bullous impetigo. Br Med J 1981; 283:1509–1510.

Rasmussen JE, Maibach HI. Impetigo and other pyodermas. In: Dermis D, ed. Clinical Dermatology. Vol. 3. Philadelphia: Harper & Row, Unit 16–4.

Insect Bite

INTRODUCTION   Insect bites or stings result in the introduction of venom or toxins into the skin, which in turn cause the release of vasoactive amines. This results in marked swelling and erythema of the thin tissues of the eyelid. Unless secondary infection occurs, these reactions tend to resolve rapidly. *Dermatitis nodosa* is a specific type of insult due to barbed cilia acquired from caterpillar contact. The barbs result in the cilia working their way into the skin where they set up a prolonged, sometimes severe inflammatory irritation. If the caterpillar hairs get into the eye, they cause a severe, painful reaction and can lead to later ocular sequelae from intractable inflammation (*ophthalmia nodosa*).

CLINICAL PRESENTATION   Insect insults result in localized eyelid inflammation with redness and swelling. Pain and pruritis can be intense. A minute skin defect at the site of insult may be present. Abscess formation may result due to secondary infection, localized tissue necrosis, or as a reaction to retained stinger or mouthpart. Severe hypersensitivity reactions with hemorrhagic bullae, chills, and fever several hours after the sting or bite may be seen. In rare cases an insect bite can lead to cellulitis and even necrotizing fasciitis. Rarely a toxic shock like syndrome can result with vomiting, fever, and circulatory collapse. Bee stings to the eye have been reported to result in demyelinating optic neuritis and blepharochalasis with recurrent episodes of eyelid edema. *Dermatitis nodosa* presents as one or more localized inflamed and tender nodules.

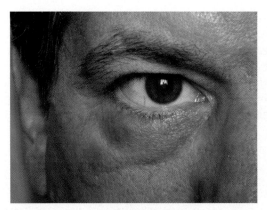

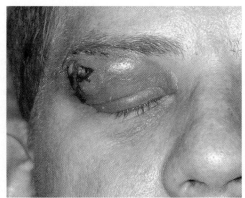

(Courtesy of Robert A. Goldberg, M.D.)   *(Courtesy of Charles S. Soparkar, M.D.)*

HISTOPATHOLOGY   The histopathological reaction to insect bites differs widely, as would be expected by the varied clinical responses. The usual reaction to an arthropod bite, such as from a mosquito, is a mixed inflammatory infiltrate containing lymphocytes, macrophages, eosinophils, and sometimes neutrophils. Variable degrees of spongiosis and dermal edema also are present. The histopathological findings in insect bites are non-specific and require clinical-pathological correlation.

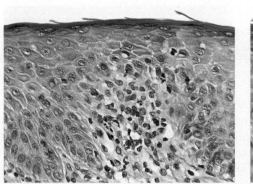

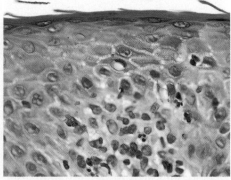

DIFFERENTIAL DIAGNOSIS   An insect bite or sting may mimic preseptal cellulitis, chalazion, orbital cellulitis, or allergic or contact dermatitis, a localized abscess nodule or ruptured inclusion cyst.

TREATMENT   If any part of the insect is left at the site of attack it should be carefully removed. Although cold compresses are usually recommended some types of venom are actually deactivated by heat. In severe cases antihistamines are sometimes useful in minimizing the reaction. Systemic anaphylaxis developing in sensitized individuals requires prompt recognition and treatment. Recent observations indicate that Dapsone (4,4'-diaminodiphenlysulfone) can be useful in reducing severe necrotizing inflammation, such as that occurring after brown recluse spider bits, and thereby reduce subsequent scarring and deformity. Antipruritics, analgesics, and in select cases steroids may be needed.

REFERENCES

Allington HV, Allington RR. Insect bites. JAMA 1954; 155:240–247.

Barnard JH. Cutaneous responses to insects, types, and mechanism of reactions. JAMA 1966; 196:159–162.

Duke-Elder S. System of Ophthalmology, Vol. 13. St. Louis: Mosby, 1974:201.

Fan PC, Chang HN. Hypersensitivity to mosquito bite: a case report. Gaoxiong Yi Xue Ke Za Zhi 1995; 11:420–424.

Finney JL, Peterson HD. Blepharochalasis after a bee sting. Plast Reconstr Surg 1984; 73:830–832.

Poitelea C, Wearne MJ. Periocular necrotizing fasciitis—a case report. Orbit 2005; 24:215–217.

Song HS, Wray SH. Bee sting optic neuritis. A case report with visual evoked potentials. J Clin Neuroophthalmol 1991; 11:45–49.

Thakur CP. The syndrome of ptosis, generalized muscular weakness and marked fasciculations of calf muscles due to insect bite. J Indian Med Assoc 1965; 45:503–504.

Intravascular Papillary Endothelial Hyperplasia

INTRODUCTION   Intravascular papillary endothelial hyperplasia (IPEH) is an unusual benign vascular lesion of proliferating endothelial cells in response to thrombus formation. It is most frequently seen in the extremities, but it can occur in other parts of the body as well. It can appear as a primary lesion developing within the lumen of a distended vessel, or it can be associated with other vascular lesions such as hemangioma, pyogenic granuloma, or lymphangioma. Lesions are typically associated with a thrombus in varying stages of development. IPEH clinically and histologically resembles soft-tissue angiosarcomas with which they are most often confused.

CLINICAL PRESENTATION   IPEH is usually seen in middle-aged adults and presents as a bluish or purple mass within the skin or subcutaneous tissues. It is confined to the intraluminal space of either an artery or vein, and the walls of the vessel form the "capsule" of the mass. This lesion is not associated with systemic or local disease. As the lesion enlarges it can compress adjacent soft tissues resulting in ptosis, ectropion or other eyelid malpositions. It can occur deep in the orbit where it can involve the ophthalmic artery and other orbital vessels.

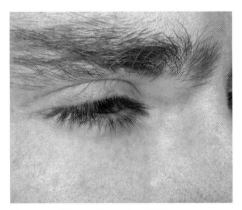

(Courtesy of Tamara Fountain, M.D.)

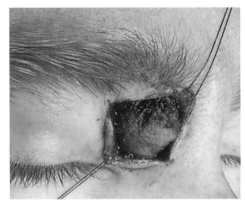

(Courtesy of Tamara Fountain, M.D.)

HISTOPATHOLOGY   This lesion lies within a blood vessel of the dermis or subcutis. It is composed of numerous, small, eosinophilic papillae covered by a layer of endothelial cells that are often flattened. The endothelial cells lack cytological atypia and mitotic activity. Thrombus is often adjacent to the lesion and is commonly in varying stages of organization.

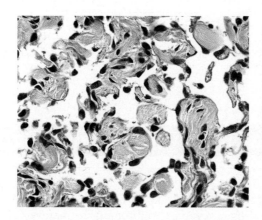 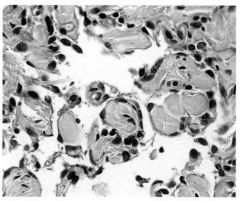

DIFFERENTIAL DIAGNOSIS   The most important lesion in the differential diagnosis is angiosarcoma from which it must be distinguished. Other similar lesions include pyogenic granuloma, hemangioma, intravascular fasciitis, and organized thrombus.

TREATMENT   Biopsy is often required for diagnosis. Management is surgical by opening the vessels and removing the mass. For lesions in areas that are not readily accessible surgically, like the deep orbit, radiosurgery has proven effective.

REFERENCES

Barras C, Olver JM, Cole C, Seet JE. Intravascular papillary endothelial hyperplasia (IPEH) mimicking a lacrimal sac mass. Eye 2001; 15:685–687.

Cagli S, Oktar N, Dalbasti T, et al. Intravascular papillary endothelial hyperplasia of the central nervous system—four case reports. Neurol Med Chir 2004; 44:302–310.

Font RL, Wheeler TM, Boniuk M. Intravascular papillary endothelial hyperplasia of the orbit and ocular adnexa. A report of five cases. Arch Ophthalmol 1983; 101:1731–1736.

Ohshima T, Ogura K, Nakayashiki N, Tachibana E. Intravascular papillary endothelial hyperplasia at the superior orbital f issure: report of a case successfully treated with gamma knife radiosurgery. Surg Neurol 2005; 64:266–269.

Patt S, Kaden B, Stoltenburg-Didinger G. Intravascular papillary endothelial hyperplasia at the fissure orbitalis superior: a case report. Clin Neuropathol 1992; 11:128–130.

Shields JA, Shields CL, Eagle RC Jr, Diniz W. Intravascular papillary endothelial hyperplasia with presumed bilateral orbital varices. Arch Ophthalmol 1999; 117:1247–1249.

Sorenson RL, Spencer WH, Stewart WB, Miller WW, Kleinhenz RJ. Intravascular papillary endothelial hyperplasia of the eyelid. Arch Ophthalmol 1983; 101:1728–1730.

Truong L, Font RL. Intravascular papillary endothelial hyperplasia of the ocular adnexa. Report of two cases and review of the literature. Arch Ophthalmol 1985; 103:1364–1367.

Weber FL, Babel J. Intravascular papillary endothelial hyperplasia of the orbit. Br J Ophthalmol 1981; 65:18–22.

Werner MS, Hornblass A, Reifler DM, Dresner SC, Harrison W. Intravascular papillary endothelial hyperplasia: collection of four cases and a review of the literature. Ophthal Plast Reconstr Surg 1997; 13:48–56.

INTRODUCTION   Pyogenic granuloma, also known as lobular capillary hemangioma, is a benign vascular tumor. The intravascular variant is an angiomatous proliferation that occurs within a blood vessel sometimes associated with an underlying arteriovenous malformation or hemangioma. The lesion is a polypoid mass projecting into the lumen of a dilated vein.

CLINICAL PRESENTATION   Intravascular pyogenic granuloma occurs within a vein such as the angular vein. It presents as a slowly enlarging deep firm nontender mass. There are no epithelial changes or erythema. The lesion is mobile and can be elongated and tubular to palpation.

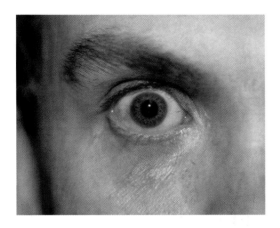

HISTOPATHOLOGY   This lesion occurs in veins and represents the intravenous analog of pyogenic granuloma of the skin or conjunctiva. There is a proliferation of blood vessels within the vessel lumen, and sometimes a stalk connecting the lesion to the vein wall can be identified. On other occasions, the lesion appears to be floating within the vessel lumen or it may completely occlude the lumen. In addition to the endothelial cells, smooth muscle cells can be demonstrated immunohisto-chemically within the tumor and are presumed to represent residua of the vein wall.

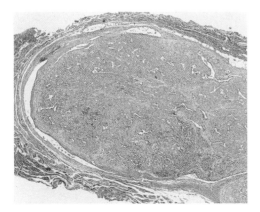
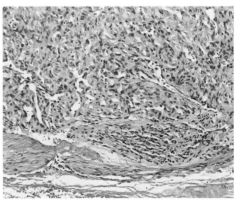

DIFFERENTIAL DIAGNOSIS   The differential diagnosis includes lesions such as intravascular papillary endothelial hyperplasia, pyogenic granuloma, angiosacoma, hemangioma, Kaposi's sarcoma, and organized thrombus.

TREATMENT Treatment is often required for diagnosis. Removal is accomplished by opening the vein with removal of the mass which shells out easily.

REFERENCES

Hung CH, Kuo HW, Chiu YK, Huang PH. Intravascular pyogenic granuloma arising in an acquired arteriovenous malformation: report of a case and review of the literature. Dermatol Surg 2004; 30:1050–1053.

Inaloz HS, Patel G, Knight AG. Recurrent intravascular papillary endothelial hyperplasia developing from a pyogenic granuloma. J Eur Acad Dermatol Venereol 2001; 15:156–158.

Truong L, Font RL. Intravascular pyogenic granuloma of the ocular adnexa. Report of two cases and review of the literature. Arch Ophthalmol 1985; 103:1364–1367.

Ulbright TM, Santa Cruz DJ. Intravascular pyogenic granuloma: case report with ultrastructural findings. Cancer 1980; 45:1646–1652.

Inverted Follicular Keratosis

INTRODUCTION Inverted follicular keratosis is a benign skin lesion that is common on the face and less frequently on the eyelids. It occurs in older individuals from the fifth decade on, and is considerably more common in males. It is frequently mistaken for a malignant tumor. These lesions arise from the infundibular epithelium of the hair follicle and therefore are related to epidermoid cysts. Inverted follicular keratosis may be an irritated form of seborrheic keratosis or verruca vulgaris.

CLINICAL PRESENTATION Inverted follicular keratosis presents as a small, solitary, well-demarcated, hyperkeratotic or wart-like keratotic mass most commonly on the upper eyelid and cheek, Rarely, it may be pigmented simulating a melanocytic tumor. This lesion may show scaling and exophytic projections presenting as a cutaneous horn. The lesion typically appears weeks to months before presentation, but sometimes may be present for many decades. Inverted follicular keratosis shows a growth pattern with epidermis extending over the base and sides of the lesion and then taking an abrupt inverted or downward turn towards the central epithelial mass.

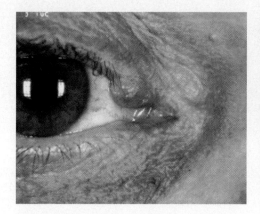
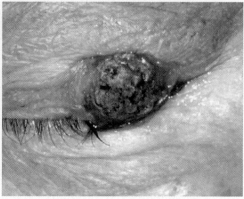

HISTOPATHOLOGY   This lesion resembles seborrheic keratosis except that the proliferating epidermis protrudes into the dermis instead of being exophytic. It is often classified as a subtype of seborrheic keratosis, distinguished by its endophytic growth and the presence of whorls of maturing squamous epithelial cells ("squamous eddies," illustrated on p. 47). There are variable numbers of horn cysts, and there may be an intense infiltrate of chronic inflammatory cells, as seen in the photomicrograph on the left.

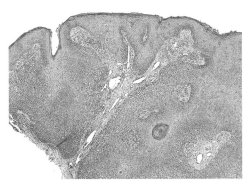 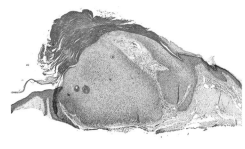

DIFFERENTIAL DIAGNOSIS   The differential diagnosis includes verruca vulgaris, papilloma, senile keratosis, seborrheic keratosis, cutaneous horn, keratoacanthoma, and squamous cell carcinoma.

TREATMENT   Complete surgical excision is recommended, as recurrences are common with incomplete removal.

REFERENCES

Azzopardi JG, Laurini R. Inverted follicular keratosis. J Clin Pathol 1975; 28:465–471.

Boniuk M, Zimmerman L. Eyelid tumors confused with squamous cell carcinoma, II: inverted follicular keratosis. Arch Ophthalmol 1963; 69:698–707.

Lever WF. Inverted follicular keratosis is an irritated seborrheic keratosis. Am J Dermatopathol 1983; 5:474.

Mehregan AH. Inverted follicular keratosis is a distinct follicular tumor. Am J Dermatopathol 1983; 5:467–470.

Sassani JW, Yanoff M. Inverted follicular keratosis. Am J Ophthalmol 1979; 87:810–813.

Schweitzer JG, Yanoff M. Inverted follicular keratosis. Ophthalmology 1987; 94:1465–1468.

Sim-Davis D, Marks R, Wilson-Jones E. Inverted follicular keratosis: surprising variant of seborrheic wart. Acta Dermatol Venereol (Stockh) 1976; 56:337–344.

Yanoff M. Most inverted follicular keratoses are probably verrucal vugares. Am J Dermatopathol 1983; 5:475.

Juvenile Xanthogranuloma

INTRODUCTION   Juvenile xanthogranuloma (JXG) is a rare systemic childhood disease of non-Langerhans cell histiocytes. It is characterized by cutaneous and, on occasion, intraocular lesions. It may be a granulomatous reaction of histiocytes to an unidentified stimulus. There is special predilection for skin and eye involvement. It affects children below the age of five years with 85% of the cases being under one year of age. Most patients are younger than two years of age at presentation. There is no sexual or racial predilection. Other sites of ocular involvement include the orbit, conjunctiva, cornea, episclera, iris, and ciliary body. Iris lesions are associated with spontaneous hyphema, unilateral glaucoma, uveitis, and heterochromia iridis. Although lesions are common on the face and neck, they may also occur on the trunk or extremities. Visceral involvement is rare, however, with a predilection for lung, spleen, testis, pericardium and gastrointestinal tract.

CLINICAL PRESENTATION   The eyelid is the most frequent site of ocular involvement. Lesions on the lid often appear quite suddenly. They typically present as a rapidly growing solitary papular or nodular lesion with a rubbery or cartilaginous consistency, varying in size from few millimeters to 1.5 cm. The lesions are typically yellow in color, frequently with an orange overtone. With time they may enlarge and become yellow-brown. New lesions can arise within a few months of the appearance of the first lesion, near or distant to the primary site. The lesions may resolve spontaneously within months or a few years, leaving a slightly atrophic area that may be hyper or hypopigmented. Very large lesions may show ulceration and crusting. Intraocular lesions can be associated with glaucoma and even blindness.

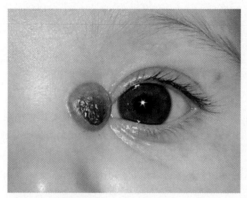
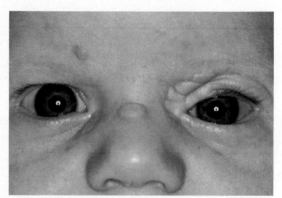

(Courtesy of Morris Hartstein, M.D.)   *(Courtesy of David Lyon, M.D.)*

HISTOPATHOLOGY   Lipid-laden macrophages (foam cells) and Touton giant cells are the distinguishing features of xanthogranulomas. The Touton giant cells have multiple nuclei forming a circle near the middle of the cell surrounding a core of brightly eosinophilic cytoplasm. The cytoplasm around the outside of the nuclei is vacuolated and clear or palely eosinophilic. Lymphocytes, plasma cells, and occasional eosinophils are scattered among the foam cells and Touton giant cells.

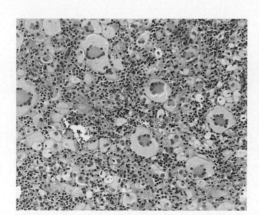
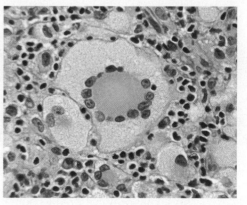

DIFFERENTIAL DIAGNOSIS   Xanthomas or xanthelasmas, syringoma, and molluscum contagiosum most commonly mimic eyelid involvement of JXG.

TREATMENT   Surgical biopsy may be necessary to establish the diagnosis. Treatment of juvenile xanthogranuloma should be tailored to the individual case. The majority of lesions are asymptomatic, and may sometimes resolve spontaneously. For isolated skin lesions limited to the eyelid or the epibulblar tissue, observation alone may be appropriate. Skin lesions may be removed surgically for improved cosmesis. For intraocular lesions subconjunctival or systemic corticosteroid therapy, irradiation, and surgery have been reported to give a good response. With systemic visceral involvement, chemotherapy is indicated.

REFERENCES

Cadera W, Silver MM, Burt L. Juvenile xanthogranuloma. Can J Ophthalmol 1983; 4:169–174.

Chalfin S, Lloyd WC. Juvenile xanthogranuloma of the eyelid in an adult. Arch Ophthalmol 1998; 116:1546–1547.

Hamdani M, El Kettani A, Rais L, et al. Juvenile xanthogranuloma with intraocular involvement. A case report. J Fr Ophtalmol 2000; 23:817–820.

Harley RD, Romayananda N, Chan GH. Juvenile xanthogranuloma. J Pediatr Ophthalmol Strabismus 1982; 19:33–39.

Nakatani T, Morimoto A, Kato R, et al. Successful treatment of congenital systemic juvenile xanthogranuloma with Langerhans cell histiocytosis-based chemotherapy. J Pediatr Hematol Oncol 2004; 26:371–374.

Nasour AM, Traboulsi E, Frangieh G. Multiple Recurrences of juvenile xanthogranuloma of the eyelid. J Pediatr Ophthalmol Strabismus 1985; 22:156–157.

Schwartz TL, Carter KD, Judisch GF, Nerad JA, Folberg R. Congenital marcronodular juvenile xanthogranuloma of the eyelid. Ophthalmology 1991; 98:1230–1233.

Kaposi's Sarcoma

INTRODUCTION   Kaposi's sarcoma is a vascular tumor that has been reported to affect up to 25% of patients with AIDS. Up to 20% of AIDS related Kaposi's sarcoma involves the conjunctiva or eyelid. In addition to HIV, Kaposi's sarcoma has been observed in three other clinical settings; the "classic" or European type more prevalent among elderly men of Mediterranean or Eastern European Jewish origin; the lymphadenopathic or visceral form, more prevalent in individuals of African origin; and the form associated with exogenous immunosuppression. Some authors have theorized that this lesion may have a viral etiology.

CLINICAL PRESENTATION   Kaposi's sarcoma usually presents as a red to brown macule that enlarges to become a more elevated, highly vascular, purple or red nodule on the cutaneous aspect of the

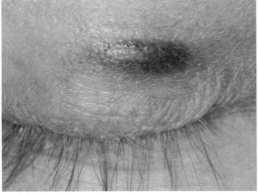
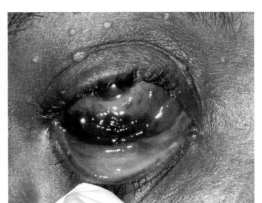

(Courtesy of Richard S. Smith, M.D.)

eyelids, the caruncle, or on the conjunctiva. Rarely, it may involve the lacrimal sac and orbit. In milder cases, skin lesions often wax and wane, with some regressing completely, leaving atrophic, pigmented scars.

HISTOPATHOLOGY   The patch stage of Kaposi's sarcoma has a proliferation of irregular, often jagged, vascular channels within the dermis. The vessels are thin walled, lined by plump or inconspicuous endothelial cells, some have perivascular lymphocytes and plasma cells, and there may be extravasated erythrocytes and hemosiderin deposits. The plaque and nodular stages of Kaposi's sarcoma have interlacing bundles of spindle cells and poorly defined, slit-like vessels within the dermis. Chronic inflammatory cells are present focally, and there are extravasated erythrocytes and deposits of hemosiderin. Small, eosinophilic hyaline globules may be intracellular or extracellular and provide a clue to the diagnosis; the globules are positive using periodic acid-Schiff (PAS) stain and they are bright red with Masson's trichrome stain.

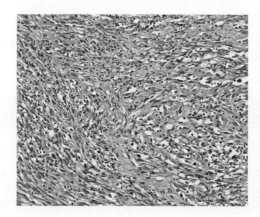 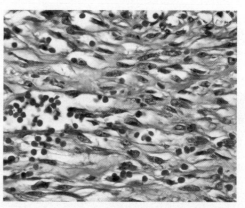

DIFFERENTIAL DIAGNOSIS   Lesions that may mimic a Kaposi's sarcoma include pyogenic granuloma, hemangiopericytoma, angiosarcoma, glomus tumor, lymphoma, metastatic tumor, cavernous hemangioma, chalazion, foreign body granuloma, and conjunctival hemorrhage.

TREATMENT   The goal of therapy is to relieve ocular irritation, mass effect, and disfigurement. Accepted treatment options include surgical excision, cryotherapy, irradiation, chemotherapy, and immunotherapy such as intralesional injection with interferon alpha-2a. For patients receiving chemotherapy or for whom chemotherapy is planned for systemic Kaposi's sarcoma, local treatment often proves unnecessary. Although therapy may reduce or clear the visible lesions, it is not curative. Low dose radiotherapy in the range of 2000 to 3000 cGy can be effective for localized lesions.

REFERENCES

Alexander C. Kaposi's sarcoma with ocular manifestations. Am J Ophthalmol 1963; 55:625.
Bookstead JH, Wood GS, Gletcher V. Evidence for the origin of Kaposi's sarcoma from lymphatic endothelium.
    Am J Pathol 1985; 119:292–300.
Brun SC, Jakobiec FA. Kaposi's sarcoma of the ocular adnexa. Int Ophthalmol Clin 1997; 37:25–38.

Dugel PU, Gill PS, Frangieh GT, Roa NA. Treatment of ocular adnexal Kaposi's sarcoma in acquired immunodeficiency syndrome. Ophthalmology 1992; 99:1127–1132.

Friedman-Kien AE, Saltzman BR. Clinical manifestations of classical, endemic African and epidemic AIDS-associated Kaposi's sarcoma. J Am Acad Dermatol 1990; 22:1237–1250.

Holecek MJ, Harwood AR. Radiotherapy of Kaposi's syndrome. Cancer 1978; 41:1733–1738.

Kalinske M, Leone CR. Kaposi's sarcoma involving eyelid and conjunctiva. Ann Ophthalmol 1982;14:497–499.

Munteanu G, Munteanu M, Giuri S. Conjunctival-palpebral Kaposi's Angiosarcoma: report of a case. J Fr Ophtalmol 2003; 26:1059–1062.

Pang C, Kong L. Kaposi's sarcoma of eyelid and conjunctiva. Zhonghua Yan Ke Za Zhi 1999; 35:262–264.

Shields JA, DePotter P, Shields CL, Komarnicky LT. Kaposi's sarcoma of the eyelids: response to radiotherapy. Arch Ophthalmol 1992; 110:1689.

Shuler JD, Holland GN, Miles SA, et al. Kaposi sarcoma of the conjunctiva and eyelids associated with the acquired immunodeficiency syndrome. Arch Ophthlamol 1989; 107:858–862.

Soll DB, Redovan EG. Kaposi's sarcoma of the eyelid as the initial manifestation of AIDS. Ophthal Plast Reconstr Surg 1989; 5:49–51.

Keloid

INTRODUCTION Keloids represent exuberant scar formation resulting from proliferation of dermal tissue following skin injury. Mechanisms for keloid formation represent abnormal wound healing and include alterations in growth factors, collagen turnover, tension alignment, and genetic and immunologic contributions. Keloids differ from hypertrophic scars in that they spread beyond the initial site of injury. Because they tend to be invasive into the surrounding normal skin both clinically and histologically, with prolongation of the proliferative phase of wound repair they have been described as "incomplete tumors." Although any body area can be affected, keloids commonly develop on the face, neck, chest, shoulders, and back. Keloids on the eyelid skin are relatively rare, even in patients who are prone to keloid formation. These scars tend to occur with greater frequency in patients with darker skin tones, but patients of any skin type can develop this exuberant clinical response.

CLINICAL PRESENTATION Keloids are generally painless proliferations of dermal collagen that appear as red or purple, raised, firm nodules which grow beyond the margins of the original sites of injury. There texture is shiny, with minimal to no epithelial markings.

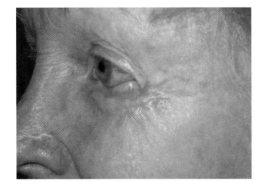 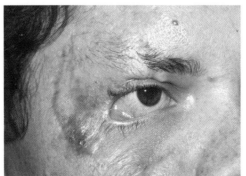

HISTOPATHOLOGY Mature keloids are composed of haphazardly arranged, broad, brightly eosinophilic, glassy, collagen bundles. The collagen bundles tend to form variably sized nodules. Fibroblasts are along the collagen bundles, but the overall cellularity is reduced compared to other scars due to the space occupied by the broad collagen bundles. Early keloids have greater cellularity, abundant fibrillary collagen, and fewer of the thick collagen bundles.

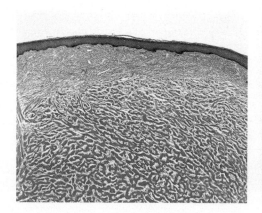 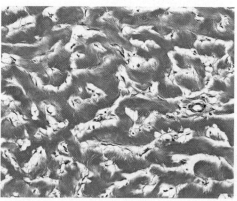

DIFFERENTIAL DIAGNOSIS Keloids are most commonly confused with hypertrophic scars.

TREATMENT The treatment of keloid can be very difficult. Traditionally keloids have been dermabraded, chemically peeled, excised, irradiated, and injected with corticosteroids. Cryotherapy has been reported to be effective in reducing the size of the scar. Although CO_2 laser resurfacing may not be suitable in darker skin types, and in fact may promote further keloid formation, the 585-nm pulsed dye laser may be helpful in eradicating these lesions. Newer treatment modalities include injections of interferon and 5-fluorouracil. Silicone gel sheeting may reduce the incidence and degree of scarring by modulating expression of basic fibroblast growth factor.

REFERENCES

Al-Attar A, Mess S, Thomassen JM, Kauffman CL, Davison SP. Keloid pathogenesis and treatment. Plast Reconstr Surg 2006; 117:286–300.

Atiyeh BS, Costagliola M, Hayek SN. Keloid or hypertrophic scar: the controversy: review of the literature. Ann Plast Surg 2005; 54:676–680.

Chen MA, Davidson TM. Scar management: prevention and treatment strategies. Curr Opin Otolaryngol Head Neck Surg 2005; 13:242–247.

Hanasono MM, Lum J, Carroll LA, Mikulec AA, Koch RJ. The effect of silicone gel on basic fibroblast growth factor levels in fibroblast cell culture. Arch Facial Plast Surg 2004; 6:88–93.

Marneros AG, Krieg T. Keloids—clinical diagnosis, pathogenesis, and treatment options. J Dtsch Dermatol Ges 2004; 2:905–913.

Meshkinpour A, Ghasri P, Pope K, et al. Treatment of hypertrophic scars and keloids with a radiofrequency device: A study of collagen effects. Lasers Surg Med 2005; 37:343–349.

O'Brien L, Pandit A. Silicone gel sheeting for preventing and treating hypertrophic and keloid scars. Cochrane Database Syst Rev 2006; CD003826.

Poochareon VN, Berman B. New therapies for the management of keloids. J Craniofac Surg 2003; 14:654–657.

Ragoowansi R, Cornes PG, Moss AL, Glees JP. Treatment of keloids by surgical excision and immediate postoperative single-fraction radiotherapy. Plast Reconstr Surg 2003; 111:1853–1859.

Tanzi EL, Alster TS. Laser treatment of scars. Skin Therapy Lett 2004; 9:4–7.

Thompson LD. Skin Keloid. Ear Nose Throat 2004; 83:519.

INTRODUCTION   Keratoacanthoma is a relatively common squamoproliferative neoplasm that occurs on sun-exposed areas of adults, the incidence increasing with advancing years. Males outnumber females by a ratio of 2:1. It resembles squamous cell carcinoma both clinically and pathologically, and in 15% to 17% of cases squamous cell carcinoma is misdiagnosed as keratoacanthoma. Some authors have argued that keratoacanthoma should be classified as a variant of well-differentiated squamous cell carcinoma. However, the two lesions have been shown to be distinct on immuno-histochemical grounds. Although multiple, aggressive and giant varieties have been described, most are solitary and self-limited. The lesion may also occur as part of Muir-Torre syndrome (skin lesion associated with an internal malignancy). The etiology is unknown but sunlight, trauma, chemical carcinogens, UVB exposure, and immunocompromised status have been implicated as etiologic factors.

CLINICAL PRESENTATION   The classic lesion appears spontaneously as a small flesh-colored papule that evolves very rapidly over three to six weeks to a 0.5 to 2.5 cm dome-shaped violaceous or brownish nodule. The nodule is usually umbilicated with a distinctive central crater filled with a keratin plug. The edges of the crater may have elevated rolled margins. Lesions have a predilection for the lower eyelid where more than half are located. It typically undergoes spontaneous involution within four to six months to leave an atrophic scar. Lesions that occur on the eyelids may produce ectropion or ptosis, and occasionally may cause destructive changes.

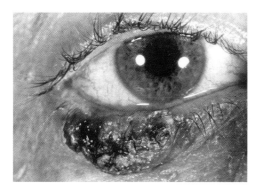 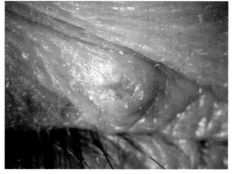

HISTOPATHOLOGY   Keratoacanthomas have a proliferation of well-differentiated, keratinizing squamous epithelium at the sides and bottom of the lesion, with a central keratin-filled crater that enlarges as the lesion matures. A key diagnostic feature is a lip of epidermis (collarette) overlapping the central crater. The lesion usually has a relatively even lower border that remains superficial to

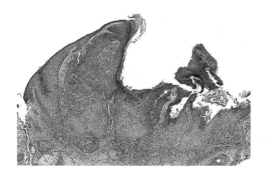

the sweat glands. The adjacent dermis contains a mixture of lymphocytes, macrophages, plasma cells, neutrophils, and varying numbers of eosinophils. Keratoacanthomas lack marked epithelial dysplasia, abnormal mitotic figures, and a marked desmoplastic reaction in the stroma, helping to distinguish them from squamous cell carcinomas.

DIFFERENTIAL DIAGNOSIS   The differential diagnosis includes squamous cell carcinoma, basal cell carcinoma, verruca vulgaris, molluscum contagiosum, and seborrheic keratosis.

TREATMENT   In the past treatment of keratoacanthoma has typically been conservative. However, because of its sometimes aggressive behavior and uncertain relationship to squamous cell carcinoma complete surgical excision is now considered the treatment of choice. In a recent study 16% of lesions clinically diagnosed as keratoacanthoma proved to be invasive squamous cell carcinoma on biopsy. Surgical excision, besides providing definitive treatment also confirms diagnosis, speeds recovery, and limits scarring. Complete excision is recommended under frozen section control or Mohs surgery since invasive variants exist with the potential for perineural and intramuscular spread. When surgery is not possible cryotherapy, radiotherapy, and chemotherapy have been effective. Both intralesional injections and topical 5-fluorouracil (5-FU) have been advocated. Intralesional methotrexate has also been used with complete resolution of the lesion after three weeks.

REFERENCES

Bergin DJ, Lamins NA, Deffer TA. Intralesional 5-fluorouracil for keratoacanthoma of the eyelid. Ophthal Plast Reconstr Surg 1986; 2:201–204.

Boniuk M, Zimmerman L. Eyelid tumors confused with squamous carcinoma, III: Keratoacanthoma. Arch Ophthalmol 1967; 77:29–40.

Boyton JR, Searl SS, Caldwell EH. Large periocular keratoacanthoma: The case for definitive treatment. Ophthalmic Surg. 1986; 17:565–569.

Burge K, Winklemann R. Keratoacanthoma associated with basal and squamous cell carcinoma. Arch Dermatol 1969; 100:306–311.

Cohen PR, Schults KE, Teller CF, Nelson BR. Intralesional methotrexate for keratoacanthoma of the nose. Skinmed 2005; 4:393–395.

Craddock KJ, Rao J, Lauzon GJ, Tron VA. Multiple keratoacanthomas arising post-UVB therapy. J Cutan Med Surg 2004; 8:239–243.

Donaldson MJ, Sullivan TJ, Whitehead KJ, Williamsom RM. Periocular keratoacanthoma: clinical features, pathology, and management. Ophthalmology 2003; 110:1403–1407.

Farina AT, Leider M, Newall J, Carella R. Radiotherapy for aggressive and destructive keratoacanthomas. J Dermatol Surg Oncol 1977; 3:177–180.

Grossniklaus HE, Wojno TH, Yanoff M, Font RL. Invasive keratoacanthoma of the eyelid and ocular adnexal. Ophthalmology 1996; 103:937–941.

Hamou S, Hochart G, Jouredel D, et al. Giant keratoacanthoma of the eyelid. J Fr Ophtalmol 2005; 28:1115–1119.

Iverson R, Vistnes L. Keratoacanthoma is frequently a dangerous diagnosis. Am J Surg 1973; 126:359.

Leibovitch I, Huilgol SC, James CL, et al. Periocular keratoacanthoma: can we always rely on the clinical diagnosis? Br J Ophthalmol 2005; 89:1201–1204.

Melton JL, Nelson BR, Stough DB, et al. Treatment of keratoacanthoma with intralesional methotrexate. J Am Acad Dermatol 1991; 25:1017–1023.

Requena L, Romero E, Sanchez M, Ambrojo P, Sanchex Yus E. Aggressive keratoacanthoma of the eyelid: malignant keratoacanthoma or squamous cell carcinoma? J Dermatol Surg Oncol 1990; 16:564–568.

Slater M, Barden JA. Differentiating keratoacanthoma from squamous cell carcinoma by the use of apoptotic and cell adhesion markers. Histopathology 2005; 47:170–178.

Tay E, Schofield JB, Rowell NP, Jones CA. Ophthalmic presentation of the Muir Torre syndrome. Ophthal Plast Reconstr Surg 2003; 19:402–404.

INTRODUCTION   Also known as *Hutchinson's melanotic freckle* or *precancerous melanosis*, lentigo maligna is a pigmented patch most often found on the sun-exposed forehead or malar areas and may involve the lower eyelid and canthal areas. It represents 4% to 5% of all cutaneous melanomas. Lentigo maligna arises from the benign lentigo senilis (solar lentigo), and represents a premalignant in situ stage of what later can become invasive lentigo cutaneous malignant melanoma. After a variable period of slow peripheral growth (up to decades), nodules of invasive melanoma develop in these lesions in 30% to 50% of cases. Lentigo maligna accounts for 90% of head and neck melanomas and has the most favorable prognosis of all tumor types. Once it becomes invasive, however, the prognosis falls significantly.

CLINICAL PRESENTATION   Lentigo maligna presents as a flat cutaneous macule with irregular borders and variable pigmentation from tan to brown. It typically presents during the fourth or fifth decades of life as a small lesion that slowly enlarges. Patients may also have primary acquired melanosis of the conjunctiva, which may be the mucous membrane equivalent. Lentigo maligna may have a long in situ (horizontal growth) phase in which the pigmentation extends for up to several centimeters in diameter over many years. This phase is associated with variable growth and sometimes with spontaneous regression of the lesion with alteration in pigmentation. Subclinical extension may be apparent as a broader area of pigmentation when the lesion is examined under a Wood's lamp. When areas become invasive lentigo maligna melanoma, nodule formation is seen within the broader flat macule. Lesions on the eyelid may progress over the eyelid margin and onto the conjunctival surface.

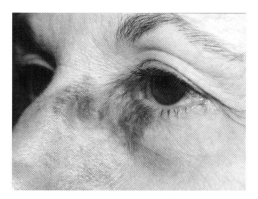

HISTOPATHOLOGY   This confusing term describes a histological spectrum ranging from slightly increased numbers of basally located melanocytes with mild cytological atypia to a confluent, often nested,

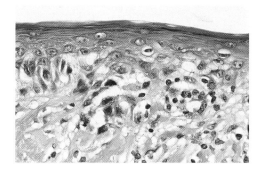

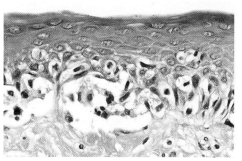

proliferation of highly atypical melanocytes. Some pathologists consider all lentigo maligna to be melanoma in situ, while others do not. Due to confusion associated with the term "lentigo maligna," Barnhill advocates classifying basal proliferations of atypical melanocytes as either "melanoma in situ" or "lentiginous melanocytic proliferation with atypia" for those lesions judged to fall short of melanoma in situ.

DIFFERENTIAL DIAGNOSIS   The differential diagnosis includes lentigo senilis, pigmented actinic keratosis, reticulated seborrheic keratosis, malignant melanoma, and cutaneous fungal infections.

TREATMENT   The treatment of choice for lentigo maligna is complete surgical excision. In general 2 to 4 mm of clear tumor-free margins may be sufficient. If there are suspected areas of invasive lentigo malignant melanoma a wider surgical excision with 1 cm of clear skin margins confirmed by histologic monitoring is recommended. Mohs micrographic surgery has been associated with the lowest recurrence rates of 4% to 5%. Alternative treatments with cryosurgery or radiotherapy are also effective with reported recurrence rates of about 8% to 10%. More recently the topical immunostimulator, imiquimod, has been shown to destroy these tumors before they become invasive.

REFERENCES

Charles CA, Yee VS, Dusza SW, et al. Variation in the diagnosis, treatment, and management of melanoma in situ: a survey of US dermatologists. Arch Dermatol 2005; 141:723–729.

Christenson LJ. Management of lentigo maligna. Dermatol Nurs 2004; 16:495–498.

Clark WH, Mihm MC Jr. Lentigo maligna and lentigo maligna melanoma. Am J Pathol 1969; 55:39–67.

Gonder JR, Wagoner MD, Albert DM: Idiopathic acquired melanosis. Ophthalmology 1980; 87:835–840.

Huilgol SC, Selva D, Chen C, et al. Surgical margins for Lentigo maligna and Lentigo maligna melanoma: the technique of mapped serial excision. Arch Dermatol 2004; 140:1087–1092.

Michalik EE, Fitzpatrick TB, Sober AJ. Rapid progression of lentigo maligna to deeply invasive lentigo maligna melanoma. Report of two cases. Arch Dermatol 1983; 119:831–834.

Naylor MF, Crowson N, Kuiwahara R, et al. Treatment of lentigo maligna with topical imiquimod. Br J Dermatol 2003; 149(suppl) 66:66–70.

Rodriquez-Sains RS, Jakobiec FA, Iwamoto T. Lentigo maligna of the lateral canthal skin. Ophthalmology 1981; 88:1186–1192.

Stevenson O, Ahmed I. Lentigo maligna: prognosis and treatment options. Am J Clin Dermatol 2005; 6:151–164.

Urist MM, Balch CM, Soong S, Shaw HM, Milton GW, Maddox WA. Head and neck melanoma in 534 clinical stage I patients. A prognostic factors analysis and results of surgical treatment. Ann Surg 1984; 200: 769–875.

Vaughn GJ, Dortzbach RK. Benign eyelid lesions. In: Yanoff M, Duker JS, eds. Ophthalmology. London: Mosby, 1999: 7–12:5–7.

Lentigo Senilis

INTRODUCTION   Also known as *senile lentigines*, *solar lentigo*, *age spots*, or *liver spots*, these are the most common lesions found on sun-exposed areas of light-skinned older individuals. They may also occur in younger individuals after prolonged sun exposure, and are common in patients with xeroderma pigmentosum. They are related to aging phenomena in light-skinned individuals where areas of hypopigmentation may be seen along side of focal hyperpigmentation (lentigo senilis). The hyperpigmentation appears to result from an increase in melanocyte proliferation or aggregation, and increased melanin accumulation.

CLINICAL PRESENTATION   Lentigo senilis presents as tan to brown to black macules with slightly irregular borders, but are evenly pigmented. They start out only 3 to 6 mm in diameter, but they slowly increase in size and number, coalescing and reaching diameters of several centimeters after many years of growth.

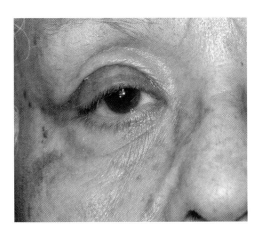

HISTOPATHOLOGY   The epidermal rete ridges extend to form bud-like processes into the papillary dermis. The epidermis between ridges may be atrophic. The number of melanocytes may be normal or increased, but there is a marked increase in the melanin content. The dermis usually exhibits actinic elastosis. Pigment incontinence is common, and there may be slight chronic inflammation in the dermis.

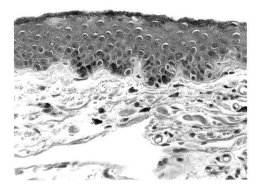 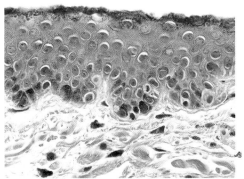

DIFFERENTIAL DIAGNOSIS   The differential diagnosis includes junctional nevi, seborrheic keratoses, and lentigo maligna.

TREATMENT   Biopsy should be performed for any suspicious-looking lesions to rule out the presence of a melanoma. When the diagnosis is not in question a light application of cryotherapy is often adequate. Melanocytes are injured at temperatures below −4°C to −7°C, whereas squamous epithelial cells can resist injury down to –20°C. Retinoids have proven useful in decreasing the cohesiveness of abnormal hypoproliferative cells and in modulating keratinocyte differentiation. Bleaching creams such as 4% hydroquinones lighten hyperpigmented lesions by suppressing melanocyte production.

REFERENCES

Braun-Falco O, Schoefinius HH. Lentigo senilis. Review and studies. Hautarzt 1971; 22:277–283.

Cawley EP, Curtis AC. Lentigo senilis. AMA Arch Derm Syphilol 1950; 62:635–641.

Haddad MM, Xu W, Madrano EE. Aging in epidermal melanocytes: cell cycle genes and melanins. J Invest Dermatol Symp Proc 1998; 3:36–40.

Hodgson C. Senile lentigo. Arch Dermatol 1963; 87:197–207.

Holzle E. Pigmented lesions as a sign of photoaging. Br J Dermatol 1992; 41:48–50.

Mehregan AH. Lentigo senilis and its evolutions. J Invest Dermatol 1975; 65:429–433.

Leukemia Cutis

INTRODUCTION   Leukemia is a result of neoplastic proliferation of bone marrow-derived leukocytes, the majority of which are of B-cell origin. The disease may be subdivided into acute or chronic forms. The acute form presents with anemia, thrombocytopenia, hemorrhage, adenopathy, hepatosplenomegaly, and a rapidly fatal course. The chronic indolent form is often incidentally diagnosed following prolonged episodes of fever, weight loss, and infection. The acute leukemias are more likely to show eye involvement than chronic leukemias. Leukemia cutis may occur concurrently with bone marrow involvement, as an isolated site of relapse, or as the initial manifestation of leukemia. Leukemia cutis occurs in 25% to 30% of infants with congenital leukemia. In older persons the incidence of leukemia cutis at diagnosis is approximately 10% in acute myeloid leukemia and 1% in acute lymphoblastic leukemia. Between 75% and 90% of patients with leukemia will show eye or adnexal involvement at some stage of the disease.

CLINICAL PRESENTATION   Leukemia cutis of the eyelid skin manifests most commonly as multiple 1 to 2.5 cm discrete nodules ranging from a solitary lesion to involvement of 70% of the body surface. These lesions rarely ulcerate, and may be associated with urticaria and pruritis. Lesions vary in color from blue to red, to purple to green, to brown, depending on the amount of myeloperoxidase present within the immature blast cells. Diffuse infiltration of the dermis by leukemic cells may be seen. Associated ocular involvement may include lesions of the retina, optic nerve, globe, or conjunctiva. The retina shows the most frequent clinical involvement in leukemia with hemorrhage, cotton-wool spots, venous dilatation, micro-aneurysms, and leukemic infiltrates.

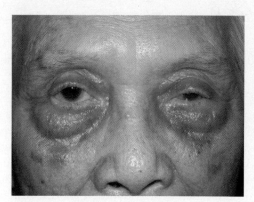

(Courtesy of Charles S. Soparkar, M.D.)

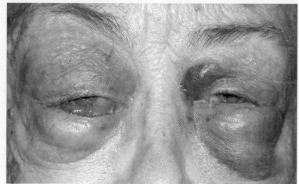

(Courtesy of Charles S. Soparkar, M.D.)

Associated orbital disease is not uncommon and presents with pain, lid edema, and exophthalmos. Systemic manifestations include purpura due to thrombocytopenia, urticaria, pruritis, erythema multiforme, leonine facies, alopecia, exfoliative dermatitis, and infection with opportunistic organisms may be seen. Death may result from infection or hemorrhage.

HISTOPATHOLOGY   The appearance of the leukemic infiltrate is a reflection of the underlying form of leukemia. An example of acute monocytic leukemia is illustrated, demonstrating neoplastic cells with folded, monocytoid nuclei.

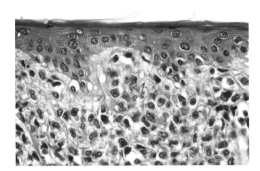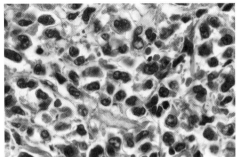

DIFFERENTIAL DIAGNOSIS   The differential diagnosis includes syphilis, dermatitis, leprosy, erythema multiforme, exfoliative dermatitis, and infection.

TREATMENT   The treatment of leukemia depends upon the stage of the disease, the cell type, site of involvement, and clinical symptoms. Systemic disease is best treated with chemotherapy, and bone marrow transplants following total irradiation of the myelopoietic tissues. Central nervous system leukemia may be treated with intrathecal methotrexate, and cutaneous nodules may be palliated with local X-ray irradiation. Death may result from infection or hemorrhage.

REFERENCES

Agnew KL, Ruchlemer R, Catovsky D, et al. Cutaneous findings in chronic lymphocytic leukemia.
    Br J Dermatol 2004; 150:1129–1135.
Allen R, Straatsma B. Ocular involvement in leukemia and allied disorders. Arch Ophthalmol 1961; 66:490–508.
Broder S, Bunn PA, Jaffe ES, et al. NIH Conference. T-cell lymphoma-proliferative syndrome associated with human T-cell
    leukemia/lymphoma virus. Ann Intern Med 1984; 100:543–557.
Ikeda T, Sakurane M, Uede K, Furukawa F. A case of symmetrical leukemia cutis on the eyelids complicated by
    B-cell chronic lymphocytic lymphoma. J Dermatol 2004; 31:560–563.
Ogunbiyi AO, Shokunbi WA, Fasola FA, Ogunbiyi JO. Leukemia cutis in a patient with acute myelogenous leukemia: case
    report. East Afr Med J 2003: 80:606–608.
Yen A, Sanchez R, Oblender M, Raimer S. Leukemia cutis: Darier's sign in a neonate with acute lymphoblastic leukemia.
    J Am Acad Dermatol 1996; 34:375–377.
Zhang IH, Zane LT, Braun BS, et al. Congenital leukemia cutis with subsequent development of leukemia.
    J Am Acad Dermatol 2006; 54:S22–S27.
Zweegman S, Vermeer MH, Bekkink MW, et al. Leukemia cutis: clinical features and treatment strategies. Haematologica
    2002; 87:ECR 13.

Lupus Erythematosus

INTRODUCTION   Lupus erythematosus is a chronic inflammatory autoimmune disease with a spectrum of clinical forms ranging from a benign chronic cutaneous variety (*discoid lupus erythematosus*) to an often-fatal systemic type with nephritis (*systemic lupus erythematosus*). Intermediate types, variously known as *disseminated discoid lupus erythematosus* and *subacute cutaneous lupus erythematosus*, are characterized by various combinations of widespread cutaneous lesions and mild to severe systemic manifestations. The role of immune complexes in the inflammatory manifestations of lupus is well recognized, and in about 4% of cases an associated vasculitis may be seen from small vessel involvement. Lupus erythematosus occurs most commonly in women in the third to fifth decades. When skin lesions occur they typically appear in areas exposed to the ultraviolet rays of the sun. Rarely discoid lupus can degenerate into squamous cell carcinoma.

CLINICAL PRESENTATION   Eyelid lesions may be acute or chronic, and either scarring or nonscarring. Common nonscarring eyelid lesions include a pruritic eruption of the lower eyelids. Scarring lesions often present as sharply demarcated purple-red, slightly raised, circumscribed plaques covered with thin adherent whitish scales and telangiectasias. Often such lesions are localized to the lateral aspect of the lower eyelids. Such lesions may enlarge to reach a size of about 5 to 10 mm. The major disfigurement of discoid lupus occurs as the lesions involute where atrophic scarring may lead to trichiasis and entropion. Often, pronounced hypopigmentation or hyperpigmentation occurs. Other common skin manifestations include the classic butterfly rash, cutaneous vasculitic foci, urticaria, vesiculobullous lesions, and nonscarring alopecia. Ocular manifestations include retinal hemorrhages, cotton wool spots, retinal vasculitis, papillitis, diffuse retinal edema, keratoconjunctivitis sicca, and band keratopathy. Associated systemic findings in lupus erythematosus include arthralgia, nephritis, pleurisy, pericarditis, vasculitis, CNS problems, and hematologic abnormalities.

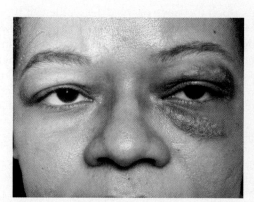
(Courtesy of Robert A. Goldberg, M.D.)

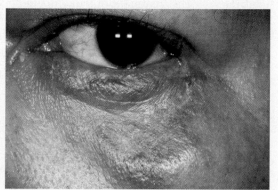
(Courtesy of Charles S. Soparkar, M.D.)

HISTOPATHOLOGY   Active lesions of discoid lupus erythematosus (DLE) exhibit hyperkeratosis, follicular dilation with keratin plugging, epidermal atrophy, hydropic degeneration of the basal layer of epidermis with variable degrees of pigmentary incontinence, basement membrane thickening, occasional apoptotic (cytoid) bodies in the epidermis, dermal edema, mucin deposition in the reticular dermis, and a predominantly perivascular and periappendageal infiltrate of lymphocytes and macrophages. Healing lesions of DLE have hyperkeratosis, atrophic or slightly thickened epidermis, markedly thickened epidermal basement membrane, dermal fibrosis, and marked follicular plugging. Histological features of subacute cutaneous lupus erythematosus and systemic lupus erythematosus overlap and may be indistinguishable from those of DLE.

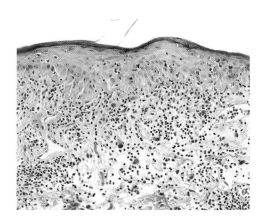
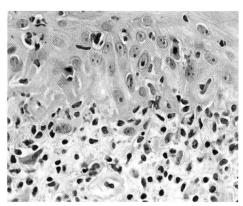

DIFFERENTIAL DIAGNOSIS   The differential diagnosis includes blepharitis, eczema, psoriasis, rosacea, allergic dermatitis, granuloma faciale, polymorphic light eruption, vitiligo, seborrheic dermatitis, and fungal dermatitis.

TREATMENT   Important diagnostic laboratory studies may include lupus band test (LBT), fluorescent antinuclear antibody test (ANA), anti-native DNA (n DNA), and anti-double stranded DNA (ds DNA). ANA is very sensitive, but not specific for SLE. The most specific autoantibody for SLE is n DNA or ds DNA antibody. Antibody titers tend to increase with flare-ups. Elevated sedimentation rates, elevated IgG levels and abnormal complement level abnormalities can be seen, however they may be normal in purely cutaneous forms of the disease. Patients with cutaneous lupus are often treated to prevent late pigmentary changes and scarring, as well as the rare sequelae of skin cancers arising from these lesions. Early skin lesions can often be treated effectively with oral, topical, or intralesional corticosteroids. Systemic antimalarial agents (chloroquine and hydroxychloroquine) are helpful adjuvants in treating all the cutaneous manifestations of lupus. Surgical correction of eyelid malpositions may be necessary, but should be delayed until after quiescence of the disease.

REFERENCES

Acharya N, Pineda R 2nd, Uy HS, Foster CS. Discoid lupus erythematosus masquerading as chronic blepahroconjunctivitis. Ophthalmology 2005; 112:e19–e23.

Calamia KT, Balabanova M. Vasculitis in systemic lupus erythematosus. Clin Dermatol 2004; 22:148–156.

Donzis PB, Insler MS, Buntin DM, Gately LE. Discoid lupus erythematosus involving the eyelids. Am J Ophthalmol 1984; 98:32–36.

Dubois EL, Tuffanelli DL. Clinical manifestations of systemic lupus erythematosus. JAMA 1964; 190:104–111.

Feiler-Ofry V, Isler Z, Hanau D, Godel V. Eyelid involvement as the presenting manifestation of discoid lupus erythematosus. J Pediatr Ophthalmol Strabismus 1979; 16:395–397.

Frith P, Burge SM, Millard PR, Wojnarowska F. External ocular findings in lupus erythematosus: A clinical and immunopathological study. Br J Ophthalmol 1990; 74:163–167.

Huey C, Jakobiec FA, Iwamoto T, et al. Discoid lupus erythematosus of the eyelids. Ophthalmology 1983; 90:1389–1398.

Kearns W, Wood W, Marchese A. Chronic cutaneous lupus involving the eyelid. Ann Ophthalmol 1982; 11:1009–1010.

Pianigiani E, Andreassi A, De Aloe G, Rubegni P, Rufia A, Motolese E. "Chronic erythematous desquamative plaques of the eyelids" discoid lupus erythematosus (DLE). Arch Dermatol 2002; 138:527–532.

Rony Z. Discoid lupus erythematosus of the eyelids. J Am Acad Dermatol 1986; 15:112–113.

Tosti A, Tosti G, Giovannini A. Discoid lupus erythematosus solely involving the eyelids: report of three cases. J Am Acad Dermatol 1987; 6:1259–1260.

Tumulty PA. The clinical course of systemic lupus erythematosus. JAMA 1954; 156:947–953.

Lymphangioma

INTRODUCTION   Lymphangiomas are lymphatic malformations that may involve the eyelid, conjunctiva, or orbit. This condition is divided into three different types: capillary, or lymphangioma circumscripta, cavernous lymphangioma, and cystic hygroma. Sometimes more than one type will coexist in the same patient. Lesions often present at birth or early in childhood, and only occasionally present in adulthood. The condition may appear as a simple dilatation of lymphatic vessels (lymphangiectasia), or a formed multilobulated tumor (lymphangioma).

CLINICAL PRESENTATION   Eyelid involvement may present as a superficial lesion with multiple cyst-like excrescences, or as a complex of channels that cause lid thickening and distortion of the eyelid. Lymphangioma circumscripta reside near the skin surface and present as one or more crops of small, vesicle-like lesions which may become hyperkeratotic or verrucous and can become hemorrhagic especially following manipulation. Cavernous lymphangiomas present as spongy, vermiform lesions. Extensive involvement may be complicated by elephantiasis of the eyelid. Cystic hygroma is the most massive form of lymphangioma and usually involves the neck or extremities, and while seldom directly affecting the eyelid it may be associated with separate vascular lid abnormalities. Hemorrhage into any of these lesions may occur forming a clotted hematoma (chocolate cyst). Lesions may enlarge with upper respiratory infection due to proliferation of lymphoid aggregates within the tumor.

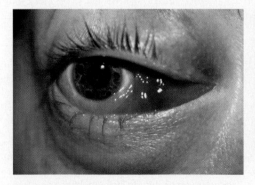 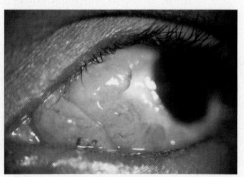

HISTOPATHOLOGY   Lymphangiomas are infiltrative lesions having wide variation in the size of the lymphatic channels. The channels in a given lesion vary from the size of capillaries to cavernous spaces. The channels are lined by attenuated endothelium resembling that in normal lymphatics.

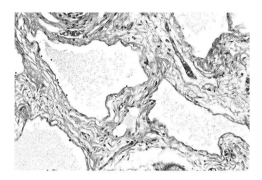 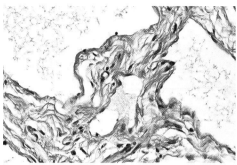

The adventitial coat of the lymphatic spaces is inconspicuous in most eyelid lymphangiomas. The lymphatic spaces contain proteinaceous (eosinophilic) fluid with occasional lymphocytes, or erythrocytes may be present if there has been spontaneous hemorrhage into the tumor. The stroma between lymphatic channels begins as loose fibrous connective tissue with a variable number of lymphoid aggregates. Older or re-operated lesions have a fibrotic stroma, often with hemosiderin deposits from prior bleeding.

DIFFERENTIAL DIAGNOSIS   The differential diagnosis includes herpetic disease, papillomas, papillomatous verrucae, nevi, cavernous hemangioma, and plexiform neurofibromas.

TREATMENT   Lesions isolated to the eyelid are best left undisturbed. Partial surgical excision may be indicated for severe proptosis or optic nerve compromise due to orbital extension, severe cosmesis concerns, or eyelid malpositions that threaten amblyopia. Caution must be taken as these lesions are particularly prone to hemorrhage during surgery which may compromise vision. Larger lesions may be difficult to manage due to extensive infiltration into normal tissues. Carbon dioxide laser has been advocated as a useful modality when excision is required.

REFERENCES

Dryden RM, Wulc AE, Day D. Eyelid ecchymosis and proptosis in lymphangioma. Am J Ophthalmol 1985; 100:486–487.

Flanagan BP, Helwig EB. Cutaneous lymphangioma. Arch Dermatol 1977; 113:24–30.

Goble RR, Frangoulis MA. Lymphangioma circumscriptum of the eyelids and conjunctiva. Br J Ophthalmol 1990; 74:574–575.

Goto H, Usui M, Okada S. Histopathological study of orbital lymphangioma in an infant. Jpn J Ophthalmol 2004; 48:594–597.

Harkins GA, Sebastion DC Jr. Lymphangioma in infancy and childhood. Surgery 1960; 47:811–822.

Iliff WJ, Green WR. Orbital lymphangiomas. Ophthalmology 1979; 86:914–929.

Jakobiec F, Jones I. In: Duane T, ed. Clinical Ophthalmology. Vol. 2. Philadelphia: Harper & Row, 1983; 37:8.

Pang P, Jakobiec FA, Iwamoto T, Hornblass A. Small lymphangiomas of the eyelids. Ophthalmology 1984; 91:1278–1284.

Peachey RD, Liu CC, Whimster IW. Lymphangioma of the skin. A review of 65 cases. Br J Dermatol 1970; 83:519–527.

Rootman J, Hay E, Graeb D, Miller R. Orbital-adnexal lymphangiomas. A spectrum of hemodynamically isolated vascular hamartomas. Ophthalmology 1986; 93:1558–1570.

Russo PE, Dewar JP. Congenital Lymphangioma. Am J Roentgenol 1961; 85:726–728.

Vineyard W. In: Demis D, ed. Clinical Dermatology. Vol. 2. Philadelphia: Harper & Row, 1984. Unit 7–74.

Lymphoma

INTRODUCTION   B-cell lymphoma is a systemic malignancy of lymphoid tissue. Lymphoma more typically involves the orbit, and eyelid involvement is usually due to forward extension of the tumor. Most orbital lymphomas are of the non-Hodgkin's variety, and most are low-grade proliferations of small, monoclonal lymphocytes. In many cases lymphoma may be confined to the periocular region without obvious systemic involvement. In some instances both orbits may be involved. The majority of these primary orbital adnexal lymphomas are believed to be mucosal-associated lymphoid tissue (MALT)—type tumors arising from extranodal mucosal tissues, and they may be associated with acquired immune deficiency syndrome (AIDS). About 5% of patients with systemic lymphoma develop orbital or adnexal metastases. Lymphomas are seen primarily in patients 50 to 70 years of age. Individuals who initially have well-differentiated localized disease have a 15% chance of developing systemic disease; whereas 50% to 60% of those with less well differentiated disease may manifest systemically within five years. Therefore, patients who present with isolated orbital disease should be re-examined at periodic intervals for systemic disease.

CLINICAL PRESENTATION   The clinical onset of lymphoma is typically insidious and most often painless. Eyelid involvement presents as swelling, mechanical ptosis, and presence of a subcutaneous palpable mass. A salmon-colored lesion may extend beneath the conjunctiva. The most common signs of orbital involvement are proptosis and often a downward displacement of the globe since these lesions have a predilection for the superior orbit. Limitation of ocular motility and decreased vision are late signs, occurring only in advanced cases. In 40% of patients with orbital lymphoma there is evidence of systemic involvement at presentation.

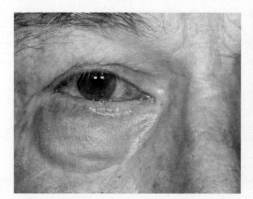 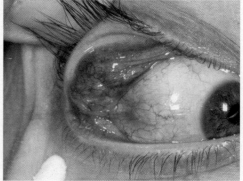

HISTOPATHOLOGY   The eyelid may be involved in primary cutaneous lymphoma or as part of a generalized lymphoma. Both B-cell and T-cell lymphomas may occur as primary cutaneous processes or spread secondarily to the eye, and the histopathology reflects the specific entity. The lymphomatous infiltrate in systemic lymphomas is typically in the dermis and subcutis, while primary cutaneous lymphomas may have both dermal and epidermal components. An example of an anaplastic large cell lymphoma localized to the eyelid is illustrated on p. 193.

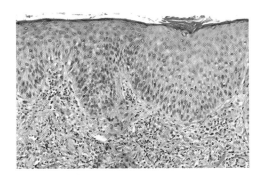 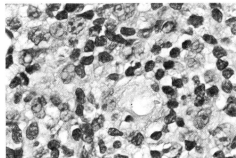

DIFFERENTIAL DIAGNOSIS   The differential diagnosis includes reactive lymphoid hyperplasia, plasmacytoma, lacrimal gland tumors, and chloroma.

TREATMENT   Biopsy is recommended to establish a diagnosis. Once the diagnosis is confirmed, a general physical examination, complete blood count, bone marrow biopsy, liver and spleen scan, bone scan, chest X ray, serum immuno-protein electrophoresis, and CT scanning of the thorax and abdomen, for the detection of mediastinal and retro peritoneal lymph node involvement is recommended. Treatment includes observation, radiation, and/or chemotherapy. Observation without treatment for low-grade tumors with only local orbital involvement may be appropriate. Radiotherapy at 2500 to 3000 cGy has been reported to achieve excellent local control for isolated orbital lymphoma. For less well-differentiated tumors and for systemic disease, chemotherapy is indicated. For individuals with low-grade tumors that are confined to the eyelid and orbit, prognosis is excellent even without treatment. Overall, the five-year survival rate is 93%.

REFERENCES

Copeland SE, Krause L, Delecluse HJ, et al. Lymphoproliferative lesions of the ocular adnexa: analysis of 112 cases. Ophthalmology 1998; 105:1430–1441.

Dutton JJD, Byrne SF, Proia AD. Diagnostic Atlas of Orbital Dieases. Philadelphia: WB Saunders, 2000:100–101.

Ellis JH, Banks PM, Campbell J, Liesgang TJ. Lymphoid tumors of the ocular adnexa. Ophthalmol Clin 1993; 33:163–173.

Jakobiec FA, Iwamoto T, Patell M, Knowles DM 2nd. Ocular adnexal monoclonal lymphoid tumors with a favorable prognosis. Ophthalmology 1986; 93:1547–1557.

Jakobiec FA, Knowles DM. An overview of ocular adnexal lymphoid tumors. Trans AM Ophthalmol Soc 1989; 87:420–442.

Jakobiec FA, McLean I, Font RL, Clinicopathologic characteristics of orbital lymphoid hyperplasia. Ophthalmology 1979; 86:948–966.

Jakobiec FA, Neri A, Knowles DM II. Genotypic monoclonality in immunophenotypically polyclonal orbital lymphoid tumors. A model of tumor progression in the lymphoid system. The 1986 Wendell Hughes lecture. Ophthalmology 1987; 94:980–994.

Keleti D, Flickinger JC, Hobson SR, Mittal BB. Radiotherapy of lymphoproliferative diseases of the orbit. Surveillance of 65 cases. Am J Clin Oncol 1992; 15:422–427.

Kennerdell JS, Johnson BL, Deutsch M. Radiation treatment of orbital lymphoid hyperplasia. Ophthalmology 1979; 86:942–947.

Knowles DM II, Jakobiec FA, NcNally L, Burke JS. Lymphoid hyperplasia and malignant lymphoma occurring in the ocular adnexa (orbit, conjunctiva, and eyelids): A prospective multiparametric analysis of 108 cases during 1977 to 1987. Hum Pathol 1990; 21:959–973.

Knowles DM II, Jakobiec FA. Orbital lymphoid neoplasms: a clinicopathologic study of 60 patients. Cancer 1980; 46:576–589.

Liesegang TJ. Ocular adnexal lymphoproliferative lesions. Mayo Clin Proc 1993; 68:1003–1010.

Rootman J, Patel S, Jewell L. Polyclonal orbital and systemic infiltrates. Ophthalmology 1984; 91:1112–1117.

Westacott S, Garner A, Moseley IF, Wright JE. Orbital lymphoma versus reactive lymphoid hyperplasia: an analysis of the use of computed tomography in the differential diagnosis. Br J Ophthalmol 1991; 75:722–725.

White WL, Ferry JA. Ocular adnexal lymphoma: a clinicopathologic study with identification of lymphomas of mucosa-associated lymphoid tissue type. Ophthalmology 1995; 102:1994–2006.

Malignant Melanoma

INTRODUCTION   Cutaneous malignant melanoma is an invasive proliferation of malignant melanocytes, and accounts for 1% of all eyelid malignancies. The incidence increases with age, but remains relatively stable from the fifth to the seventh decades. Cutaneous malignant melanoma may be classified into four different types: *lentigo maligna melanoma* (5%), *superficial spreading melanoma* (70%), *nodular melanoma* (16%), and *acral lentiginous melanoma* (9%). Nodular melanoma and lentigo maligna melanomas are the most common types affecting the eyelids. In all types, initially, a noninvasive horizontal growth phase occurs, which is followed by an invasive vertical growth phase. Changes in outline and color are features that tend to distinguish melanoma from benign pigmented lesions. Risk factors for the development of malignant melanoma include congenital and dysplastic nevi, changing cutaneous moles, excessive sun exposure and sun sensitivity, family history, age greater than 20 years, and Caucasian race. Patients with the dysplastic nevus syndrome (B-K mole syndrome) have a high risk of developing malignant melanoma. Prognosis and metastatic potential are linked to the depth of invasion and thickness of the tumor. Lesions less than 0.75 mm have a five-year survival rate of 98%, while those greater than 4 mm have a less than 50% survival rate. Additionally, malignant melanoma involving the eyelid margin has a poorer prognosis.

CLINICAL PRESENTATION   Superficial spreading melanoma presents as a small, pigmented lesion with mild elevation and irregular borders. It may go through a phase of horizontal growth, in which the pigmentation extends in diameter, but eventually tends to become nodular and indurated, signifying invasive growth. Nodular melanoma may present as a markedly pigmented or amelanotic

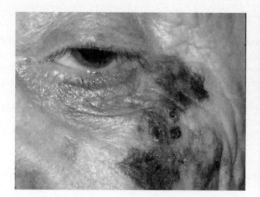
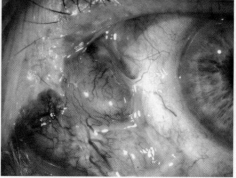

nodule that rapidly increases in size with associated ulceration and bleeding. Any lesion that develops hues of white, gray, blue, black, red, or pink is suspect. Variation in brown pigment especially if in an asymmetric fashion is suspicious. Other factors such as papule or nodule formation of a previously flat pigmented lesion, bleeding, ulceration, or loss of fine skin lines should raise concern for possible melanoma.

HISTOPATHOLOGY   Superficial spreading malignant melanoma features a proliferation of atypical melanocytes, singly and in nests, within all levels of the epidermis. The atypical melanocytes may be confined to the epidermis (in situ melanoma) or they may be associated with tumor cells invading the dermis. The tumor cells may be epithelioid, nevus-cell like, or spindle-shaped. Nodular melanoma lacks an intraepidermal component of atypical melanocytes adjacent to the infiltrative tumor, but there is usually epidermal invasion by malignant cells directly over the tumor. Nodular malignant melanoma is commonly composed of round to oval epithelioid cells with varying amounts of melanin pigment.

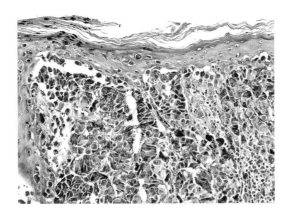 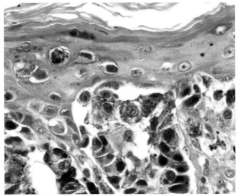

DIFFERENTIAL DIAGNOSIS   The differential diagnosis for malignant melanoma includes nonmalignant pigmented nevocellular nevi, pigmented basal cell carcinoma, pigmented seborrheic keratosis, dysplastic nevi, Kaposi's sarcoma and hemangioma.

TREATMENT   The treatment of choice for cutaneous malignant melanoma of the eyelid is surgical excision with wide margins of 1 cm confirmed by histologic monitoring. Often, a 1 cm clear margin may not be possible. In such cases Mohs' micrographic surgery may be helpful, but some Moh's surgeons do not feel that frozen sections are accurate enough for melanomas. Regional lymph node dissection should be performed for tumors greater than 1.5 mm depth and/or for tumors that show evidence of vascular or lymphatic spread. A metastatic evaluation also is recommended for patients diagnosed with any malignant melanoma.

REFERENCES

Balch CM, Murad TM, Soong SJ, et al. Tumor thickness as a guide to surgical management of clinical stage I melanoma patients. Cancer 1979; 43:883–888.

Bondi EE, Elder DE, Guerry D 4th, Clark WH Jr. Skin markings in malignant melanoma. JAMA 1983; 25:503–505.

Breslow A. Tumor thickness, level of invasion, and node dissection in stage I cutaneous melanoma. Ann Surg 1975; 182:572–575.

Clark WH Jr, Reimer RR, Greene MH, Ainsworth AH, Mastrangelo MJ. Origin of familial malignant melanoma from heritable melanocytic lesions. The B-K mole syndrome. Arch Dermatol 1978; 114:732–738.

Cosimi AB, Sober AJ, Mihm MC Jr, Fitzpatrick CB. Conservative surgical management of superficially invasive cutaneous melanoma. Cancer 1984; 53:1256–1244.

Day CL, Mihm MC Jr, Sober AJ, Fitzpatrick CB, Malt RA. Narrower margins for clinical stage I malignant melanoma. N Engl J Med 1982; 306:479–482.

Garner A, Koornneef L, Levine A, Collin JR. Malignant melanoma of the eyelid skin: histopathology and behavior. Br J Ophthalmol 1985; 69:180–186.

Gonder JR, Wagoner MD, Albert DM. Idiopathic acquired melanosis. Ophthalmology 1980; 87:835–840.

Greene MH, Clark WH Jr, Tucker MA, et al. Acquired precursors of cutaneous malignant melanoma: the familial dysplastic nevus syndrome. N Engl J Med 1985; 312:91–97.

Grossnilklaus HE, McLean IW. Cutaneous melanoma of the eyelid: clinicopathologic features. Ophthalmology 1991; 98:1867–1873.

Michalik EE, Fitzpatrick TB, Sober AJ. Rapid progression of lentigo maligna to deeply invasive lentigo maligna melanoma. Arc Dermatol 1983; 119:831–835.

Mihm MC Jr, Fitzpatrick TB, Brown MML, et al. Early detection of primary cutaneous malignant melanoma: a color atlas. N Engl J Med 1973; 289:989–996.

Rhodes AR, Weinstock MA, Fitzpatrick TB, Mihm MC Jr, Sober AJ. Risk factors for cutaneous melanoma: a practical method of recognizing predisposed individuals. JAMA 1987; 258:3146–3154.

Rogers GS, Kopf AW, Rigel DS, et al. Effect of anatomical location on prognosis in patients with clinical stage I melanoma. Arch Dermatol 1983; 119:644–649.

Sober AJ, Fitzpatrick TB, Mihm MC Jr. Primary melanoma of the skin: recognition and management. J Am Acad Dermatol 1980; 2:179–197.

Tahery DP, Goldberg RA, Moy RL. Malignant melanoma of the eyelid: a report of eight cases and a review of the literature. J Am Acad Dermatol 1992; 27:1237–1250.

Urist MM, Balch CM, Soong SJ, et al. Head and neck melanoma in 534 clinical stage I patients; a prognostic factors analysis and results of surgical treatment. Ann Surg 1984; 200:769–775.

Zimmerman LE. Melanocytic tumors of interest to the ophthalmologist. Ophthalmology 1980; 87:497–502.

Zoltie N, O'Neill TJ. Malignant melanoma of the eyelid skin. Plast Reconstr Surg 1989; 83:994–996.

Melanocytic Nevus

INTRODUCTION   Also known as *nevocellular or nevomelanocytic nevi,* these common benign neoplasms or hamartomas are composed of melanocytes. Nevi are nests of melanocytes that may be congenital or acquired. Congenital nevi probably represent malformations or errors in development and migration of these neural crest elements. When nevocytes are sequestered along the palpebral fissure of the embryo, this results in the presence of a nevus on both the upper and lower eyelid margin, so-called kissing nevi. Acquired nevi are not present at birth and the incidence increases during the first 3–4 decades of life with a peak incidence in the third to fourth decades. They are especially common in individuals with fair complexion and frequently occur on the sun-exposed areas of eyelid skin. Occasionally they arise in an eruptive fashion, usually following some generalized insult to the skin such as erythema multiforme or burns. Melanocytic nevi can take on several distinct forms. In lentigo simplex proliferating melanocytes are confined to the basal epidermal layer. In junctional nevi nested proliferations of melanocytes are located in the basal epidermis and extend into the tips of the rete ridges. Compound nevi have both a nested junctional location and an intradermal component. The intradermal nevus is confined to the dermis without any junctional component.

CLINICAL PRESENTATION   The clinical appearance of melanocytic nevi is often predictive of the histologic type. The majority of nevi found in young children are junctional nevi. Clinically these are oval or round, light to dark brown macules that gradually enlarge in size. On the lid margin intradermal nevi are frequently amelanotic. When large they may cause amblyopia. After this radial expansion is completed they gradually become elevated, evolving into compound nevi found in older children and young adults. Nevi on the eyelid margin characteristically mold to the ocular surface. Occasionally they may extend deep into the eyelid tissues. The finding of coarse dark hairs is not unusual. As the raised component increase the nevus sinks into the dermis and becomes dome shaped, sessile, verrucous, or even polypoid. At this point they are referred to as intradermal nevi, which are more prevalent in adults. In this last stage of development, fine skin lines are lost and pigmentation is decreased to a light brown or flesh tone. Individuals living beyond age 70 years often see most of or all their nevi disappear.

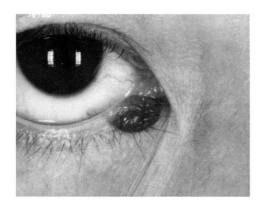
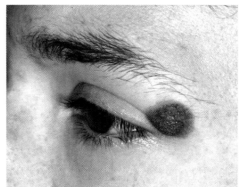

(Courtesy of Richard L. Anderson, M.D.)

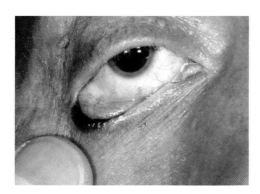
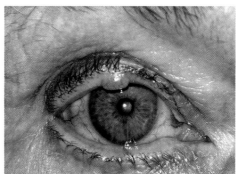

HISTOPATHOLOGY Melanocytic nevi are composed of nevus cells, which are melanocytes that have lost their long dendritic processes. Nevus cells are oval to cuboidal, have clear to pale eosinophilic cytoplasm, and contain a variable amount of melanin. The nevus cells form nests, which often coalesce when they are in the dermis. Melanocytic nevi may have discrete nests of nevus cells at the dermoepidermal junction ("junctional melanocytic nevus"), both at the dermoepidermal junction and within the dermis ("compound melanocytic nevus"), or confined within the dermis ("intradermal melanocytic nevus," shown below). On the eyelid, compound nevi may be papillomatous with a seborrheic keratosis-like appearance to their epidermis.

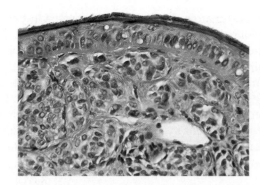 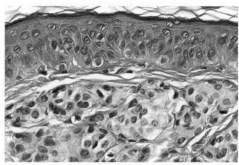

DIFFERENTIAL DIAGNOSIS   The differential diagnosis includes lentigo maligna, malignant melanoma, neurofibroma, balloon cell nevus, papilloma, seborrheic keratosis, inverted follicular keratosis, oculodermal melanocytosis, dermatofibroma, pigmented basal cell carcinoma, and fibrous histiocytoma.

TREATMENT   Malignant transformation may rarely occur, generally in the junctional or compound stages, thus suspicious lesions should be excised. Warning signs for which biopsy is indicated include irregular borders, variation in pigmentation, onset after 40 years of age, change in size or color, pain or irritation, and bleeding or ulceration. Otherwise, removal of common nevi is not required unless desired for cosmesis or relief of mechanical irritation. Shave biopsy without complete removal is acceptable for clearly benign lesions, especially those involving the eyelid margin. However, recurrence from incompletely removed lesions may occur. For non-marginal lesions, simple excision is effective.

REFERENCES

Amann J, Spraul CW, Mattfield T, Lang GK. Deep penetrating nevus of the eyelid. Klin Monatsbl Augenheilkd 1999; 215:376–377.

Groh MJ, Holbach LM. Congenital divided compound nevi of the eyelids. Klin Monatsbl Augenheilkd 1999; 215:263–265.

Margo CE. Pigmented lesions of the eyelid. In: Albert DM, Jakobiec FA, eds. Principles and Practice of Ophthalmology Philadelphia: W.B. Saunders, 1994:1797–1812.

Margo CE, Habal MB. Large congenital melanocytic nevus: light and electron microscopic findings. Ophthalmology 1987; 94:960–965.

Putterman AM. Intradermal nevi of the eyelid. Ophthalmic Surg 1980; 11:584–587.

Ribuffo D, Cavalieri L, Sonnino M, et al. Divided nevus of the eyelid: a case report. Ophthal Plast Reconstr Surg 1996; 12:186–189.

Shaffer B. Pigmented nevi: a clinical appraisal in the light of present-day histopathologic concepts. Arch Dermatol 1955; 72:120–132.

Sigg C, Pelloni F. Frequency of acquired melanonevocytic nevi and their relationship to skin complexion in 939 schoolchildren. Dermatologica 1989; 179:123–128.

Solomon LM. The management of congenital melanocytic nevi. Arch Dermatol 1980; 116:1017.

INTRODUCTION   This tumor is a rare aggressive neuroendocrine neoplasm composed of Merkel cells, nondendritic, and nonkeratinocytic epithelial clear cells of neural crest origin. Merkel cells appear to stimulate dermal nerve plexuses and to be involved in the release of various bioactive substances to the dermis. Merkel cell carcinoma accounts for less than 1% of cutaneous malignancies, and an etiologic role for chronic sun exposure has been proposed. It occurs most commonly in elderly Caucasian patients with a mean age at presentation of 75 years and there is an equal incidence among men and women.. The tumor is seen on the head and neck in 50% of cases. Merkel cell tumors show a predilection for perifollicular areas of the skin. Metastases occur initially to the regional lymph nodes, and the overall 2-year mortality rate is 30% to 50%.

CLINICAL PRESENTATION   Merkel cell tumor presents as a solitary, vascularized, nontender red or violaceous dome-shaped nodule or firm plaque. The epidermal surface is usually shinny, and fine telangiectasias may be seen. It is usually rapidly growing, hard and painless. The upper eyelid is the most common site of involvement and may lead to mechanical ptosis.

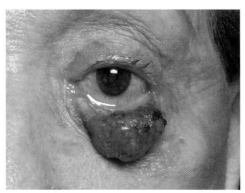
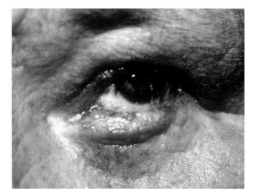

(Courtesy of Robert A. Goldberg, M.D.)

HISTOPATHOLOGY   Merkel cell (neuroendocrine) carcinomas are composed of small, round to oval tumor cells with vesicular nuclei and multiple small nucleoli. Mitoses are abundant, and there is scant amphophilic cytoplasm. The tumor cells may form nests, sheets, or trabeculae. The tumor is located in the dermis, with ulceration of the overlying epidermis in about 20% of cases. Most tumors express neuron-specific enolase, epithelial membrane antigen, and have neurofilament protein (shown below on right) and cytokeratin present as paranuclear globules. The tumor cells do not express thyroid transcription factor-1, which assists in differentiating Merkel cell carcinoma from metastatic carcinoma of the lung.

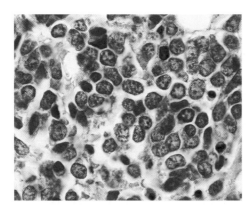
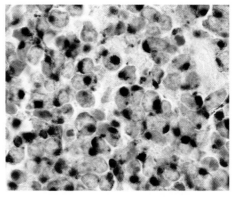

DIFFERENTIAL DIAGNOSIS   The differential diagnosis includes malignant melanoma, glomus tumor, lymphoma, metastatic tumors, sebaceous cell carcinoma, keratoacanthoma, plasmacytoma, squamous cell carcinoma, and fungal infection.

TREATMENT   Merkel cell carcinoma is treated with wide surgical excision with margins of 3 mm. Mohs microsurgery with histologic control of margins is preferred, but this tumor may be discontiguous histologically making Mohs surgery less effective than for many other tumors. Selective lymphadenectomy with sentinel node biopsy may be useful. Prophylactic node dissection combined with local excision and adjuvant radiotherapy is reported to improve survival rates. The role of chemotherapy remains unclear but so far it has not been shown to improve survival. Partial or complete regression has been reported but is very rare. Local recurrence is expected in 30% to 40% of cases, sometimes with invasion of adjacent tissues.

REFERENCES

Beyer CK, Goodman M, Dickerson GR, Dougherty M. Merkel cell tumor of the eyelid. A clinicopathologic case report. Arch Ophthalmol 1983; 101:1098–1101.

Font RL. Eyelids and lacrimal drainage system. In: Spencer WH, ed. Ophthalmic Pathology: An Alas and Textbook. 4th ed. Vol. 4. Philadelphia: WB Saunders, 1996:2218–2433.

Haag ML, Glass IF, Fenske NA. Merkel cell carcinoma. Diagnosis and treatment. Dermatol 1995; 21:669–683.

Kivela T, Tarkkanen A. The Merkel cell and associated neoplasms in the eyelids and periocular regions. Surv Ophthalmol 1990; 35:171–187.

Lamping K, Fischer MJ, Vareeska G, et al. A Merkel cell tumor of the eyelid. Ophthalmology 1983; 90:1399–1402.

Mamalis N, Medlock RD, Holds JB, Anderson RL, Crandall AS. Merkel cell tumor of the eyelid: a review and report of an unusual case. Ophthal Surg 1989: 20:410–414.

Pitale M, Session RB, Husain S. An analysis of prognostic factors in cutaneous neuroendocrine carcinoma. Laryngoscope 1992; 102:44–49.

Rubsamen PE, Tanenbaum M, Grove AS, Gould E. Merkel cell carcinoma of the eyelid and periocular tissues. Am J Ophthalmol 1992; 113:674–680.

Searl SS, Boynton JR, Markowitch W, di Sant'Agnese PA. Malignant Merkel cell neoplasm of the eyelid. Arch Ophthalmol 1984; 102:907–911.

Singh AD, Eagle RC Jr, Shields CL. Merkel cell carcinoma of the eyelids. In: Shields JA, ed. Update on Malignant Ocular Tumors: International Ophthalmology Clinics. Boston: Little Brown & Co., 1993; 33:11–17.

Wick MR, Millns JL, Sibley RK, Pittelkow MR, Winklemann RK. Secondary neuroendocrine carcinomas of the skin: an immunohistochemical comparison with primary neuroendocrine carcinoma of the skin ('Merkel cell' carcinoma). J Am Acad Dermatol 1985; 13:134–142.

Yanoff M, Fine BS, eds. Skin. In: Ocular Pathology: A Text and Atlas, 3rd ed. Philadelphia: JB Lipponcott, 1989:164–213.

Metastatic Tumors

INTRODUCTION   Eyelid metastases from distant sites are uncommon and account for less than 1% of eyelid tumors. When they do occur the most frequent sites for the primary tumor are breast, cutaneous melanoma, lung, colon, and prostate malignancies. Other primary sites including kidney, thyroid, parotid and trachea, have been reported. Females are affected more than males in a ratio of 4:1 reflecting the fact that breast carcinoma represents more than a third of eyelid metastases. Eyelid metastases usually occur in the setting of a known primary cancer elsewhere in the body, but in rare cases an eyelid tumor can be the presenting sign of an occult carcinoma.

CLINICAL PRESENTATION   The clinical presentation falls into three main categories: the first and most common is a diffuse, painless, noninflammatory, full-thickness, often leathery induration of the lid that may cause ptosis, lid lag, or epiphora. These lesions usually represent scirrhous or desmoplastic metastases from primary lesions such as breast carcinoma. The second pattern is that of an uninflamed, nontender subcutaneous nodule. The third pattern is a solitary ulcerated lesion. These last two patterns are generally seen with metastatic malignant melanoma, squamous cell carcinoma of respiratory origin, and adenocarcinomas from gastro-intestinal or genito-urinary sites. Similar lesions may be present in other areas of the body. Rarely, multiple metastatic lesions may be seen in one or more eyelids.

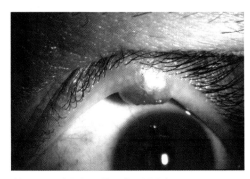 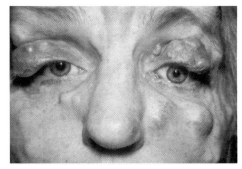

(Courtesy of Arthur Chandler, M.D.)

HISTOPATHOLOGY   Adenocarcinoma of the breast is the primary tumor that most frequently metastasizes to the eyelid (shown below). Metastatic breast adenocarcinoma resembles the primary tumor, with formation of islands and cords of tumor cells within the dermis. Vacuolation of tumor cells reflects their glandular differentiation, and "signet ring" cells may be present (cell in bottom right corner of the photomicrograph on the right). Cutaneous melanomas metastatic to the eyelid may be recognizable by the presence of melanin, or they can be identified using immunohistochemistry. Immunohistochemistry is also crucial in narrowing the possible primary sites for other tumors metastatic to the eyelid when the primary site is uncertain.

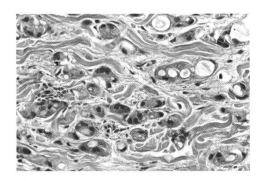 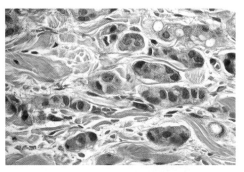

DIFFERENTIAL DIAGNOSIS   The differential diagnosis includes chalazion, infection, or other benign conditions, xanthomas, squamous cell carcinoma, and basal cell carcinoma.

TREATMENT   Biopsy is required for diagnosis. Debulking of large symptomatic tumors may be necessary to restore eyelid function while systemic treatment may be directed towards the underlying primary disease. If the metastatic eyelid lesion does not respond to chemotherapy, 3000 to 5000 cGy of external beam irradiation will often reduce the size of the tumor.

REFERENCES

Albert DM, Rubenstein RA, Scheie HG. Tumor metastasis to the eye, Part 1: Incidence in 213 adult patients with generalized malignancy. Am J Ophthalmol 1967; 63:723–726.

Aurora AL, Blodi FC. Lesions of the eyelids. A clinicopathologic study. Surv Ophthalmol 1970; 15:94–104.

Avert B, Haye C, Laurent M, Dufier JL. Metastatic tumours of the lid. J Fr Ophthalmol 1978; 1:317–320.

Char DH, Miller T, Kroll S. Orbital metastases: diagnosis and course. Br J Ophthalmol 1997; 81:386–390.

Ferry AP, Font RL. Carcinoma metastatic to the eye and orbit: I. A clinicopathologic study of 227 cases. Arch Ophthalmol 1974; 92:276–286.

Graham J, Young SE, Luna M. An unusual case of metastatic carcinoma to the eyelid. Am J Ophthalmol 1978; 86:400–402.

Kinderman WR, Shields JA, Eiferman RA, Stephens RF, Hirsch RE. Metastatic renal cell carcinoma to the eye and adnexae: a report of three cases and review of the literature. Ophthalmology 1981; 88:1347–1350.

Mansour AM, Hidayat AA. Metastatic eyelid disease. Ophthalmology 1987; 94:667–670.

Riley FC. Metastatic tumors of the eyelids. Am J Ophthalmol 1970; 69:259–264.

Rosenblum GA. Metastatic breast cancer in the eyelid. Cutis 1983; 31:411–415.

Salvado MC, Alberrto MJ, Goncalves LP, Procenca R. Palpebral metastasis revealing a gastric adenocarcinoma. Acta Med Port 1998; 11:87–90.

Shields, JA, Shields CL, Ausburger JJ, Negrey JN Jr. Solitary metastasis of choroidal melanoma to contralateral eyelid. Ophthal Plast Reconstr Surg 1987; 3:9–12.

Microcystic Adnexal Carcinoma

INTRODUCTION   Also known as *combined adnexal tumor of the skin*, *sclerosing sweat duct carcinoma*, *microcystic carcinoma*, *sweat gland carcinoma with syringomatous features*, and *malignant syringoma*, microcystic adnexal carcinoma is a rare cutaneous malignant tumor of sweat gland origin. Microcystic adnexal carcinoma typically appears in the fourth decade of life, both sexes being equally affected. In 88% of cases the lesions occur on the face. Growth is typically indolent, but the tumor is usually locally aggressive, extending into dermal, subcutaneous, and perineural planes. There is a 50% rate of local recurrence. The tumor occasionally spreads to the regional lymph nodes, but metastases are rare, amounting to only about 2%. There seems to be an association with prior radiation, and there may be an association with immunosuppression therapy.

CLINICAL PRESENTATION   The lesion is solitary and usually appears as a slowly growing, flesh-colored indurated plaque or nodule, sometimes with an overlying whitish to pink discoloration. This tumor may be more diffusely infiltrative with wide perineural spread. Lesions are typically present for several years prior to diagnosis. In some cases it may be present without symptoms for decades before a diagnosis is made. The size ranges from 1 to 3 cm. The lesion may be fixed to deep tissues because of its tendency to infiltrate tissue planes. Very rarely this tumor may be multiple and bilateral. These tumors are very rare in blacks, with only a few cases having been described.

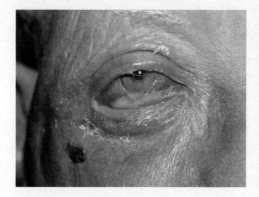 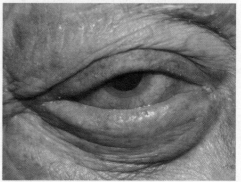

HISTOPATHOLOGY   These tumors usually involve the dermis and subcutaneous tissue and may extend into muscle. The more superficial tumor has numerous keratinous cysts along with islands and strands of squamous and basaloid epithelium with variable differentiation into ductules. The deeper portion of the tumor has nests and strands of tumor and small ductules in a dense fibrous stroma. Perineural invasion is frequent and helps to distinguish microcystic adnexal carcinoma from a syringoma.

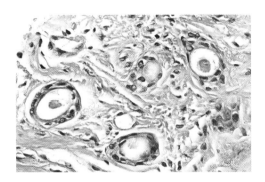

DIFFERENTIAL DIAGNOSIS   Microcystic adnexal carcinoma is difficult to distinguish clinically from other malignant conditions, even on histopathology. The differential diagnosis includes syringoma, chalazion, basal cell carcinoma, squamous cell carcinoma, and sebaceous cell carcinoma.

TREATMENT   While the standard of care for this tumor has not yet been established, complete surgical excision with wide tumor-free margins appears to be the treatment of choice to prevent the typical recurrences seen with this lesion. Mohs micrographic surgery is preferred but resection under frozen section control is a good alternative. Uncontrolled excision should include at least 4 to 5 mm of margin around the visible tumor. Once clear margins are obtained, additional wide excision is recommended. Radiotherapy is a useful adjunct in recurrent cases.

REFERENCES

Brookes JL, Bentley C, Verma S, Oliver JM, McKee PH. Microcystic adnexal carcinoma masquerading as a chalazion. Br J Ophthalmol 1998; 82:196–197.

Chiller K, Passaro D, Scheuller M, et al. Microcystic adnexal carcinoma: forty-eight cases, their treatment, and their outcome. Arch Dermatol 2000; 136:1355–1359.

Clement CI, Genge J, O'Donnell BA, Lochhead AG. Orbital and periorbital microcystic adnexal carcinoma. Ophthal Plast Reconstr Surg 2005; 21:97–102.

Delshad E, Ratner D. Microcystic adnexal carcinoma. Skinmed 2004; 3:341–343.

Eisen DB, Zloty D. Microcystic adnexal carcinoma involving a large portion of the face: when is surgery not reasonable? Dermatol Surg 2005; 31:1472–1477.

Fischer S, Breuninger H, Metzler G, Hoffmann J. Microcystic adnexal carcinoma: an often misdiagnosed, locally aggressive growing skin tumor. J Craniofac Surg 2005; 16:53–58.

Hesse RJ, Scharfenberg JC, Ratz JL, Griener E. Eyelid Microcystic adnexal carcinoma. Arch Ophthalmol 1995; 113:494–495.

Hunts JH, Patel BCK, Langer PD, Anderson RL, Gerwels JW. Microcystic adnexal carcinoma of the eyebrow and eyelid. Arch Ophthalmol 1995; 113:1332–1333.

Khachemoume A, Olbricht SM, Johnson DS. Microcystic adnexal carcinoma: report of four cases treated with Mohs' micrographic surgical technique. Int J Dermatol 2005; 44:507–512.

Leibovitch I, Huilgol SC, Selva D, et al. Microcystic adnexal carcinoma: treatment with Mohs micrographic surgery. J Am Acad Dermatol 2005; 52:295–300.

Ohtsuka H, Nagamatsu S. Microcystic adnexal carcinoma: review of 51 Japanese patients. Dermatology 2002; 204:190–193.

Ong T, Liew SH, Mulholland B, Davis P, Calonje E. Microcystic adnexal carcinoma of the eyebrow. Ophthal Plast Reconstr Surg 2004; 20:122–125.

Schwarze HP, Loche F, Lamant L, Kutchta J, Baze J. Microcystic adnexal carcinoma induced by multiple radiation therapy. Int J Dermatol 2000; 39:369–372.

Snow S, Madjar DD, Hardy S, et al. Microcystic adnexal carcinoma: report of 13 cases and review of the literature. Dermatol Surg 2001; 27:401–408.

Milia

INTRODUCTION   Milia are common tiny keratin-filled epidermoid cysts that occur as a result of occlusion of pilosebaceous units. Milia commonly occur in patients of all ages. Primary milia are seen in infants, and are believed to arise in sebaceous glands that are not fully developed. They occur on the face, associated with vellus hair follicles. They are so common as to be considered normal. In adults they may occur spontaneously or secondary to damage to the pilosebaceous unit as from trauma, radiotherapy, skin infections, surgery, or bullous diseases. A rare variant of primary milia, milia en plaque, is a distinct entity with multiple lesions arising from a base of inflammatory epithelium.

CLINICAL PRESENTATION   Milia on the eyelids are asymptomatic except for cosmetic concerns. They present as multiple, superficial, uniform, firm, pearly white to yellowish lesions. They range in size from 1 to 3 mm in diameter and usually appear on the face, commonly affecting the eyelids. Milia en plaque usually occurs in the preauricular region, but can occur on the eyelids. Multiple small papules arise on an erythematous plaque.

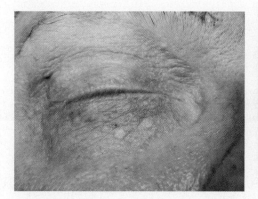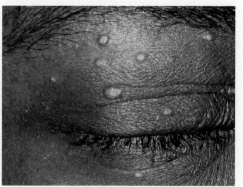

HISTOPATHOLOGY   Milia are miniature epidermoid cysts present in the superficial dermis, usually measuring 1 to 3 mm in diameter. As with epidermoid cysts, the lining is keratinized, stratified squamous epithelium and keratohyaline granules are often prominent in the cells nearer the cyst lumen. Laminated keratin fills the cyst lumen.

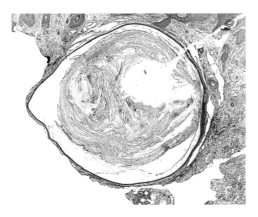 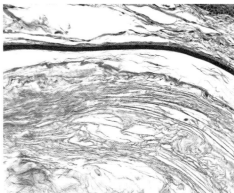

DIFFERENTIAL DIAGNOSIS   The lesions most commonly confused with milia are acne vulgaris, syringoma, and trichoepithelioma.

TREATMENT   No topical or systemic medications are effective. Primary milia tend to resolve spontaneously within the first few weeks of life. Lesions in older children and in adults tend to persist. Although they can safely be left alone, if treatment is desired then simple incision with the cutting edge of a needle with expression of the contents is very effective. Electrodessication and cryotherapy have also been advocated. Milia en plaque is treated with manual expression and minocycline.

REFERENCES

Alapati U, Lynfield Y. Multiple papules on the eyelids. Primary milia. Arch Dermatol 1999; 135:1545–1548.
Bridges AG, Lucky AW, Hanley G, Mutasim DF. Milia en plaque of the eyelids in childhood: case report and review of the literature. Pediatr Dermatol 1998; 15:282–284.
Ratnavel RC, Handfield-Jones SE, Norris PG. Milia restricted to the eyelids. Clin Exp Dermatol 1995; 20:153–154.
Thami GP, Kaur S, Kanwar AJ. Surgical pearl: enucleation of milia with a disposable hypodermic needle. J Am Acad Dermatol 2002; 47:602–603.

Molluscum Contagiosum

INTRODUCTION   Molluscum contagiosum is a common viral skin disease caused by a large intracytoplasmic DNA poxvirus that causes the epidermal cells to undergo decreased transit time. Infection usually arises from direct contact or fomites in children, and by sexually transmitted routes in young adults. The incubation period is usually about two weeks. Specific antibodies are present in 87% of affected patients by immunofluorescence.

CLINICAL PRESENTATION   The characteristic molluscum lesion appears as a raised, smooth, shiny, dome-shaped, white-to-pink nodule 1 to 5 mm in diameter with a central umbilication filled with cheesy material that is easily expressed. Rarely a single lesion will grow as large as 3 cm in diameter (a so-called giant molluscum). Lesions may be single, but more typically are multiple (less than 50) because of the autoinoculable nature of the infection. Lesions may occur in the periocular region and, if found on the eyelid margin, may produce a follicular conjunctival reaction. Other ocular manifestations include epithelial keratitis, pannus formation, conjunctival scarring, and punctal occlusion. Primary conjunctival or limbal lesions may rarely occur. Patients who have acquired immunodeficiency syndrome often have an atypical presentation of molluscum contagiosum. Disseminated disease may be present and lesions are often more confluent. Such patients may have 30 to 40 lesions on each eyelid.

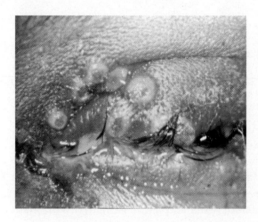 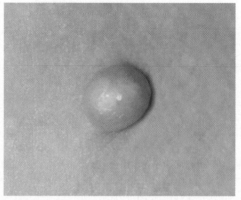

HISTOPATHOLOGY   Lesions of molluscum contagiosum consist of inverted lobules of hyperplastic epidermis expanding into the underlying dermis. Fine septa of dermis separate lobules. Infected keratinocytes have eosinophilic inclusions that occupy almost the entire cell. The inclusion bodies begin to form in keratinocytes just above the basal layer, and they progressively enlarge towards the epidermal surface. The inclusions may become basophilic near the skin surface. The viral inclusion bodies (molluscum bodies) and keratinous debris are extruded into dilated ostia leading to the skin surface.

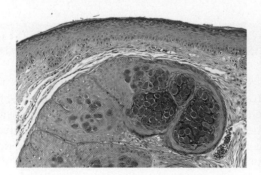 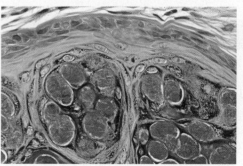

DIFFERENTIAL DIAGNOSIS   The differential diagnosis includes intradermal nevus, verruca vulgaris, milia, syringoma, keratoacanthoma, sarcoid, trichoepithelioma, and basal cell carcinoma.

TREATMENT   Molluscum may frequently resolve spontaneously in immunocompetent hosts within 3 to 12 months. However, some form of treatment is generally required to prevent corneal complications, reduce transmission, and speed recovery. Various treatment options are available including simple unroofing and curettage, chemical cautery with trichloractetic acid, cryosurgery, and electrodessication. Treatment is more difficult in AIDS patients because of extensive involvement and recurrences. Hyperfocal cryotherapy may be effective in this setting.

REFERENCES

Epstein W, Senecal I, Mossing A. An antigen in lesions of Molluscum contagiosum. Nature 1961; 191:509.

Friedman-Kien A. In: Demis D, ed. Clincial Dermatology. Vol. 3. Philadelphia: Harper & Row, 1984, Unit 14–13.

Gonnering RS, Kronish JW. Treatment of periorbital molluscum contagiosum by incision and curettage. Ophthalmic Surg 1988; 19:325–327.

Gottlieb SL, Myskowski PL. Molluscum contagiosum. Int J Dermatol 1994; 33:453–461.

Ingraham HJ, Schoenleber DB. Epibulbar molluscum contagiosum. Am J Ophthalmol 1998; 125:394–396.

Neva FA. Studies on molluscum contagiosum. Arch Intern Med 1972; 110:720–725.

North RD. Presumptive viral keratoconjunctivitis, mononucleosis, and the oncogenic viruses. Intl Ophthalmol Clin 1975; 15:211–227.

Vannas S, Lapinleimn K. Molluscum contagiosum in the skin, caruncle, and conjunctiva. Acta Ophthalmol 1967; 45:314–321.

Zacarian SA. Cryosurgery in the management of cutaneous disorders and malignant tumors of the skin. Comp Ther 1994; 20:329–340.

Mucoepidermoid Carcinoma

INTRODUCTION   Mucoepidermoid carcinoma, also known as *adenosquamous carcinoma*, is a tumor of low- and high-grade malignancy. Low-grade tumors can appear at any age and grow slowly. The high-grade lesions are more infiltrative and metastasize aggressively to the regional lymph nodes and to distant sites. They typically arise from the major and minor salivary gland epithelium and ductal elements, where they account for 10% to 30% of all primary carcinomas. However, they can also arise within the lacrimal and accessory lacrimal gland tissues, lung, esophagus, and upper respiratory tract. It can also rarely present primarily in the skin or arise from the lacrimal sac.

CLINICAL PRESENTATION   On the eyelids, mucoepidermoid carcinomas involve the lacrimal and accessory glands and present as a subconjunctival or less commonly a subcutaneous nodule. The lid margin may be red, thickened, and indurated with telangiectasias and foci of ulceration. The overlying skin can be involved through direct extension and may occasionally be ulcerated. Pain, when present, is more often associated with the high-grade type. If the lacrimal sac is involved presentation is with a medial canthal mass simulating dacryocystitis. In some cases the tumor may arise within the skin from sweat gland epithelium. In such cases a well-circumscribed subepithelial cystic mass is palpable without fixation to the overlying epithelium. Tumor can extend backward into the orbit. Enlarged preauricular lymph nodes may be palpable.

Mucoepidermoid Carcinoma (Contd.)

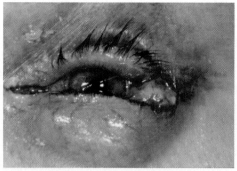

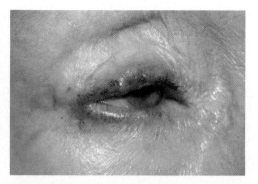

(Courtesy of Seymour Brownstein, M.D. Source: From JW Robinson, S. Brownstein, et al. Conjunctival mucoepidermoid carcinoma in a patient with ocular cicatricial pemphigoid and a review of the literature. Surv Ophthalmol 2006; 51:513–519, with permission of Elsevier.)

(Courtesy of Charles S. Soparkar, M.D.)

HISTOPATHOLOGY   This tumor is composed of a mixture of squamous epithelial cells and mucus-producing goblet cells forming lobules. Goblet cells predominate in well-differentiated tumors and squamous epithelium in poorly-differentiated neoplasms. Mucicarmine stain can be used to highlight the goblet cells, as shown on the right.

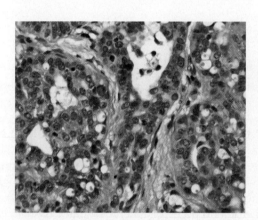

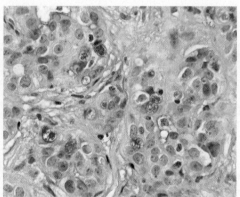

DIFFERENTIAL DIAGNOSIS   The differential diagnosis should include chalazion, squamous cell carcinoma, sebaceous cell carcinoma, mucinous cystadenoma, metastatic tumors, and dacryocystitis.

TREATMENT   Treatment is by complete surgical excision, preferably with Mohs' microsurgery or under frozen section control. Mucoepidermoid carcinoma can have a variety of clinical outcomes but the overall prognosis appears to be related to the tumor grade. For high-grade tumors the five-year survival rate is 25% to 30%, but for low-grade tumors the survival rate climbs to 80% to 95%. Sentinel node biopsy may be useful in cases of high-grade lesions.

REFERENCES

Amara H, Sriha B, Bakir D, et al. Mucoepidermoid carcinoma appearing synchronously in the lacrimal and salivary glands. Rev Stomatol Chir Maxillofac 2001; 102:119–122.

Biswas J, Datta M, Subramaniam N. Mucoepidermoid carcinoma of the conjunctiva of the lower lid—report of a case. Indian J Ophthalmol 1996; 44:231–233.

Dithmar S, Wojno TH, Washyington C, Grossniklaus HE. Mucoepidermoid carcinoma of an accessory lacrimal gland with orbital invasion. Ophthal Plast Reconstr Surg 2000; 16:162–166.

Guzzo M, Andreola S, Sirizzoti G, Cantu B, Cantu G. Mucoepidermoid carcinoma of the salivary glands: clinicopathologic review of 108 patients treated at the National Cancer Institute of Milan. Ann Surg Oncol 2002; 9:688–695.

Herschorn BJ, Jakobiec FA, Hornblass A, Iwamoto T, Harrison WG. Mucoepidermoid carcinoma of the palpebral mucocutaneous junction. A clinical, light microscopic and electron microscopic study of an unusual tubular variant. Ophthalmology 1983; 90:1437–1446.

Johnson DS, Solomon AR, Washngton CV. Mucoepidermoid/adenosquamous carcinoma of the skin: presentation of two cases. Dermatol Surg 2001; 27:1046–1048.

Nouri K, Trent J, Lowell B, Vaitla R, Jimenez GP. Mucoepidermoid carcinoma (adenosquamous carcinoma) treated with Mohs micrographic surgery. Int J Dermatol 2003; 42:957–959.

Riedlinger WF, Hurley MY, Dehner LP, Lind AC. Mucoepidermoid carcinoma of the skin: a distinct entity from adenosquamous carcinoma: a case study with a review of the literature. Am J Surg Pathol 2005; 29:131–135.

Vogel MH. Mucoepidermoid carcinoma of the lid. A clinico-pathologic report of two cases. Ophthalmologica 1977; 174:171–175.

Williams JD, Agrawal A, Wakely PE Jr. Mucoepidermoid carcinoma of the lacrimal sac. Ann Diagn Pathol 2003; 7:31–34.

Wilson MW, Fleming JC, Fleming RM, Haik BG. Sentinel node biopsy for orbital and ocular adnexal tumors. Ophthal Plast Reconstr Surg 2001; 17:338–344.

Zhang C, Ticho KE, Ticho BH, et al. Mucoepidermoid carcinoma of the eyelid skin. Ophthal Plast Reconstr Surg 1999; 15:369–372.

Mucormycosis

INTRODUCTION   Mucormycosis is a rapidly progressive fungal infection that occurs in patients in an immunocompromised state. It is most commonly seen in patients with diabetes complicated by ketoacidosis, leukemia, lymphoma, and severe neutropenia. Occasionally, mucormycosis may be the first manifestation of diabetes. The causative agent of mucormycosis is ubiquitous in nature. The fungus is characterized by the presence of large, pauciseptate hyphae that branch at 90° angles within the involved tissue. The fungus has a propensity towards invasion of blood vessels with infarction of the involved tissue. In ocular adnexal involvement the infection usually starts in the nose, followed by involvement of the paranasal sinuses and then the orbit. If left untreated ocular and brain invasion follows, and the patient succumbs in 7 to 10 days.

CLINICAL PRESENTATION   Orbital involvement is seen in 80% of patients with mucormycosis, and 11% will progress to cavernous sinus thrombosis. Patients usually present with impaired ocular movement, loss of vision, proptosis, chemosis, and periorbital cellulitis. An orbital apex syndrome with blindness and total ophthalmoplegia may be seen. Serous retinal detachment may result from inflammation of the sclera. Rare cases of fungal enophthalmitis result from angioinvasion by fungal hyphae. With eyelid involvement cutaneous lesions may appear as large necrotic and ulcerating lesions with erythematous borders, and oozing black pus. Sinusitis and nasal discharge occur and nasal exam reveals a thick, dark blood-tinged discharge and reddish black necrotic eschar on the turbinates and septum. Cerebral involvement and hemiparesis can be seen in 15% to 20% of cases. Major systemic signs and symptoms include lethargy and headache.

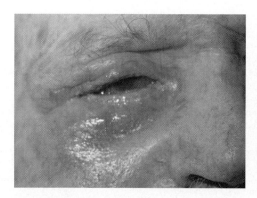 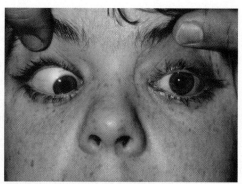

HISTOPATHOLOGY   The hyphae of mucormycosis are broad (5–20 μm), irregularly contoured, pleomorphic, and typically branch at right angles. The hyphae are pauciseptate (not nonseptate, as often described), but septa are only rarely seen in tissue sections and may be simulated by folds in the hyphae. Hyphal walls are thin and usually basophilic in H&E stained sections (shown below on left). The hyphae are often twisted, folded, and collapsed due to their thin walls. Many hyphae have absent cytoplasm and appear clear. Vascular invasion and thrombosis are common with mucormycosis. Gomori's methenamine silver stain highlights the cell walls (shown below on right), but H&E staining is often adequate for diagnosis.

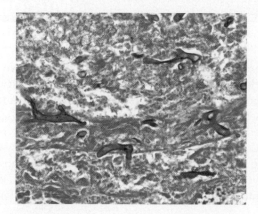 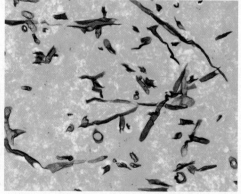

DIFFERENTIAL DIAGNOSIS   The differential diagnosis includes Aspergillosis, orbital cellulitis, preseptal cellulitis, and impetigo.

TREATMENT   The organism grows rapidly on routine laboratory media without cycloheximide; therefore cutaneous lesions should be cultured. Treatment of mucormycosis requires early diagnosis and aggressive surgical debridement of the sinuses and involved orbital and eyelid tissues. Orbital exenteration may be required to prevent extension into the cavernous sinus, but in many cases a more conservative surgical approach with orbital irrigation of amphotericin can be successful. Systemic amphotericin B, and control of the underlying immunocompromised state are necessary for control of the disease. Even then, prognosis is very guarded. Poor prognosis is associated with delayed diagnosis, bilateral involvement, hemiparesis, and renal disease.

REFERENCES

Ali S, Ahmad I. Mucormycosis causing palatal necrosis and orbital apex syndrome. J Coll Physicians Surg Pak 2005; 15:182–183.

Bhansali A, Sharma A, Kashyap A, Gupta A, Dash RJ. Mucor endophthalmitis. Acta Ophthalmol Scand 2001; 79:88–90.

Doty CI, Lucchesi M. Mucormycosis manifesting as proptosis and unilateral blindness. Acad Emerg Med 2000; 7:944–946.

Kim IT, Shim JY, Jung BY. Serous retinal detachment in a patient with rhino-orbital mucormycosis. Jpn J Ophthalmol 2001; 45:301–304.

Paques M, Wassef M, Faucon B, Erginay A, Gaudric A. Bilateral sino-orbital mucormycosis. A case report. J Fr Ophtalmol 2000; 23:1023–1025.

Pelton RW, Peterson EA, Patel BC, Davis K. Successful treatment of rhino-orbital mucormycosis without exenteration: the use of multiple treatment modalities. Ophthal Plast Reconstr Surg 2001; 17:62–66.

Talmi YP, Goldschmied-Reouven A, Bakon M, et al. Rhino-orbital and rhino-orbital-cerebral mucormycosis. Otolaryngol Head Neck Surg 2002; 127:22–31.

Yohai RA, Bullock JD, Aziz AA, Markert RJ. Survival factors in rhino-orbital-cerebral mucormycosis. Surv Ophthalmol 1994; 39:3–22.

Mycosis Fungoides

INTRODUCTION   Mycosis fungoides is a cutaneous T-cell lymphoma with ophthalmic involvement in 30% of cases. The disease typically progresses through three characteristic phases. The first is a pruritic, disseminated, eczematous dermatitis that ultimately progresses to infiltrating and plaque forming lesions and terminates in a tumor phase. Eyelid lesions are usually seen in the later tumor phase. However, the disease may start with skin tumors without a preceding dermatitis. The Sezary syndrome with skin involvement, adenopathy and hepatosplenomegaly represents a leukemic form of mycosis fungoides. In all types, this disease is characterized by a slowly progressive indolent course with episodes of remissions and exacerbations. Ultimately the disease can prove fatal due to involvement of lymph nodes, bone marrow, and visceral organs. Survival ranges from seven months to two years. Death usually results from sepsis or from systemic involvement with lymphoma.

CLINICAL PRESENTATION   The disease begins as a chronic, pruritic, scaling dermatitis. This premycotic stage is represented by an erythematous, eczematous, or psoriasiform dermatitis that slowly progresses into the second, or plaque, stage. In this stage discrete plaques with bizarre configurations and a variable degree of scaling arise on a background of otherwise normal skin. Pruritius and excoriation are common. The third, or tumor, stage is characterized by eyelid tumors and plaques that are indistinguishable from lesions that occur on other body areas. Full-thickness eyelid ulceration with cicatricial ectropion is the most common sequel affecting 40% of patients with ophthalmic involvement. In addition conjunctival and lacrimal tumors, keratitis, corneal ulceration, uveitis, secondary glaucoma, optic atrophy, and papilledema have been reported. Nonspecific findings include cataracts, dry eyes, glaucoma, and ectropion.

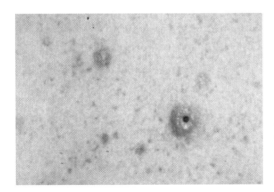 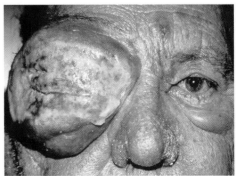

HISTOPATHOLOGY   The patch stage of mycosis fungoides (MF) has subtle histological changes that may include mild hyperkeratosis with focal parakeratosis, basal cell hydropic degeneration, small numbers of atypical irregularly shaped lymphocytes (mycosis cells) in the epidermis surrounded by a halo, atypical lymphocytes palisading ("tagging") along the epidermal-dermal junction, and a superficial perivascular lymphohistiocytic infiltrate. The plaque stage of MF (shown below) usually has compact hyperkeratosis often with patchy parakeratosis, acanthosis, large numbers of atypical lymphocytes in the epidermis, and a predominantly superficial and band-like infiltrate of atypical lymphocytes in the dermis. The tumor stage of MF has a very dense infiltrate of atypical lymphocytes in the dermis and sometimes the subcutis, and there may be epidermal ulceration or slight to absent infiltration of the epidermis by mycosis cells.

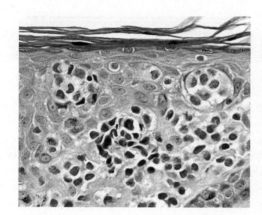 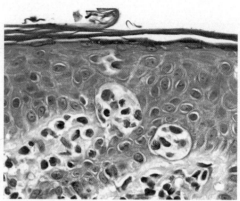

DIFFERENTIAL DIAGNOSIS   The differential diagnosis includes psoriasis, contact dermatitis, discoid lupus, atopic dermatitis and lymphoma.

TREATMENT   Current forms of therapy include topical corticosteroids, systemic chemotherapy, ionizing radiation (x-ray or electron beam), and ultraviolet light with or without psoralen (PUVA). Both topical and systemic steroids are frequently of benefit. Superinfections, viral, bacterial, or fungal, should be watched for and treated appropriately. Eyelid necrosis and ectropion are repaired with standard eyelid reconstructive techniques.

REFERENCES

Cook BE Jr, Barltley GB, Pittelkow MR. Ophthalmic abnormalities in patients with cutaneous T-cell lymphoma. Ophthalmology 1999; 106:1339–1344.

Deutsch AR, Duckworth JK. Mycosis fungoides of upper lid. Am J Ophthalmol 1968; 65:884–888.

Game JA, Davies R. Mycosis fungoides causing severe lower eyelid ulceration. Clin Experimental Ophthalmol 2002; 30:369–371.

Goldberg DF, Negvesky GJ, Butrus SI, Goodglick TA. Ulcerative keratitis in mycosis fungoides. Eye Contact Lens 2005; 31:219–220.

Ing E, Hsieh E, Macdonald D. Cutaneoud T-cell lymphoma with bilateral full-thickness eyelid ulceration. Can J Ophthalmol 2005; 40:467–468.

Patel SP, Holtermann OA. Mycosis fungoides: an overview. J Surg Oncol 1983; 22:221–227.

Probst LE, Burt WL, Heathcote JG. Mycosis fungoides causing lower eyelid ectropion. Can J Ophthalmol 1993; 28:333–338.

Stenson S, Ramsay DL. Ocular findings in mycosis fungoides. Arch Ophthalmol 1981; 99:272–277.

Thiers BH: Controversies in mycosis fungoides. J Am Acad Dermatol 1982; 7:1–16.

INTRODUCTION   Cutaneous myxomas are benign adnexal mesenchymal tumors that may occur in isolation or be associated with Carney syndrome. The latter is a familial disorder characterized by multiple neoplasias including a variety of nonendocrine and endocrine tumors, blue nevi, schwannomas and other neoplasms. CNS aneurysms may be part of the syndrome in some cases. Skin myxomas are seen in 33% of cases, and these often involve the eyelids. Skin lesions are benign with no metastatic potential. The myxoma occurs within the dermis and in 30% of cases basaloid proliferation can be seen in the overlying epidermis.

CLINICAL PRESENTATION   Myxomas present as well-circumscribed usually solitary skin papules that may be sessile or pedunculated. They measure 2–6 mm in size and are flesh-colored to erythematous. They may superficially look like a pyogenic granuloma. When multiple, they are more likely to be associated with Carney syndrome. In this syndrome spotty pigmented lentigines are often present on the face and eyelids which tend to fade with age, generally after the fourth decade. Blue nevi and systemic endocrine abnormalities are also a significant finding in Carney syndrome. Multiple eyelid myxomas may also be seen without any findings suggestive of Carney syndrome and have also been associated with scleromyxedema characterized by myalgias and fatigue along with diffuse cutaneous myxomas. Occasionally the skin lesion may present as a vasculitis due to embolic manifestations.

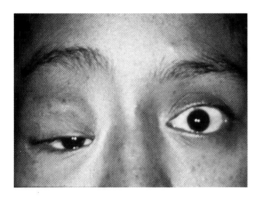 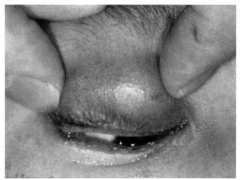

HISTOPATHOLOGY   Myxomas contain scattered small spindle-shaped or stellate-shaped cells within a loose, lightly basophilic to clear, myxoid matrix. The matrix is thought to result from exuberant

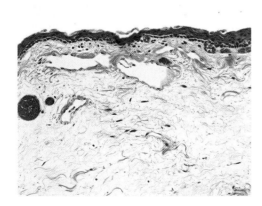 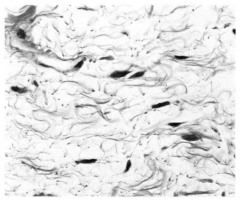

glycosaminoglycan production by the associated fibroblasts. Eyelid myxomas are not encapsulated, and a paucity of blood vessels helps to distinguish them from myxoid liposarcomas and myxoid malignant fibrous histiocytomas. Most eyelid myxomas occur in people with Carney's complex, which includes cardiac myxomas, spotty cutaneous pigmentation, and endocrine overactivity.

DIFFERENTIAL DIAGNOSIS   The differential diagnosis should include lesions that result in cutaneous nodules. These include neurofibroma, fibromyxoid tumors, fibrous histiocytoma, liposarcoma, lipoma, dermatofibroma, and pyogenic granuloma.

TREATMENT   Most eyelid myxomas are associated with Carney syndrome so that these patients are at risk for developing cardiac myxomas which are responsible for a significant mortality rate. Therefore, any patient with a cutaneous myxoma requires a thorough initial and periodic cardiac evaluation with echocardiography. In the absence of a systemic syndrome, cutaneous lesions can be removed surgically. In the context of Carney syndrome excision of the lesion is not curative and new lesions may recur. Excisional biopsy is usually required for diagnosis and to rule out malignancy.

REFERENCES

Abraham Z, Rozenbaum M, Rosner I, Odeh M, Oliver A. Cutaneous eruption in a patient with cardiac myxoma. J Dermatol 1995; 22:276–278.

Allen PW. Myxoma is not a single entity: a review of the concept of myxoma. Ann Diagn Pathol 2000; 4:99–123.

Almeida MQ, Villares MC, Mendonca BB. Carney complex: a case report and literature review. Arq Bras Endocrinol Metabol 2004; 48:544–554.

Craig NM, Putterman AM, Roenigk RK, Wang TD, Roenigk HH. Multiple periorbital cutaneous Myxomas progressing to scleromyxedema. J Am Acad Dermatol 1996; 34:298–230.

Daicker BC. Multiple Myxoma of the eyelid. Ophthalmologica 1979; 179:125–128.

Grossniklaus HE, McLean IW, Gillespie JJ. Bilateral eyelid myxomas in Carney's complex. Br J Ophthalmol 1991; 75:251–252.

Mehregan DR, Thomas L, Thomas JE. Epidermal basaloid proliferation in cutaneous myxomas. J Cutan Pathol 2003; 30:499–503.

Murphy CM, Grau-Massanes M, Snachez RL. Multiple cutaneous Myxomas. Report of a case without other elements of Carney's complex. J Cutan Pathol 1995; 22:556–562.

Srivastava M. Carney complex. Dermatol Online J 2004; 30:10.

Yuen HK, Cheuk W, Luk FO, et al. Solitary superficial angiomyxoma in the eyelid. Am J Ophthalmol 2005; 139:1141–1142.

Necrobiotic Xanthogranuloma

INTRODUCTION   Necrobiotic xanthogranuloma is associated with paraproteimia and with histocytic proliferative disorders. It may be associated with the presence or subsequent development of multiple myeloma or leukemia. Laboratory findings show dysproteinemia due to an IgG paraprotein, leukopenia, greatly elevated ESR, hyperlipidemia, cryoglobulinemia, and depressed complement levels. Most patients have ophthalmic manifestations, mainly affecting the eyelid skin.

CLINICAL PRESENTATION   These lesions present as painless nonpruritic indurated nodules or plaques, which typically extend into the anterior orbital fat, and sometimes involve the extraocular muscles and the lacrimal gland. They may appear either as firm superficial waxy yellowish plaques with prominent telangiectasia, as deeper violaceous plaques, or as flesh-colored nodules. The lesions are usually inflamed and become ulcerated and undergo some degree of scarring. The nodules can cause loss of function of the eyelid with secondary lagophthalmos and corneal exposure and subsequent ulceration. Associated ocular findings include episcleritis, scleritis, keratitis, uveitis, and proptosis.

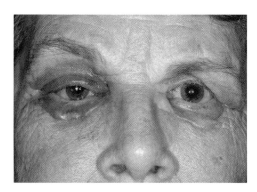
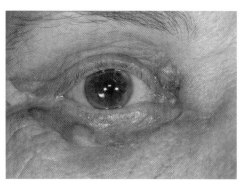

HISTOPATHOLOGY   Necrobiotic xanthogranuloma has areas of diffuse xanthogranulomatous inflammation along with foci of necrotic collagen and other components of the connective tissue ("necrobiosis"). In some areas, there are well-formed granulomas with central necrosis. The necrotic center is amorphous compared to the surrounding tissue and may contain cholesterol clefts. Altered (necrobiotic) collagen often has a hyaline appearance. Palisading epithelioid cells (histiocytes), foam cells (lipid-laden macrophages), Touton giant cells, lymphocytes, and plasma cells surround the necrotic centers. Plasma cells are conspicuous in some biopsies.

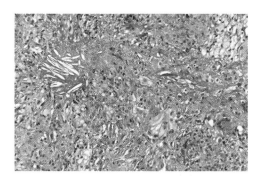
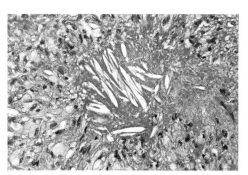

DIFFERENTIAL DIAGNOSIS   The differential diagnosis includes xanthelasma, juvenile xanthogranuloma, and mycosis fungoides.

TREATMENT   Treatment options include local excision, radiotherapy, plasmapheresis, locally injected, topical, or systemic steroids. Systemic or topical chemotherapy, such as chlorambucil, nitrogen mustard, cyclophsphamide, or melphalan may be necessary for the control of any underlying hematologic abnormality. Currently, surgical removal is not recommended because the tumors usually recur with a greater tendency to ulceration and necrosis. Low dose periorbital radiotherapy coupled with high doses of corticosteroids has been used to successfully manage the eyelid lesions.

REFERENCES

Codere F, Lee RD, Anderson RL. Necrobiotic xanthogranuloma of the eyelid. Arch Opthalmol 1983; 101:60–63.

Jakobiec FA, Mills MD, Hidayat AA, et al. Periocular xanthogranulomas associated with sever adult-onset asthma. Trans Am Ophthalmol Soc 1993; 91:99–125.

Kossard S, Winkelmann RK. Necrobiotic xanthogranuloma with paraproteinemia. J Am Acad Dermatol 1980; 3:257–270.

Robertson DM, Winkelmann RK. Ophthalmic features of necrobiotic xanthogranuloma with paraproteinemia. Am J Ophthamol 1984; 97:173–183.

Rodriquez J, Ackerman AB. Xanthogranuloma in adults. Arch Dermatol 1976; 112:43–44.

Rose, GE, Patel BC, Garner A, Wright JE. Orbital xanthogranuloma in adults. Br J Ophthalmol 1991; 75:680–684.

Necrotizing Fasciitis

INTRODUCTION   Necrotizing fasciitis is an uncommon and severe invasive soft tissue infection characterized by cutaneous gangrene, suppurative fasciitis, and vascular thrombosis. The disease is usually preceded by penetrating trauma in patients that have systemic problems, most commonly diabetes, alcoholism, and immunosupression, but may occur after blepharoplasty or other eyelid surgery. Necrotizing fasciitis represents a synergistic polymicrobial soft tissue infection with the release of endogenous cytokines and bacterial toxins. The disease is most frequently attributed to group A *Streptococcus* and *Staphylococcus aureus*. The mortality rate overall is 34%, and for those cases with periorbital involvement it is 12.5%. Death usually results from a fulminant course that may lead to septic shock, respiratory distress syndrome, and renal failure. The average age at time of infection is 57 years, but it may be seen in all age groups.

CLINICAL PRESENTATION   Clinical features include presence of cellulitis with dusky, violaceous discoloration of the eyelid skin, often with bullae formation. Infection of the superficial and deep tissue results in thrombosis of subcutaneous vessels and subsequent necrosis of the overlying skin. Gas crepitation with copious foul-smelling drainage may be present. The patient is febrile and may appear septic. Hypotension, hypercalcemia, and disorientation may also be seen. Complications include

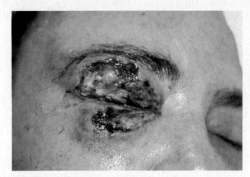

(Courtesy of John Holds, M.D.)

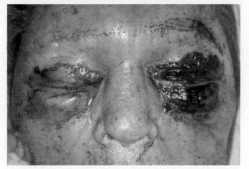

(Courtesy of Grant Gilliland, M.D.)

cicatricial ectropion and subsequent corneal ulceration, and visual loss from orbital invasion and ophthalmic artery occlusions.

HISTOPATHOLOGY   Necrotizing fasciitis is manifest histologically by edema, severe necrosis, and mixed acute and chronic inflammation involving the skin and subcutaneous tissue, including fascial planes. Vasculitis and vascular thrombosis are common, as are skeletal muscle necrosis and colonies of bacteria (illustrated below). Necrotizing cellulitis differs from necrotizing fasciitis by lack of extension of the inflammation and necrosis into the subcutaneous tissue planes.

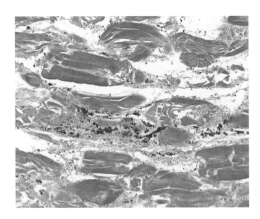 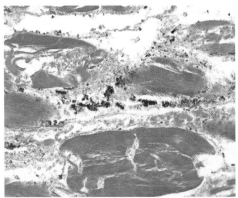

DIFFERENTIAL DIAGNOSIS   The differential diagnosis includes preseptal cellulitis, erysipelas, thermal injury, frostbite, electrical burn, trauma, venom reaction, mucormycosis, anthrax infection, embolic event, or pressure necrosis.

TREATMENT   Treatment necessitates prompt wide surgical debridement of all necrotic fascia, subcutaneous tissue, and muscle. Multiple debridements may be necessary in up to 30% of cases. Broad spectrum parenteral antimicrobial therapy, including penicillin and clindamycin, has been shown to produce higher survival rates. In some cases with only eyelid involvement a more conservative nondestructive debridement and antimicrobial therapy may give good results. Ancillary treatment includes hyperbaric oxygen therapy and intravenous immunoglobulin therapy which can reduce wound morbidity and the overall mortality. Reconstruction usually requires skin grafts to repair the cutaneous defects and resulting cicatricial ectropion.

REFERENCES

Brook I, Frazier EH. Clinical and microbiological features of necrotizing fasciitis. J Clin Microbiol 1995; 33:2382–2387.

Giuliano A, Lewis F Jr, Hadley K, Blaisdell FW. Bacteriology of necrotizing fasciitis. Am J Surg 1977; 134:52–57.

Jordan DR, Mawn L, Marshall DH. Necrotizing fasciitis caused by group A streptococcus infection after laser blepharoplasty. Am J Ophthalmol 1998; 125:265–266.

Kaul R, McGeer A, Low DE, Green K, Schwartz B. Population-based surveillance for group A streptococcal necrotizing fasciitis: clinical features, prognostic indicators, and microbiologic analysis of seventy-seven cases. Ontario Group A Streptococcal Study. Am J Med 1997; 103:18–24.

Knudtson KJ, Gigantelli JW. Necrotizing fasciitis of the eyelids and orbit. Arch Ophthalmol 1998; 116:1548–1549.

Kronish JW, McLeish WM. Eyelid necrosis and periorbital necrotizing fasciitis. Report of a case and review of the literature. Ophthalmology 1991; 98:92–98.

Luksich JA, Holds JB, Hartstein ME. Conservative management of necrotizing fasciitis of the eyelids. Ophthalmology 2002; 109:2118–2122.

Marshall DH, Jordan DR, Gilberg SM, et al. Periocular necrotizing fasciitis. A review of five cases. Ophthalmology 1997; 104:1857–1862.

Poitelea C, Wearne MJ. Periocular necrotizing fasciitis – a case report. Orbit 2005; 24:215–217.

Riseman UJA, Zamboni WA, Curtis A, et al. Hyperbaric oxygen therapy for necrotizing fasciitis reduces mortality and the need for debridement. Surgery 1990; 108:847–850.

Shayegani A, MacFaralane D, Kazim M, Grossman ME. Streptococcal gangrene of the eyelids and orbit. Am J Ophthalmol 1995; 120:784–792.

Suner, IJ, Meldrum ML, Johnson TE, Tse DT. Necrotizing fasciitis after cosmetic blepahroplasty. Am J Ophthalmol 1999; 128:367–68.

Walters R. A fatal case of necrotizing fasciitis of the eyelid. Br J Ophthalmol 1988; 72:428–431.

Neurofibroma

INTRODUCTION   Neurofibromas are neural tumors composed of a proliferation of axons, Schwann cells, and endoneural fibroblasts. They are most commonly considered in the context of neurofibromatosis where patients develop multiple skin lesions in association with other stigmata of the disease, usually apparent by adolescence. Here they are typically multiple, often occurring in large numbers. The neurofibromas may present on any cutaneous surface, and are common on the face. They typically slowly enlarge over many years. Isolated cutaneous neurofibromas may occur in individuals with no other associated systemic abnormalities. In this setting they typically present between 20 and 30 years of age, but have been described in young children as well. They can occur on any part of the body, but are relatively rare in the head and neck.

CLINICAL PRESENTATION   Solitary neurofibromas appear as painless soft, fleshy, slowly enlarging, nodular or occasionally pedunculated masses. They tend to be single, but can also present as multiple masses. Occasionally solitary lesions can occur on the conjunctiva or in the orbit without any cutaneous involvement. In about 25% of solitary lesions there will be a history of systemic neurofibromatosis (NF-1). When associated with NF-1 ocular findings may also include pigmented iris hamartomas (Lisch nodules), glaucoma, retinal astrocytic hamartoma, optic nerve glioma or

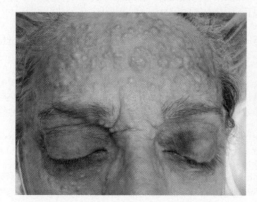
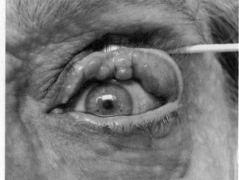

meningioma, pulsating exophthalmos due to defects of the sphenoid wing, and orbital schwannoma. In the absence of neurofibromatosis, there are no other associated findings.

HISTOPATHOLOGY   Cutaneous neurofibromas are nonencapsulated dermal tumors that often extend into the subcutis. A zone of normal dermis usually separates the tumor from the overlying epidermis. Delicate, wavy fascicles, often one-cell thick, comprise the tumor. The tumor cells have oval or elongated nuclei, often undulating, and indistinct cytoplasm. Mild nuclear pleomorphism is sometimes apparent, but mitoses are rare. The tumor matrix usually consists of delicate, wavy collagen fibers, though it may have myxoid or hyalinized areas. If the diagnosis is in doubt, then silver stains or immunohistochemical stains using antibodies to S100 protein or neurofilament protein can be confirmatory.

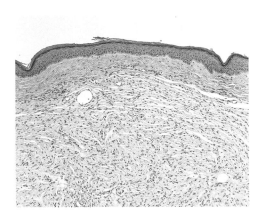 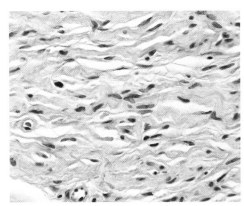

DIFFERENTIAL DIAGNOSIS   The differential diagnosis includes chalazion, intradermal nevus, schwannoma, leiomyoma, granular cell tumor, chondroid syringoma, phakomatous choristoma, fibrous histiocytoma, cysticercosis, dermatofibroma, neurothekeoma, and cutaneous malignancies.

TREATMENT   Isolated cutaneous lesions unrelated to neurofibromatosis may be surgically excised if they are of cosmetic concern, or if they are large enough to cause functional problems with eyelid movement. Since these are benign lesions resection should be subtotal if nerve function is at risk from the surgery. When present in the orbit, proptosis, motility restriction, and visual loss might prompt earlier intervention. Malignant degeneration has not been reported with solitary neurofibromas. In patients with neurofibromatosis, the plexiform and intraneural types of neurofibroma can be precursors of malignant peripheral nerve sheath tumor.

REFERENCES

Brownstein S, Little JM. Ocular neurofibromatosis. Ophthalmology 1983; 90:1595–1599.
Berney C, Spahn B, Oberhansli C, Uffer S, Borruat FX. Multiple intraorbital neurofibromas: a rare cause of proptosis. Klin Monatsbl Augenheilkd 2004; 221:418–420.
Chick G, Alnot JY, Sibermann-Hoffman O. Benign solitary tumors of the peripheral nerves. Rev Chir Orthop Reparatrice Appar Mot 2000; 86:825–834.

Ing EB, Kennerdell JS, Olson PR, Ogino S, Rothfus WE. Solitary fibrous tumor of the orbit. Ophthal Plast Reconstr Surg 1998; 14:57–61.

Kalina PH, Bartley GB, Campbell RJ, Buettner H. Isolated neurofibromas of the conjunctiva. Am J Ophthalmol 1991; 111:694–698.

Lewis RA, Riccardi VM. Von Recklinghausen neurofibromatosis. Ophthalmology 1981; 88:348–354.

Rose GE, Wright JE. Isolated peripheral nerve sheath tumors of the orbit. Eye 1991; 5:668–673.

Shields JA, Shields CL. The systemic hamartomatoses ("Phakomatoses"). In: Mannis MJ, Macsai MS, Huntley AC, eds. Eye and Skin Diseases. Philadelphia: Lippincott-Raven, 1996:367–380.

Woog JJ, Albert DM, Solt LC, Hu DN, Wang WJ. Neurofibromatosis of the eyelid and orbit. Int Ophthalmol Clin 1982; 22:157–187.

Yanoff M, Fine BS. Ocular Pathology, 2nd ed. Philadelphia: Harper & Row, 1984:34.

Nevus Flammeus

INTRODUCTION   Also known as a *port-wine stain*, nevus flammeus is not a vascular neoplasm but a vascular capillary malformation composed of mature telangiectatic vessels. It can be seen commonly at birth as a discrete median and symmetrical vascular lesion that disappears within the first year of life. A more striking form of congenital nevus flammeus is asymmetric and persists throughout life. It can be isolated and unilateral, or associated with ocular and leptomeningeal vascular hamartomas as in the Sturge-Weber syndrome. A lighter-colored pink variant has been called nevus roseus and may be a distinct entity.

CLINICAL PRESENTATION   Nevus flammeus presents as a flat purple or deep red vascular lesion that can vary from only a few millimeters in size to those covering vary large areas. On the face it is usually unilateral and in the distribution of one or more branches of the trigeminal nerve. Unlike other congenital eyelid vascular lesions it does not undergo spontaneous regression. In older adults nevus flammeus can undergo cavernous changes making them elevated and rather prominent. Pyogenic granuloma may arise within a nevus flammeus without any predisposing factors, as can rare cases of basal cell carcinoma. In the presence of Sturge-Weber syndrome associated ocular manifestations include diffuse choroidal hemangioma, ipsilateral glaucoma, and serous retinal detachment. Cases of acquired nevus flammeus have been described following trauma.

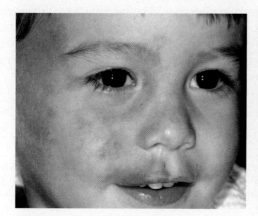
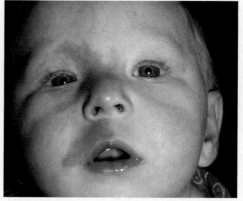

HISTOPATHOLOGY   Both the salmon patch and port wine stains, encompassed by the term nevus flammeus, are characterized histologically by ectatic vessels of variable caliber within the dermis.

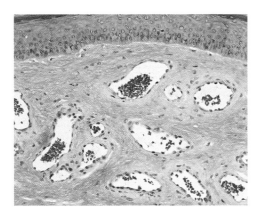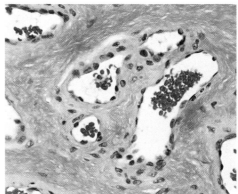

DIFFERENTIAL DIAGNOSIS   The differential diagnosis includes capillary hemangioma, lymphangioma, Nevus of Ota, nevoid telangiectasia syndrome, and eruptive spider nevi.

TREATMENT   Treatment for light colored lesions may be limited to covering them with occlusive make-up. However, Nd:YAG and pulsed dye laser therapy has been successful in treatment of these lesions. While complete eradication of the lesion is rarely accomplished, it can be made significantly lighter and less obvious. Intense pulsed light treatment has proven useful in cases resistant to laser therapy. The effectiveness of laser treatment is related to variations in skin thickness, being less beneficial in areas of thicker skin such as the midface area. Tissue hypertrophy that is sometimes associated with these lesions will remain. Surgical resection with full-thickness grafts are used less often than in the past.

REFERENCES

Bjerring P, Christiansen K, Troilius A. Intense pulsed light source for the treatment of dye laser resistant port-wine stains. J Cosmet Laser Ther 2003; 5:7–13.

Cosman B. Experience in the argon laser therapy of port-wine stains. Plas Reconst Surg 1980; 65:119–129.

Font RL, Ferry AP. The phakomatosis. Int Ophthalmol Clin 1972; 12:1–50.

Goldman L, Dreffer R. Laser treatment of extensive mixed cavernous port-wine stains. Arch Dermatol 1977; 113:504–505.

Happle R. Nevus roseus: a distinct vascular birthmark. Eur J Dermatol 2005; 15:231–234.

Jacobs AH, Walton RG. The incidence of birthmarks in the neonate. Pediatrics 1976; 58:218–222.

Levy R, Fisher M. In: Demis D, ed. Clinical Dermatology. Vol. 2. Philadelphia: Harper & Row, 1984, Unit 7–63.

Lindsey PS, Shields JA, Goldberg RE, Augsburger JJ, Frank PE. Bilateral choroidal hemangiomas and facial nevus flammeus. Retina 1981; 1:88–95.

Noe JM, Barsky SH, Geer DE, Rosen S. Port-wine stains and the response to argon laser therapy: successful treatment and predictive role of color, age, and biopsy. Plast Reconstr Surg 1980; 65:130–136.

Pence B, Aybey B, Ergenekon G. Outcomes of 532 nm frequency-doubled Nd:YAG laser use in the treatment of port-wine stains. Dermatol Surg 2005; 31:509–517.

Senti G, Trueb RM. Acquired naevus flammeus (Fegeler syndrome) Vasa 2000; 29:225–228.

Sheehan DJ, Lesher JL Jr. Pyogenic granuloma arising within a port-wine stain. Cutis 2004; 73:175–180.

Tan OT, Gilchrest BA. Laser therapy for selected cutaneous vascular lesions in the pediatric population: a review. Pediatrics 1988; 82:652–662.

Nodular Fasciitis

INTRODUCTION   Nodular fasciitis is a benign reactive proliferation of fibroblasts in the subcutaneous tissues. It is also referred to as *subcutaneous pseudosarcomatous fibromatosis* or *proliferative fasciitis*. It is seen most commonly in young individuals between 30 and 40 years of age, with about 10% occurring in children. The cause is unknown, but in some cases there may be a history of trauma. It is believed that they may be triggered by a local injury or inflammatory process. Because of the rich cellularity, mitotic activity, and rapid growth these lesions are often misdiagnosed as a sarcoma. Occasionally metaplastic bone formation may occur within the lesion in which case they may be referred to as ossifying fasciitis.

CLINICAL PRESENTATION   Nodular fasciitis presents as a small rapidly growing, solitary, grey to white solid lesion in the subcutaneous tissue that may be flat or slightly elevated. In about one-third of cases there may be associated pain or tenderness. Rarely, they may arise in Tenon's capsule or conjunctiva, or in the deep orbit.

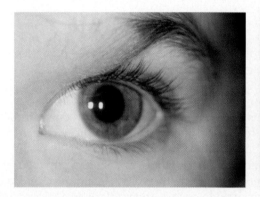 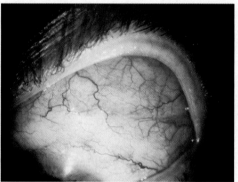

(Courtesy of Gordon K. Klintworth, M.D.)

HISTOPATHOLOGY   Nodular fasciitis is characterized by a proliferation of spindle-shaped to plump fibroblasts that tend to be haphazardly arranged. A vague storiform (cartwheel) pattern is sometimes present focally. Mitoses are frequent, but atypical mitotic figures are rare. Cleft-like spaces between fibroblasts may be seen (shown below). Capillaries within the lesion commonly have plump endothelial cells. The tumors are very cellular and collagen is typically sparse. Lymphocytes are scattered throughout the tumor, though they are not abundant.

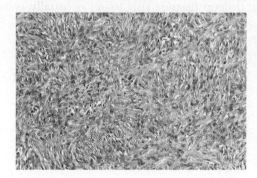 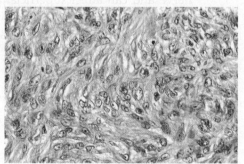

DIFFERENTIAL DIAGNOSIS   The differential diagnosis includes benign tumors such as fibrous histiocytoma, epidermal hyperplasia, neurofibroma, and spindle cell lipoma. They can also be mistaken for malignant lesions including leiomyosarcoma, fibrosarcoma, and malignant peripheral nerve sheath tumors.

TREATMENT   Treatment is not necessary since these are benign with no potential for metastatic spread. However, because of their rapid initial growth, biopsy or excision is usually performed. Spontaneous resolution has been reported, and intralesional steroid injection has been reported to result in rapid regression.

REFERENCES

Graham BS, Barrett TL, Goltz RW. Nodular fasciitis: response to intralesional corticosteroids. J Am Acad Dermatol 1999; 40:490–492.

Haas AF. Nodular fasciitis of the forehead. Dermatol Surg 1999; 25:140–142.

Handa Y, Asai T, Tomita Y. Nodular fasciitis of the forehead in a pediatric patient. Dermatol Surg 2003; 29:867–868.

Hymas DC. Mamalis N, Pratt DV, Scott MH, Anderson RL. Nodular fasciitis of the lower eyelid in a pediatric patient. Ophthal Plast Reconstr Surg 1999; 15:139–142.

Meffert JJ, Kennard CD, Davis TL, Quinn BD. Intradermal nodular fasciitis presenting as an eyelid mass. Int J Dermatol 1996; 35:548–552.

Novakova FN, Hejemanova D, Nozicka Z. Nodular fasciitis—rare localization on the eye (a case report). Cesk Slov Oftalmol 2004; 60:368–372.

Perry RH, Ramani PS, McAllister V, Kalbag RM, Kanagasundaram CR. Nodular fasciitis causing unilateral proptosis. Br J Ophthalmol 1975; 59:404–408.

Ruoppi P, Vornanen M, Nuutinen J. A rapidly progressing periorbital mass in an infant: fasciitis nodularis. Acta Otolaryngol 2004; 124:324–327.

Schmidt JG, Krueger GR, Brusis T. Nodular fasciitis of the orbit. Klin Monatsbl Augenheilkd 1984; 184:213–215.

Silva P, Bruce IA, Malik T, Homer J, Banerjee S. Nodular fasciitis of the head and neck. J Laryngol Otol 2005; 119:8–11.

Stone DU, Chodosh J. Epibulbar nodular fasciitis associated with floppy eyelids. Cornea 2005; 24:361–362.

Vestal KP, Bauer TW, Berlin AJ. Nodular fasciitis presenting as an eyelid mass. Ophthal Plast Reconstr Surg 1990; 6:130–132.

Oculodermal Melanocytosis

INTRODUCTION   Also known as *nevus of Ota* or *nevus fuscocaeruleus ophthalmomaxillaris*, this lesion arises from dermal melanocytes. It typically affects tissues along the distribution of the trigeminal nerve and can affect superficial and deep tissues. This lesion is usually congenital, but later onset in puberty or during pregnancy has been reported. Women, especially Asian or black, are most commonly affected. Malignant degeneration may occur, particularly in whites, with the intraocular choroidal tissue being the most common site of involvement. Isolated ocular involvement without skin discoloration may occur and is termed *ocular melanocytosis* (*melanosis oculi*).

CLINICAL PRESENTATION   The lesion appears as a flat blue-to-purple mottled pigmentation of the skin. It tends to follow the distribution of the ophthalmic and maxillary divisions of the trigeminal nerve. It is associated with ipsilateral ocular melanocytosis that can variously involve the conjunctiva, sclera, and uveal tract. Other ipsilateral involved tissues may be orbital fat and muscles, bone, periorbita, dura, and brain. The nevus tends to be unilateral, but bilateral involvement may occur. Pigmentation is irregular and may occur in small isolated disconnected patches. It may be so pale as to be overlooked on casual observation. Glaucoma can be an associated finding. Intraocular nevi, choroidal malignant melanoma, and orbital melanoma may occur.

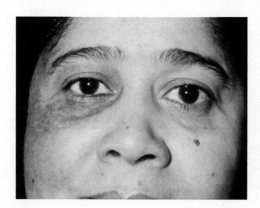
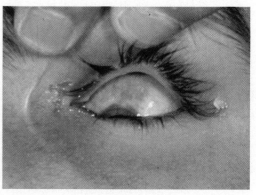

HISTOPATHOLOGY   Heavily-pigmented melanocytes in the upper and mid-dermis characterize oculodermal melanocytosis. The melanocytes are spindle-shaped, bipolar, or dendritic, and they tend to be oriented parallel to the skin surface but may also surround epidermal appendages. The epidermis may also be hyperpigmented.

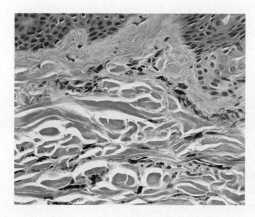
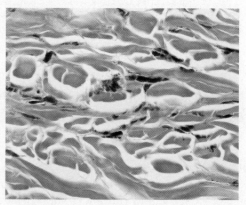

DIFFERENTIAL DIAGNOSIS   The differential diagnosis includes lentigo, malasma, malignant melanoma, osteogenesis imperfecta, ochronosis, and blue nevus.

TREATMENT   Camouflage make-up may mask the lesion when limited and pale in color. Intense pulsed light therapy or pulsed dye lasers may diminish the degree of pigmentation. Periodic dilated fundus examination is important to rule out uveal melanoma.

REFERENCES

Dutton JJ, Anderson RL, Schelper RL, Purcell JJ, Tse DT. Orbital malignant melanoma and oculodermal melanocytosis: report of two cases and review of the literature. Ophthalmology 1984; 91:497–507.

Foulks GN, Shields MB. Glaucoma in oculodermal melanocytosis. Ann Ophthalmol 1977; 9:1299–1304.

Gonder JR, Shields JA, Albert DM, Augsburger JJ, Lavin PT. Uveal malignant melanoma associated with ocular and oculodermal melanocytosis. Ophthalmology 1982; 89:953–960.

Gonder JR, Shields JA, Albert DM. Malignant melanoma of the choroid associated with oculodermal melanocytosis. Ophthalmology 1981; 88:372–376.

Hamilton RF, Weiss JS, Gelender H. Posterior corneal pigmentation in melanosis oculi. Arch Ophthalmol 1983; 101:1909–1911.

Pomeranz GA, Bunt AH, Kalina RE. Multifocal choroidal melanoma in ocular melanocytosis. Arch Ophthalmol 1981; 99: 857–863.

Sagar HJ, Ilgren LB, Adams CB. Nevus of Ota associated with meningeal melanosis and intracranial melanoma. Case Report. J Neurosurg 1983; 58:280–283.

Sang DN, Albert DM, Sober AJ, McMeekin TO. Nevus of Ota with contralateral cerebral melanoma. Arch Ophthalmol 1977; 95:1820–1824.

Skalka H. Bilateral oculodermal melanocytosis. Ann Ophthalmol 1976; 5:565–567.

Papilloma

INTRODUCTION

A papilloma is any lesion that is papillomatous in growth pattern: that is a smooth, rounded, or pedunculated elevation. The squamous papilloma is a generic term for any papilloma of nonviral origin. Also known as a *fibroepithelial polyp, acrochordon,* or *skin tag*, this neoplasm commonly occurs on the eyelid, neck, axilla, and groin. This is a benign tumor of squamous epithelial origin, and this is the most common benign lesion found on the eyelid, representing 15% to 30% of all benign lesions on the lids. It can be seen at any age but occurs most frequently in patients over the age of 30 years.

CLINICAL PRESENTATION

Papillomas on the eyelid present as small 2 to 3 mm flesh-colored sessile or pedunculated masses. They may be single or multiple. Occasionally they can develop on the palpebral or bulbar conjunctiva. They typically have thickened hyperkeratotic epithelium and may show multiple finger-like projections. On close examination it may be possible to identify a central vascular core.

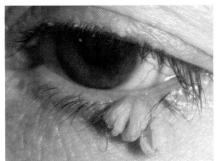
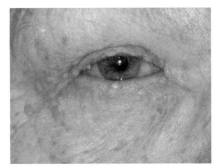
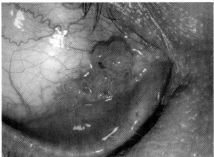

(Courtesy of Charles S. Soparkar, M.D.)

HISTOPATHOLOGY   Papillomas (acrochordons; skin tags) are highly variable histologically. Furrowed papules are most common on the eyelids and are characterized histologically by epidermal hyperplasia with a seborrheic keratosis-like appearance, as illustrated here. The hyperplastic epidermis forms interdigitating cords. Horn cysts may be present, though they are not common.

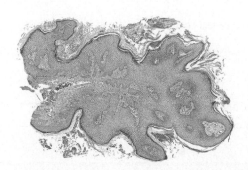 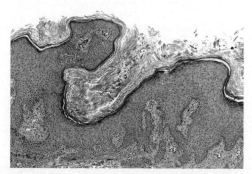

DIFFERENTIAL DIAGNOSIS   The differential diagnosis includes seborrheic keratosis, actinic keratosis, verruca vulgaris, intradermal nevus, keratoacanthoma, and sebaceous carcinoma. Occasionally malignant lesions can look like a papilloma, but these more often have telangiectatic vessels or are associated with lash loss or ulceration.

TREATMENT   Treatment may be indicated for large lesions that interfere with vision or cause ocular irritation, or for lesions of cosmetic concern. Removal is by simple surgical excision or light electrodessication. If the base is broad, a shave biopsy may be appropriate in order to preserve the lid margin and lash line, even though recurrence may be expected over several years.

REFERENCES

Abdi U, Tyagi N, Maheshwari V, Gogi R, Tyagi SP. Tumours of eyelid: a clinicopathologic study. J Indian Med Assoc 1996; 94:405–409.

D'hermies F, Morel X, Bourgade JM, et al. Hyperkeratosis papilloma of the eyelid. An anatomic clinical case. J Fr Ophtalmol 2001; 24:558–561.

Domonkos AN, Arnold HL, Odom RB, eds. Andrew's Diseases of the Skin. Philadelphia: Saunders, 1982:773.

Khong JJ, Leibovitch I, Selva D, Dodd T, Muecke J. Sebaceous gland carcinoma of the eyelid presenting as a conjunctival papilloma. Clin Experiment Ophthalmol 2005; 33:197–198.

Ni Z. Histopathological classification of 3,510 cases with eyelid tumor. Zhonghua Yan Ke Za Zhi 2006; 32:435–437.

Older JJ. Eyelid tumors. Clinical Diagnosis and Surgical Treatment. New York: Raven Press, 1987:37–38.

INTRODUCTION   Pemphigus vulgaris is an acquired autoimmune disease in which IgG antibodies are targeted against desmosomal proteins. This results in intraepithelial mucocutaneous blistering. It occurs at all ages but with a peak frequency in the third to sixth decades. Lesions almost always begin on mucous membranes and then spread to involve the skin. Any part of the body can be involved with the eye and eyelids being rather rare.

CLINICAL PRESENTATION   Lesions present with mucocutaneous erosions or blisters. In the majority of cases the oral mucosa is the first site of involvement. It extends to involve the skin within several months. Ocular involvement almost always follows involvement of the skin and mucosa elsewhere on the body and is usually limited to the conjunctiva, the eyelids, or both. The eyelid is thickened and indurated with erosions, papules, or blisters on the lid margin and the conjunctiva. These may be associated with conjunctival injection, reflex epiphora, and pain. Skin lesions can appear as yellowish crusted areas. Visual acuity may not be affected, but in severe cases corneal opacity can occur. Late sequelae can include conjunctival cicatrization, corneal ulceration, and perforation.

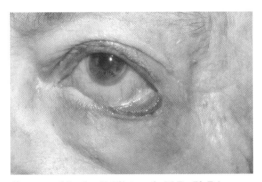

(Courtesy of Gordon K. Klintworth, M.D., Ph.D.)

HISTOPATHOLOGY   The earliest changes in pemphigus vulgaris are epidermal edema and disappearance of the intercellular bridges between keratinocytes in the lower epidermis. Keratinocytes dissociate (acantholysis) with resultant formation of suprabasal bullae, which are characteristic of established lesions. Basal epidermal cells separate from each other due to loss of intracellular bridges, but they remain attached to the dermis. The dermis has a mild mixed acute and chronic inflammatory infiltrate that usually includes scattered eosinophils. The diagnosis is established by the direct immunofluorescence demonstration of IgG in the intercellular regions of the epidermis, creating a basket-weave pattern (shown below).

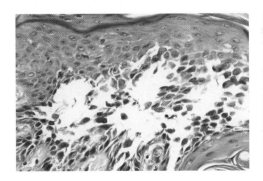
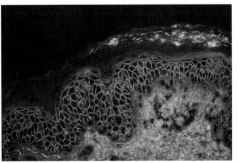

DIFFERENTIAL DIAGNOSIS   In the differential diagnosis one should consider bullous pemphigoid, cicatricial pemphigoid, actinic keratosis, and malignant skin tumors.

TREATMENT   Initial treatment is aimed at inducing a clinical remission, and then to establish a maintenance therapy to minimize outbreaks. Systemic corticosteroids are the mainstay of treatment in doses of 40 to 100 mg per day of prednisone depending on the severity of the disease. Cessation of blisters is seen within two to three weeks and healing of lesions within eight weeks. Adjuvant drugs such as azathioprine and cyclophosphamide have been advocated to reduce the steroid dose. Rarely, for disease confined to mucosal surfaces topical therapy alone may be useful. Recurrences are common.

REFERENCES

Baykal HE, Pleyer U, Sonnichsen K, Thiel HJ, Zierhut M. Severe eye involvement in pemphigus vulgaris. Ophthalmologie 1995; 92:854–857.

Bianciotto C, Herreras Cantalapiedra JM, Alvarez MA, Mendez Diaz MC. Conjunctival blistering associated with pemphigus vulgaris: report of a case. Arch Soc Esp Oftalmol 2005; 80:365–368.

Daoud YJ, Cervantes R, Foster CS, Ahmed AR. Ocular pemphigus. J Am Acad Dermatol 2005; 53:585–590.

Harman KE, Albert S, Black MM. Guidelines for the management of pemphigus vulgaris. Br J Dermatol 2003; 149:926–937.

Lifshitz T, Levy J, Cagnano E, Halevy S. Severe conjunctival and eyelid involvement in pemphigus vulgaris. Int Ophthalmol 2004; 25:73–74.

Lisch K. Bullous dermatoses with special reference to the symptomatology of the eyelids in pemphigus vulgaris. Klin Monatsbl Augenheilkd 1983; 183:493–496.

Marinovic B, Bukvic Mokos ZB, Basta-Juzbasic A, et al. Atypical clinical appearance of pemphigus vulgaris on the face: case report. Acta Dermatolvenerol Croat 2005; 13:233–236.

Sehgal VN, Sharma S, Sardana K. Unilateral refractory (erosive) conjunctivitis: a peculiar manifestation of pemphigus vulgaris. Skinmed 2005; 4:250–252.

Seishima M, Oyama Z, Shimizu H, et al. Pemphigus of the eyelids. Eur J Dermatol 2001; 11:141–143.

Phakomatous Choristoma

INTRODUCTION   Phakomatous choristoma, also known as *Zimmerman's tumor,* is a benign congenital adnexal hamartoma of lens tissue. It is seen at birth or shortly thereafter and three-fourths of patients are male. It likely develops from an abnormal migration of cells from the lenticular anlage into the mesodermal structures of the eyelid. Inferior cells of this presumptive lens tissue may become displaced as choristomatous elements into the embryonic mesenchyme destined to become the lower eyelid or anterior orbit. Alternatively, it may represent an additional locus of lens vesicle in the primitive surface ectoderm. The lesion may initially enlarge in an abortive attempt to form a lens.

CLINICAL PRESENTATION   Phakomatous choristoma appears in newborns or in young children usually within the first few months of life and not associated with other developmental abnormalities. It presents as a circumscribed firm to rubbery subcutaneous mass in the medial lower eyelid near the inner canthus and can occasionally occur in or extend to the anterior orbit. They may range up to several centimeters in size. When large there may be concern about amblyopia or astigmatism.

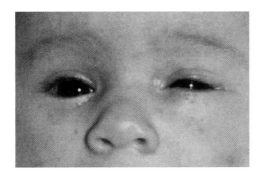

(Courtesy of Stefan Seregard, M.D. Source: From Seregard S. Phakomatous choristoma may be located in the eyelid or orbit or both. Acta Ophthal Scand 1999; 77: 343–346, with permission of Wiley-Blackwell Publishing, Oxford, U.K.)

HISTOPATHOLOGY   Within dense collagenous tissue are nests and irregular islands of polygonal epithelial cells having lightly eosinophilic cytoplasm and round to oval nuclei without nucleoli. The nests and islands of epithelial cells are surrounded by basement membrane material that stains positively with periodic acid-Schiff reagent (PAS stain), and thick strands of PAS-positive material often accumulate between cells (shown below on the right). Swollen epithelial cells may resemble "bladder cells" occurring in cataractous crystalline lenses, and brightly eosinophilic material resembling cataractous lens fibers forms pools within the epithelial islands. Dystrophic calcification and psammoma bodies may be present.

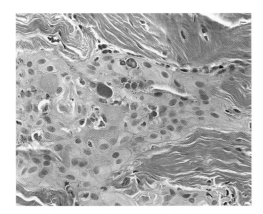 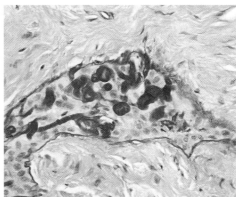

DIFFERENTIAL DIAGNOSIS   The differential diagnosis should consider any mass lesion that can occur in the medial canthus of young children. These include dacryocystocele, dermoid cyst, adnexal neoplasms, or cutaneous carcinomas.

TREATMENT   Since phakomatous choristomas are completely benign and frequently stable in size, aggressive and potentially damaging surgery to the lacrimal drainage system is not indicated. Excision is usually performed for diagnostic purposes to rule out more serious conditions. Conservative excision is warranted in most cases. Even when incompletely removed lesions do not recur.

REFERENCES

Baggesen LH, Jensen OA. Phakomatous choristoma of lower eyelid. A lenticular anlage tumour. Ophthalmologica 1977; 175:231–235.

Blenc AM, Gomez HA, Lee MW, Torres FX, Linder JS. Phakomatous choristoma: a case report and review of the literature. Am J Dermatopathol 2000; 22:55–59.

Dithmar S, Schmack I, Volcker HE, Grossniklaus HE. Phakomatous choristoma of the eyelid. Graefes Arch Clin Exp Ophthalmol 2004; 242:40–43.

Ellis FJ, Eagle RC Jr, Shields JA, et al. Phakomatous choristoma (Zimmerman's tumor). Immunohistochemical confirmation of lens-specific proteins. Ophthalmology 1993; 100:955–960.

Eustis HS, Karciogly ZA, Dharma S, Hoda S. Phakomatous choristoma: clinical, histopathologic, and ultrastructural findings in a 4-month-old boy. J Pediatr Ophthalmol Strabismus 1990; 27:208–211.

Filipic M, Silva M. Phakomatous choristoma of the eyelid: a tumor of lenticular anlage. Arch Ophthalmol 1972; 88:172–175.

Greer CH. Phakomatous choristoma of the eyelid. Aust J Ophthalmol 1975; 3:106–107.

Kamada Y, Sakata A, Nakadomari S, Takehana M. Phakomatous choristoma of the eyelid: immunohistochemical observation. Jpn J Ophthalmol 1998; 42:41–45.

Leatherbarrow B, Nerad JA, Carter KD, Pe'er J, Spencer J. Phakomatous choristoma of the orbit: a case report. Br J Ophthalmol 1992; 76:507–508.

McMahon RT, Font RL, McLean IW. Phakomatous choristoma of eyelid: electron microscopical confirmation of lenticular derivation. Arch Ophthalmol 1996; 94:1778–1781.

Mencia-Gutierrez E, Gutierrez-Diaz E, Ricoy JR, Sarmiento-Torres B. Eyelid phakomatous choristoma. Eur J Ophthalmol 2003; 13:482–485.

Peres LC, da Silva AR, Belluci AD, Cruz AA. Phakomatous choristoma of the orbit. Orbit 1998; 17:47–53.

Rosenbaum PS, Kress Y, Slamovits TL, Font L. Phakomatous choristoma of the eyelid. Immunohistochemical and electron microscopic observations. Ophthalmology 1992; 99:1779–1784.

Seregard S. Phakomatous choristoma may be located in the eyelid or orbit or both. Acta Ophthalmol Scand 1999; 77:343–346.

Shin HM, Song HG, Choi MY. Phakomatous choristoma of the eyelid. Korean J Ophthalmol 1999; 13:133–137.

Sinclair-Smith CC, Emms M, Morris HB. Phakomatous choristoma of the lower eyelid. A light and ultrastructural study. Arch Pathol Lab Med 1989; 113:1175–1177.

Szyfelbein K, Kozakewicz HP, Syed NA, Zemowicz A. Phakomatous choristoma of the eyelid: a report of a case. J Cutan Pathol 2004; 31:506–508.

Thaung C, Bonshek RE, Leatherbarrow B. Phakomatous choristoma of the eyelid: a case with associated eye abnormalities. Br J Ophthalmol 2006; 90:245–246.

Tripathi RC, Tripathi BJ, Ringus J. Phakomatous choristoma of the lower eyelid with psammoma body formation: a light and electron microscopic study. Ophthalmology 1981; 88:1198–1206.

Zimmerman LE. Phakomatous choristoma of the eyelid. A tumor of lenticular anlage. Am J Ophthalmol 1971; (1 Pt 2):169–177.

Pilomatrixoma

INTRODUCTION   Also known as a *calcifying epithelioma of Malherbe*, pilomatrixoma is a benign tumor of the hair cortical cells. The lesion tends to occur in children and young adults, with 75% less than 10 years of age. The head and upper extremities are the most common sites of involvement with a significant proportion occurring in the periorbital region, particularly the upper eyelid and brow. Most lesions are misdiagnosed as epidermoid and dermoid cysts, and are unsuspected until histopathologic examination.

CLINICAL PRESENTATION   Usually solitary, these slowing growing lesions appear as a solid or cystic, mobile, subcutaneous nodule with normal overlying skin. They are firm, irregular, masses with the overlying skin showing a pink or blue discoloration. In 15% to 18% of cases the lesion can be associated with pain or inflammation. Stretching the overlying skin taut may reveal a whitish, multifaceted tumor, the so-called "tent sign." Dilated vessels may be seen on the tumor surface.

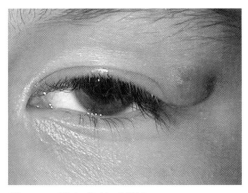 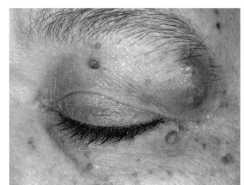

(Courtesy of Peter Rubin, M.D.)

HISTOPATHOLOGY   Pilomatrixomas are composed of islands of basophilic cells surrounding eosinophilic shadow cells. The basophilic cells have little cytoplasm, indistinct cell borders, hyperchromatic nuclei, and abundant mitoses. Eosinophilic shadow cells represent mummified basophilic cells and have more cytoplasm and distinct, though faint, cell borders. There may be abrupt transition from the basophilic cells to the eosinophilic shadow cells, or there may be an intermediate zone of transitional cells that develop progressively more eosinophilic cytoplasm while the nucleus becomes pyknotic. Foci of calcification are very common. Pilomatrixomas are dermal lesions that often extend into the subcutis.

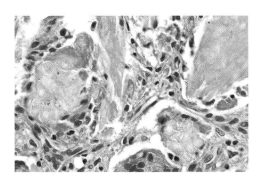 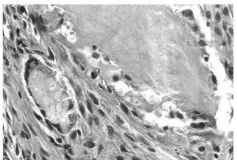

DIFFERENTIAL DIAGNOSIS   Differential diagnosis includes epidermoid and dermoid cysts, sebaceous cyst, squamous cell carcinoma, and vascular lesions.

TREATMENT   These lesions do not regress. Treatment is with surgical excision including the overlying skin. Incomplete removal is associated with recurrence.

REFERENCES

Agarwal RP, Handler SD, Matthews MR, Carpentieri D. Pilomatrixoma of the head and neck in children. Otolaryngol Head and Neck Surg 2001; 125:510–515.

Cahill MT, Moriarty PM, Mooney DJ, Kennedy SM. Pilomatrixoma carcinoma of the eyelid. Am J Ophthalmol 1999; 127:463–464.

Duflo S, Nicollas R, Roman S, Magalon G, Triglia JM. Pilomatrixoma of the head and neck in children: a study of 38 cases and a review of the literature. Arch Otolaryngol Head Neck Surg 1998; 124:1239–1242.

Huerva V, Sanchez MC, Asenjo J. Large, rapidly growing pilomatrixoma of the upper eyelid. Ophthal Plast Reconstr Surg 2006; 22:401–403.

Jang HS, Park JH, Kim MB, Kwon KS, Oh CK. Two case of multiple giant pilomatrixoma. J Dermatology 2000; 24:276–279.

Mathen LC, Olver JM, Cree IA. A large rapidly growing pilomatrixoma on a lower eyelid. Br J Ophthalmol 2000; 84:1203–1204.

Moehlembeck FW. Pilomatrixoma. Arch Dermatol 1973; 108:532–534.

O'Grady R, Spoerl G. Pilomatrixoma (benign calcifying epithelioma of Malherbe). Ophthalmology 1981; 88:1196–1197.

Orlando RG, Rogers GL, Bremer DL. Pilomatrixoma in a pediatric hospital. Arch Ophthalmol 1983; 101:1209–1210.

Perez RC, Nicholson DH. Malherbe's calcifying epithelioma (pilomatrixoma) of the eyelid. Clinical features. Arch Ophthalmol 1979; 97:314–315.

Shields JA, Shields CL, Eagle RC JR, Mulvey L. Pilomatrixoma of the eyelid. J Pediatr Ophthalmol Strabismus 1995; 32: 260–261.

Yap EY, Hoberger GG, Bartley GB. Pilomatrixoma of the eyelids and eyebrows in children and adolescents. Ophthal Plast Reconstruct Surg 1999; 15:185–189.

Plasmacytoma

INTRODUCTION   Malignant plasma cell tumors are divided according to site of origin. They may be multicentric such as multiple myeloma, or localized originating within bone or soft tissue. The latter form is a malignant tumor that is thought to be a separate neoplasm from multiple myeloma with a much better prognosis. Extramedullary plasmacytomas represent 2% to 10% of plasma cell tumors and males are affected three times more often than females. The age at presentation usually lies between the sixth and seventh decades of life. This tumor is more commonly localized in the nasopharynx, oropharynx, gastrointestinal tract, skin, and more rarely in lymph nodes and the spleen. In general, primary plasmacytomas in the eye or periocular region are extremely rare and may be the first manifestation of multiple myeloma. When eyelid lesions do occur the majority are cutaneous.

CLINICAL PRESENTATION   Eyelid lesions appear as a painless, firm, discrete nodule that may be violaceous or reddish-blue in color. Sometimes more diffuse eyelid swelling may be seen. Ecchymosis can be an initial finding. The lesion may be infiltrated into deeper eyelid structures such as the tarsal plate. Rarely ulceration may occur. Extension into the orbit may be associated with diplopia, decreased vision, and increased intraocular pressure.

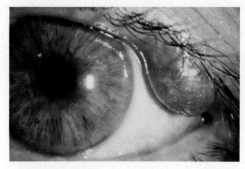
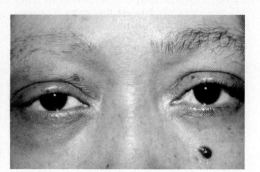
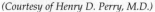

(Courtesy of Henry D. Perry, M.D.)

HISTOPATHOLOGY   Sheets of normal appearing and atypical plasma cells are the constituents of a plasmacytoma. Normal plasma cells are oval with an eccentrically placed round nucleus and abundant basophilic cytoplasm. Nuclear chromatin is clumped and often arranged in a distinctive radial ("cart wheel") pattern. Atypical plasma cells are enlarged, may have a prominent nucleolus, and they are often binucleate or multinucleate. Inclusions may be seen in the plasma cells, including Dutcher bodies (intranuclear vacuolation due to invagination of dilated Golgi cisternae), Russell bodies (globular cytoplasmic eosinophilic inclusions of immunoglobulin), and rarely rhomboidal crystalline immunoglobulin inclusions. The neoplastic plasma cells express either kappa or lambda light chain, confirming their clonal origin.

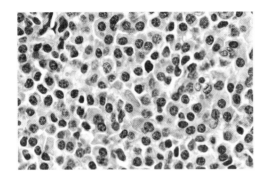

DIFFERENTIAL DIAGNOSIS   The differential diagnosis includes lymphoma and Kaposi's sarcoma.

TREATMENT   Treatment of solitary extramedullary plasmacytoma is usually local radiotherapy and/or surgery. Extensive systemic evaluation is required to rule out multiple myeloma or other lymphoproliferative conditions. This should include a complete blood cell count with differential, serum and urine protein electrophoresis, bone marrow biopsy, skeletal survey, and CT scan of the chest and abdomen. Systemic disease may respond to melphalan alone or in combination with cyclophosphamide and prednisone.

REFERENCES

Adkins JW, Shields JA, Shields CL, et al. Plasmacytoma of the eye and orbit. Intl Ophthalmol 1997; 20:339–343.

Benjamin I, Taylor H, Spindler J. Orbital and conjunctival involvement in multiple myeloma. Am J Clin Pathol 1975; 63:811–817.

Choi WJ, Tchah H, Kim YJ. Plasmacytoma presented as a lid mass – a case report. Korean J Ophthalmol 1991; 5:92–95.

De Smet MD, Rootman J. Orbital manifestations of plasmacytic lymphoproliferations. Ophthalmology 1987; 94:995–1003.

Kremer I, Flex D, Manor R. Solitary conjunctival extramedullary plasmacytoma. Ann Ophthalmol 1990; 22:126–130.

Olivieri L, Ianni MD, Giansanti M, Falini B, Tabilio A. Primary eyelid plasmacytoma. Medical Oncology 2000; 17:74–75.

Ria R, Di Ianni M, Sporotoletti P, et al. Recurrent primary plasmacytoma of the eyelid with rapid regional matastasis. Leuk Lymphoma 2006; 47:549–552.

Rodman HI, Font RL. Orbital involvement in multiple myeloma: Review of the literature and report of 3 cases. Arch Ophthalmol 1972; 87:30–35.

Seddon JM, Corwin JM, Weiter JJ, Brisbane JU, Sutula FC. Solitary extramedullary plasmacytoma of the palpebral conjunctiva. Br J Ophthalmol 1982; 66:450–454.

UCEDA-Montanes AU, Blanco G, Saornil MA, et al. Extramedullary plasmacytoma of the orbit. Acta Ophthalmol Scand 2000; 78:601–603.

Plexiform Neurofibroma

INTRODUCTION   Plexiform neurofibromas are the most common benign peripheral nerve tumor occurring in the eyelid and are considered pathognomonic for type 1 neurofibromatosis (NF-1). The lesion arises from and grows along any peripheral nerve. Plexiform neurofibromas typically present in children during the first decade of life. Mechanical ptosis can be profound, and in younger children may cause deprivation amblyopia. Associated systemic and ocular findings in patients with neurofibromas are related to underlying neurofibromatosis. Systemic findings may include hamartomas of the CNS, and cranial and peripheral nerves. Patients are at increased risk of developing pheochromocytoma, breast carcinoma, medulllary thyroid carcinoma, and gastrointestinal tumors. Ocular findings may include iris nodules (Lisch nodules), glaucoma, retinal astrocytic hamartoma, optic nerve glioma or meningioma, pulsating exophthalmos due to defects of the sphenoid wing, and orbital schwannoma. Rarely an eyelid neurofibroma may be seen in segmental neurofibromatosis without systemic manifestations of NF-1.

CLINICAL PRESENTATION   The plexiform neurofibroma often presents as a diffuse infiltration of the eyelid and orbit. The upper eyelid is involved in almost all cases and the lower lid in more than half. Brow infiltration is seen in about 20% of cases. The upper eyelid is usually ptotic and often develops an S-shaped curvature due to thickening and horizontal redundancy. On palpation the individual thickened nerves have the feel of a "bag of worms." Congenital glaucoma has been reported in some children with NF-1 and plexiform neurofibromas.

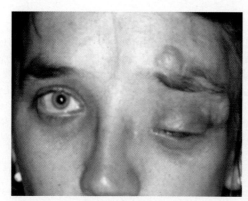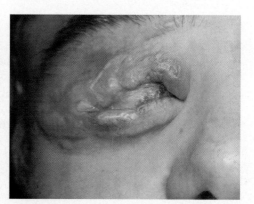

(Courtesy of Richard L. Anderson, M.D.)

HISTOPATHOLOGY   Plexiform neurofibromas are the most common form of eyelid neurofibroma. In plexiform neurofibromas large segments of peripheral nerve become convoluted and appear like a "bag of worms" macroscopically. Microscopically there is a tortuous mass of expanded nerve branches, each surrounded by a perineurium. In early lesions, the nerve is swollen by endoneurial accumulation of myxoid (glycosaminoglycan-rich) matrix. As the lesions age, Schwann cells proliferate and collagen accumulates within the nerves.

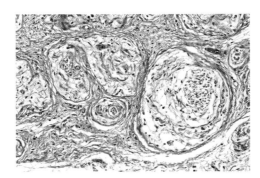 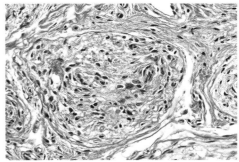

DIFFERENTIAL DIAGNOSIS   The differential diagnosis includes capillary hemangioma, lymphangioma, and dermoid cyst.

TREATMENT   Because of the infiltrative nature and vascularity of this tumor, therapeutic management is usually frustrating and disappointing. Recurrences are typical. Repeated surgical debulking may be necessary to maintain visual function and to offer some cosmetic improvement.

REFERENCES

Avisar R, Leshem Y, Savir H. Unilateral congenital ptosis due to plexiform neurofibroma, causing refraction error and secondary amblyopia. Metab Pediatr Syst Ophthalmol 1991; 14:62–63.

Dailey RA, Sullivan SA, Wobig JL. Surgical debulking of eyelid and anterior orbital plexiform neurofibromas by means of the carbon dioxide laser. Am J Ophthalmol 2000; 130:117–119.

Dutton JD, Byrne SF, Proia AD. Diagnostic Atlas of Orbital Diseases. Philadelphia: WB Saunders, 2000:132–133.

Farris SR, Grove AS Jr. Orbital and eyelid manifestations of neurofibromatosis: a clinical study and the literature review. Ophthal Plast Reconstr Surg 1996; 12:245–259.

Kobrin JL, Blodi FC, Weingeist TA. Ocular and orbital manifestations of neurofibromatosis. Surv Ophthalmol 1979; 24:5–50.

Lapid-Gortzak R, Lapid O, Monos T, Lifshitz T. CO2-laser in the removal of a plexiform neurofibroma from the eyelid. Ophthalmic Surg Lasers 2000; 31:432–434.

Listernick R, Mancini AJ, Charrow J. Segmental neurofibromatosis is childhood. Am J Med Genet A 2003; 121:132–135.

McCarron KF, Goldblum JR. Plexiform neurofibroma with and without associated malignant peripheral nerve sheath tumor: A clinicopathologic and immunohistochemical analysis of 54 cases. Mod Pathol 1998; 11:612–617.

Wood JJ, Albert DM, Solt LC, Hu DN, Wang WJ. Neurofibromatosis of the eyeball and orbit. Int Ophthalmol Clin 1982; 22:157–187.

Zimmerman RA, Bilaniuk LT, Metzger RA, et al. Computed tomography of orbital facial neurofibromatosis. Radiology 1983; 146:113–116.

Primary Mucinous Carcinoma

INTRODUCTION   Also known as *cutaneous adenocystic adenocarcinoma*, this lesion is a rare and relatively undifferentiated adenocarcinoma of eccrine sweat gland origin that arises de novo in the skin, especially in the eyelids of middle-aged or elderly males, and more often in blacks. These tumors have a low metastatic potential but tend to recur locally. When they do spread it is to the regional lymph nodes following multiple recurrences. Neglected tumors may invade the orbital tissues and adjacent bone.

CLINICAL PRESENTATION   The tumor usually presents as a painless firm, discrete skin-colored nodule, cyst, or ulcer on the eyelid or in the head and neck region. On occasion it may have a red-blue cystic appearance. They grow slowly and may be associated with lash loss, lid swelling, and fine telangiectasis.

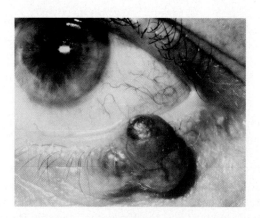

(Courtesy of Richard B. O'Grady, M.D. Source: From Gardner TW, O'Grady RB. Mucinous adenocarcinoma of the eyelid. A case report. Arch Ophthal 1984; 102:912, with permission of the American Medical Association.)

HISTOPATHOLOGY   This rare neoplasm, with a predilection for the eyelids, is situated in the dermis and often extends into the subcutaneous adipose tissue. Islands of tumor cells suspended in pale-staining mucin are separated by fibrous septa. Glandular differentiation is common, and there may be a cribriform pattern resembling that of primary cutaneous adenoid cystic carcinoma. Primary mucinous carcinoma must be distinguished from adenocarcinoma metastatic to the eyelid, and this requires thorough systemic evaluation of the patient.

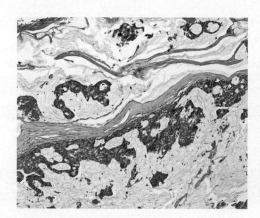 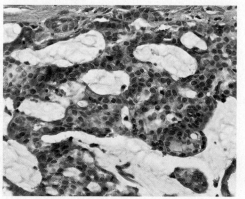

DIFFERENTIAL DIAGNOSIS   The differential diagnosis includes basal cell carcinoma, metastatic carcinoma, hydrocystoma, pilomatrixoma, epidermal inclusion cyst, and keratoacanthoma.

TREATMENT   Recommended treatment is wide en bloc excision of the tumor with frozen section control of the margins. Mohs microsurgery is particularly effective in reducing recurrences.

REFERENCES

Bellezza G, Sidoni A, Bucciarelli E. Primary mucinous carcinoma of the skin. Am J Dermatol 2000; 22:166–170.

Grizzard WS, Torczinski E, Edwards WC. Adenocarcinoma of eccrine sweat glands. Arch Ophthlamol 1976; 94:2119–2123.

Rosen Y, Kim B, Yermakov VA. Eccrine sweat gland origin involving the eyelids. Cancer 1975; 36:1034–1041.

Santa-Cruz DJ, Meyers JH, Gnepp DR, Perez BM. Primary mucinous carcinoma of skin. Br J Dermatol 1978; 98:645–653.

Thomas JW, Fu YS, Levine MR. Primary mucinous sweat gland carcinoma simulating metastatic carcinoma. Am J Ophthalmol 1979; 87:29–33.

Vaughn JG, Dortzbach RK. Benign eyelid lesions. In: Yanoff M, Duker JS, eds. Ophthalmology. London: Mosby, 1999; 8:7–12.

Weber PJ, Hevia O, Gretzula JC, Rabinovitz HC. Primary mucinous carcinoma. J Dermatol Surg Oncol 1988; 14:170–172.

Wright JD, Font RL. Mucinous sweat gland adenocarcinoma of the eyelid: a clinicopathologic study of 21 cases with histochemical and electron microscopic observations. Cancer 1979; 44:1757–1768.

Pyogenic Granuloma

INTRODUCTION   Also known as *granuloma pyogenicum*, the pyogenic granuloma is a common benign vascular lesion of the skin and mucosa. Its name is a misnomer since it is neither infectious nor granulomatous in nature. These lesions often follow trauma or surgery along the areas of injury, and may also develop in association with inflammatory processes such as chalazia. They may be seen in children and young adults without antecedent events, and are prone to arise on the head, neck, upper trunk, and extremities. Several variants have been described including the disseminated, subcutaneous, and intravascular types. They can occur within the canalicular system in the presence of silicone tubes, and beneath an ocular prosthesis associated with irritation from a poor fit, or around a motility peg. One form has been associated with systemic medications, particularly retinoids and protease inhibitors. The cause of pyogenic granuloma is not known, but roles have been postulated for viral oncogenes, underlying microscopic arteriovenous malformations, and production of angiogenic growth factor.

CLINICAL PRESENTATION   Pyogenic granuloma presents as a fast-growing fleshy, bright red-to-pink mass, 2 to 10 mm in diameter. It is very soft and friable and bleeds easily with minor contact. These lesions are frequently pedunculated and may be multilobulated. They often reach their full size in a few days, and may undergo spontaneous regression.

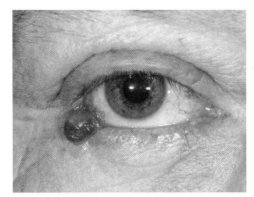
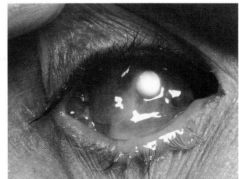

(Courtesy of Robert A. Goldberg, M.D.)

HISTOPATHOLOGY   Pyogenic granulomas may be encountered on the conjunctival surface or the epidermal surface of the eyelid. In the ophthalmological literature, these represent a form of exuberant granulation tissue usually resulting from trauma and comprised of radially arranged capillaries extending from the narrow base of the lesion towards the surface. The capillaries are within edematous stroma containing lymphocytes, plasma cells, and macrophages. The overlying epithelium or epidermis may ulcerate with a neutrophilic infiltrate in this area. In the dermatological literature, pyogenic granulomas are lobular capillary hemangiomas and only a minority follow trauma.

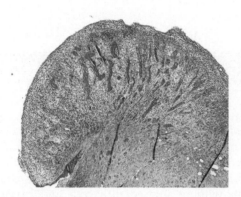 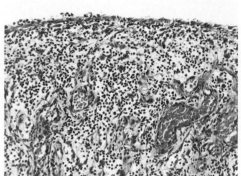

DIFFERENTIAL DIAGNOSIS   The differential diagnosis includes capillary hemangioma, Kaposi's sarcoma, basal cell carcinoma, malignant melanoma, and bacillary angiomatosis.

TREATMENT   If there is a clear inciting factor such as canalicular stents or a poorly-fitting prosthesis, these should be corrected. Topical steroids will sometimes reduce the size of the lesion and in some cases of conjunctival lesions these may resolve. For larger lesions that are of functional or cosmetic concern, treatment is by surgical excision with cautery at the base of the lesion. Chemical cautery with silver nitrate has also been reported to be effective. Recurrences are reported in up to 50% of cases regardless of the treatment modality.

REFERENCES

Allen RK, Rodman OG. Pyogenic granuloma recurrent with satellite lesions. J Dermatol Surg Oncol 1979; 5:490–493.

Cooper PH, Mills SE. Subcutaneous granuloma pyogenicum. Lobular capillary hemangioma. Arch Dermatol 1982; 118:30–33.

Davies MG, Barton SP, Atai F, Marks R. The abnormal dermis in pyogenic granuloma. J Am Acad Dermatol 1980; 2:132–142.

Font RL. Eyelids and lacrimal drainage system. In: Spencer WH, ed. Ophthalmic Pathology: An Atlas and Textbook. Vol. 4. 4th ed. Philadelphia: WB Saunders, 1996:2218–2437.

Levy R, Fisher M. In: Demis D, ed. Clinical Dermatology. Vol. 2. Philadelphia: Harper & Row, 1984, Unit 7–67.

Patrice SJ, Wiss K, Mulliken JB. Pyogenic granuloma (lobular capillary hemangioma): a clinicopathologic study of 178 cases. Pediatr Dermatol 1991; 8:267–276.

Yanoff M, Fine B. Ocular Pathology. 2nd ed. Philadelphia: Harper & Row, 1982:220–223.

INTRODUCTION   Rosacea is a common chronic condition of unknown etiology characterized by facial flushing, inflammatory papules and pustules, erythema, and telangiectasia. The onset is usually between ages 25 to 50 years, but has been reported in all age groups including children as young as two years. There is a 2:1 predilection for males. The clinical findings result from inflammation of the skin, capillary proliferation, and collagen deposition. Recent studies have shown an increase in the presence of a prostaglandin-like substance and an increase in free fatty acids in the sebaceous glands. Symptoms tend to be worsened by heat, hot or spicy foods, and alcohol. Symptoms may be caused by or worsened by potent topical steroids.

CLINICAL PRESENTATION   Skin lesions consisting of variable combinations of patchy erythema, telangiectasia, small papules, pustules, and hypertrophic sebaceous glands occur on the brow, eyelids, and midface. Heat, sunlight and possibly gastrointestinal stimuli may induce physiologic flushing. Capillary proliferation and dilatation may lead to dermal lymphatic stasis and a sterile cellulitis. Common ocular symptoms include burning, redness, itching, foreign body sensation, tearing, dryness, photophobia, and eyelid swelling. Inflammation of the meibomian glands with dilation and plugging of the gland orifices is seen along the lid margins and pressure on the tarsus results in expression of abnormally thick secretions. Greasy scales (scurf) may be present on the eyelashes. With chronic disease there is often loss of lashes and recurrent chalazia. Gland dropout and abnormally low lipid levels result in excessive evaporation of tears and a subsequent dry eye state. An associated conjunctival hyperemia, papillary conjunctivitis, episcleritis and marginal keratitis may occur in up to 5% of cases. A coexisting tear deficiency occurs in over 30% of patients.

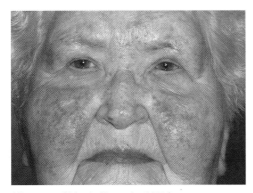 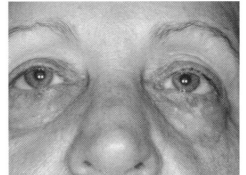

(Courtesy of Morris Hartstein, M.D.)

HISTOPATHOLOGY   The lesions of rosacea are variable. There may be only telangiectatic vessels with a mild to moderate perivascular infiltrate of lymphocytes containing a small number of plasma cells. Papulopustular rosacea lesions have more intense inflammation that is both perivascular and around hair follicles. Active pustular lesions have a superficial folliculitis, while older lesions may have loosely associated granulomas adjacent to follicles. Granulomatous rosacea has "tuberculoid" granulomas with epithelioid cells, multinucleated giant cells of Langhans and foreign-body types, and a substantial rim of lymphocytes and plasma cells. The granulomas may be centered on ruptured hair follicles. The granulomas may have central necrosis ("caseating necrosis") in approximately 10% of cases.

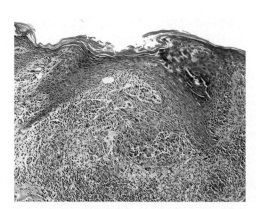
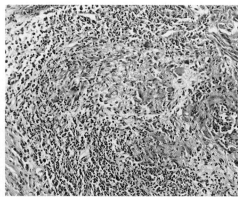

DIFFERENTIAL DIAGNOSIS   The differential diagnosis includes acne vulgaris, seborrhea, pityriasis, rubric pilaris, lupus erythematosus, syphilis, cutaneous tuberculosis, and sarcoidosis.

TREATMENT   Rosacea is often moderately to poorly responsive to therapy. Treatment usually requires a combination of topical and oral medications, and treatment for weeks to months may be necessary to prevent relapse. All patients should be advised to avoid heat, spicy and hot food and potent topical corticosteroids. Tetracycline 250 mg four times daily is an effective treatment for moderate to severe cutaneous papulo-pustular rosacea. Oral metronidazole 250 mg once or twice daily may also be as effective as oral tetracycline. Benefit begins in three to four weeks and reaches a maximum in six to eight weeks. Pustules and papules respond better than does the erythema. Mild topical corticosteroid creams (hydrocortisone 1%) twice daily may control the erythematous component. Benzoyl peroxide gel 2.5% to 5%, or a topical antibiotic solution once or twice daily may be effective for the treatment of the papulo-pustular component. For resistant cases use of a vitamin A derivative such as isotretinoin may induce a prolonged remission. A topical ocular steroid with or without antibiotic may be necessary for treatment of associated keratitis, and artificial tears are the mainstay for treatment of associated dry eyes. Lid hygiene with a dilute "no tears" shampoo following warm compresses is effective in melting the stagnant lipid secretions. Topical ophthalmic antibiotics applied to the lid margins can in some cases be useful in decreasing the bacterial flora, whose lipases may contribute to the increased free fatty acid production.

REFERENCES

Alvarenga LS, Mannis MJ. Ocular rosacea. Ocul Surf 2005; 3:41–58.

Berg M, Liden S. An epidemiologic study of Rosacea. Acta Derm Venereol 1989; 69:419–423.

Browning DJ. Tear studies in ocular rosacea. Am J Ophthalmol 1985; 99:530–533.

Diamantis S, Waldorf HA. Rosacea: clinical presentation and pathophysiology. J Drugs Dermatol 2006; 5:8–12.

Donaldson KE, Karp CL, Dunbar MT. Evaluation and treatment of children with ocular rosacea. Cornea 2007; 26:42–46.

Jenkins MS, Brown SI, Lempert SL, Weinberg RJ. Ocular rosacea. Am J Ophthalmol 1979; 88:618–622.

Lemp MH, Mahmood MA, Weiler HH. Association of rosacea and keratoconjunctivitis sicca. Arch Ophthalmol 1984; 102:556–557.

Stone DU, Chodosh J. Ocular rosace: an update on pathogenesis and therapy. Curr Opin Ophthalmol 2004; 15:499–502.

INTRODUCTION   Sarcoidosis is a noncaseating granulomatous multi-system disease of unknown etiology that most commonly affects young adults. It affects males and females equally, but females are more likely to show ocular involvement. There is a greater prevalence of sarcoidosis in the southeastern United States, and it is believed to occur more commonly among blacks. A bimodal incidence has been reported. A sub-acute presentation in patients less than 30 years of age is more likely to be self-limited, subsiding within two years. This transient variety is seldom associated with skin lesions. A more chronic form of the disease occurs in older age groups and skin lesions occur in up to 30% of patients. This form is believed to be due to a defect in T-lymphocyte suppressor function, and it frequently presents with hilar adenopathy, lung infiltrations, and more rarely with skin or eye lesions. The incidence of ocular involvement in patients with sarcoidosis is estimated to be 22% and eyelid lesions may be seen in 11%.

CLINICAL PRESENTATION   Eyelid lesions most commonly take the form of unilateral or bilateral slightly elevated, discrete, yellow-to-brown or purplish papules and plaques that eventually demonstrate central clearing. They usually evolve into annular or circinate lesions with or without central ulceration. "Millet-seed" subcutaneous nodules or confluent violaceous nodules may also occur. Associated eyelid edema and erythema is common. Occasionally sarcoid lesions can result in full-thickness destruction of eyelid tissues. Associated ocular involvement may include acute anterior uveitis, keratitis sicca, conjunctival granulomas, lacrimal gland infiltration, orbital inflammation, chorioditis, optic neuritis, and retinal vasculitis. Candle wax exudates along the retinal veins are thought to be virtually pathognomonic, but they seldom occur. Constitutional symptoms of fever and malaise are common, as is hilar adenopathy, lung infiltrations, and arthralgias. Rarely, eyelid sarcoid can be seen in the absence of any systemic manifestations. Central nervous system abnormalities occur in fewer than 10% of cases, however, this incidence doubles if there is involvement of the optic nerve or ocular fundus.

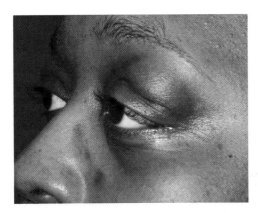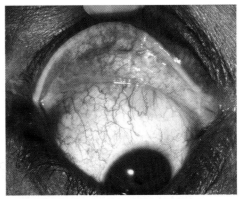

HISTOPATHOLOGY   The hallmark of sarcoidosis is the noncaseating granuloma. The granulomas have sharp borders and are formed of tightly clustered epithelioid cells, usually with Langhans or foreign body-type giant cells. Epithelioid cells are activated macrophages with oval to elongate nuclei, pale pink granular cytoplasm, and indistinct cell borders. A variable number of lymphocytes rim the granulomas. Older granulomas become surrounded by fibrous connective tissue.

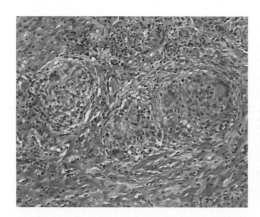 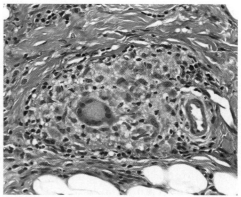

DIFFERENTIAL DIAGNOSIS   The differential diagnosis includes discoid lupus erythematosus, chalazia, hordeola, epidermal inclusion cyst, xanthelasma, lipoid proteinosis, amyloidosis, sebaceous cyst, lichen planus, erythema nodosum, tuberculosis, leprosy, syphilis and parasitic, fungal, viral (molluscum contagiosum, herpes simples and herpes zoster), or bacterial infections.

TREATMENT   Diagnosis is supported by chest X-ray (positive in 80%), tuberculin skin test anergy, increased angiotensin-converting enzyme, positive gallium scan, elevated serum protein level with elevated alph-2globulin fraction, and elevated serum calcium level. Treatment revolves around systemic steroids. The most favorable prognosis is seen in younger patients with the more acute self-limited form of sarcoidosis. Associated intraocular inflammation is controlled with topical steroids and cycloplegics. Eyelid lesions often respond to systemic corticosteroid therapy, however, they often recur when treatment is stopped. Intralesional triamcinolone for cutaneous palpebral sarcoidosis can be effective for localized eyelid disease.

REFERENCES

Bersani TA, Nichols CW. Intralesional triamcinolone for cutaneous palpebral sarcoidosis. Am J Ophthalmol 1985; 99:561–562.

Biswas J, Krishnakumar S, Raghavendran R, Mahesh L. Lid swelling and diplopia as presenting features of orbital sarcoid. Indian J Ophthalmol 2000; 48:231–233.

Browstein S, Liszauer AD, Carey WD, Nicolle DA. Sarcoidosis of the eyelid skin. Can J Ophthalmol 1990; 25:256–259.

Cacciatori M, McLaren KM, Learns PP. Sarcoidosis presenting as a cutaneous eyelid mass. Br J Ophthalmol 1997; 81:329–330.

Cook JR, Brubaker RF, Savell J, Sheagren J. Lacrimal sarcoidosis treated with corticosteroids. Arch Ophthalmol 1972; 88:513–517.

Hall JG, Cohen KL. Sarcoidosis of the eyelid skin. Am J Ophthalmol 1995; 119:100–101.

Hanno R, Neddelman A, Eiferman RA, Callen JP. Cutaneous sarcoid granulomas and the development of systemic sarcoidosis. Arch Dermatol 1981; 117:203–207.

Imes RK, Reifschneider JS, O'Connor LE. Systemic sarcoidosis presenting initially with bilateral orbital and upper lid masses. Ann Ophthalmol 1988; 20:466–467, 469.

Iwata K, Nanba K, Sobue K, Abe H. Ocular sarcoidosis: evaluation of intraocular findings. Ann NY Acad Sci 1976; 278:445–455.

Moin M, Kersten RC, Bernardini F, Kulwin DR. Destructive eyelid lesions in sarcoidosis. Ophthal Plast Reconstr Surg 2001; 17:123–125.

Pessoa de Souza Filho J, Martins MC, Sant'Anna AE, et al. Eyelid swelling as the only manifestation of ocular sarcoidosis. Ocul Immunol Inflamm 2005; 13:399–402.

Sharma OP. Cutaneous sarcoidosis. Clinical features and management. Chest 1972; 61:320–325.

Zimmerman LE, Maumenee AE. Ocular aspects of sarcoidosis. Am Rev Respir Dis 1961; 84:38–50.

INTRODUCTION   Cutaneous adnexal neoplasms showing sebaceous differentiation are difficult to classify. Because of the intimate relationship of sebaceous glands with other adnexal structures associated with the pilosebaceous unit these lesions often display complex histologic features combining sebaceous, hair follicle, and sweat gland tissues. Sebaceous neoplasms run the gamut from benign to malignant lesions. These include sebaceous gland proliferation (sebaceous hyperplasia), congenital sebaceous hamartomas (nevus sebaceum), sebaceous adenoma, and sebaceous carcinoma. Sebaceous adenoma is an uncommon, often solitary lesion usually seen in patients over 40 years of age, with a predilection for the eyelid and brow, occurring in elderly patients.

CLINICAL PRESENTATION   These present as a slowly enlarging well-demarcated firm dome-shaped lesion, generally less than 0.5 cm in diameter. They are smooth, yellow speckled papules, and sometimes may be pink to red. Fine telangiectatic vessels may be present within the lesion. Lesions are usually single, but in elderly patients may be multiple. Occasionally they may be polypoid or have a central umbilication. Occasionally they may ulcerate and bleed. Lesions may occur in combination with keratoacanthoma as part of the Muir-Torre syndrome (skin lesions occurring in association with an internal malignancy, typically adenocarcinoma of the colon), but here the sebaceous lesions tend to be cystic.

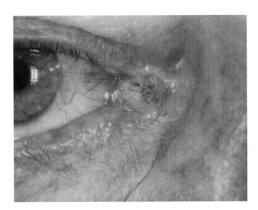 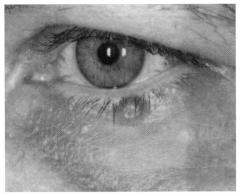

HISTOPATHOLOGY   Sebaceous adenomas are composed of multiple sharply circumscribed sebaceous lobules. The tumor is usually located in the mid dermis, but it may connect to the epidermis. The

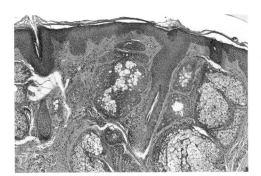 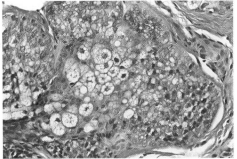

sebaceous lobules comprising the tumor have a peripheral germinative layer of small basophilic cells, then a zone of transitional cells, and finally mature sebaceous cells in the center of the lobule. Mature sebaceous cells outnumber the germinative cells.

DIFFERENTIAL DIAGNOSIS   The differential diagnosis includes benign lesions such as seborrheic keratosis, apocrine hidradenoma, nevus sebaceous, sebaceous hyperplasia, and dermoid cyst, as well as malignant tumors such as sebaceous cell carcinoma, and basal cell carcinoma.

TREATMENT   Surgical removal is indicated for diagnosis or if there is a sudden increase in size. Complete excision with clear margins is necessary as incompletely excised lesions commonly recur. Alternative treatments include electrodessication and radiotherapy.

REFERENCES

Bhattacharya AK, Nayak SR, Kirtane MV, Ingle MV. Sebaceous adenoma in the region of the medial canthus causing proptosis. J Postgrad Med 1995; 41:87–88.

Finan MC, Connolly SM. Sebaceous gland tumors and systemic disease: a clinicopathologic analysis. Medicine (Baltimore) 1984; 63:232–242.

Font RL, Rishi K. Sebaceous gland adenoma of the tarsal conjunctiva in a patient with Muir-Torre syndrome. Ophthalmology 2003; 110:1833–1836.

Prioleau PG, Santa Cruz DJ. Sebaceous gland neoplasia. J Cutan Pathol 1984; 11:396–414.

Shlopova NB, Shlopov VG. Sebaceous gland adenoma of the eyelid. Vestn Oftalmol 1989; 105:76–78.

Singh AD, Mudhar HS, Bhola R, Rundle PA, Rennie IG. Sebaceous adenoma of the eyelid in Muir-Torre syndrome. Arch Ophthalmol 2005; 123:562–565.

Spraul CW, Jakobczyk-Zmija MJ, Lang GK. Sebaceous hyperplasia of the lower eyelid. Klin Monatsbl Augenheilkd 1999; 215:319–320.

Sebaceous Cell Carcinoma

INTRODUCTION   Sebaceous cell carcinoma is a highly malignant neoplasm that arises from sebaceous glands, and the vast majority of these occur around the eyelids. It can derive from the meibomian glands, glands of Zeis, and from sebaceous glands associated with the pilosebaceous unit. Sebaceous cell carcinoma is an aggressive tumor with a high recurrence rate, a significant metastatic potential, and a notable mortality rate. Although relatively rare, sebaceous gland carcinoma represents the third most common eyelid malignancy, accounting for 1.0% to 5.5% of all eyelid cancers. It affects all races and occurs more commonly in women than in men. It usually presents in the sixth to seventh decades, but cases in younger patients, even children, have been reported. There is a clear link between sebaceous gland carcinoma and prior radiation therapy. It may invade locally into the globe, the orbit, the sinuses, or the brain. Metastases spread via local lymphatics to preauricular and submandibular lymph nodes or by hemotogenous spread to distant sites. Once metastases develop, the five-year survival rate is only 30% to 50%.

CLINICAL PRESENTATION   The upper eyelid is the site of origin in about two thirds of all cases, presumably due to a greater number of meibomian glands on the upper eyelid. The clinical appearance is varied and sebaceous cell carcinoma is very frequently misdiagnosed as a benign process. Often it presents as a firm, yellow nodule that resembles a chalazion. It can mimic a chronic blepharo-conjunctivitis or meibomianitis that does not respond to standard therapies (the so-called *masquerade syndrome*). A more worrisome presentation may be as a plaque-like thickening of the tarsal plate with destruction of meibomian gland orifices and tumor invasion of eyelash follicles leading to madarosis, or loss of lashes. Tumor tends to invade the overlying epithelium which may result in the formation of nests of malignant cells. This is known as pagetoid spread. Pagetoid spread of the tumor may result in diffuse spread of the tumor that replaces the entire thickness of the conjunctiva (intraepithelial carcinoma) and mimics conjunctivitis. This lesion can exhibit multicentric spread to the conjunctiva, corneal epithelium and even to the other eyelid. It may also spread through the caniliculus to the lacrimal excretory system and the nasal cavity.

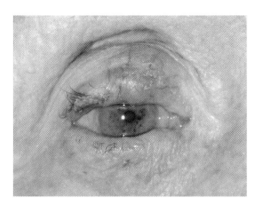 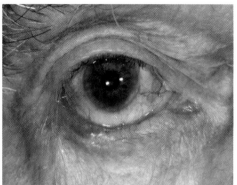

HISTOPATHOLOGY   Sebaceous carcinoma varies from well- to poorly-differentiated tumors, depending on the number of neoplastic cells with sebaceous differentiation. The cells with sebaceous differentiation have abundant, finely vacuolated cytoplasm creating a foamy appearance. The other neoplastic cells have hyperchromatic nuclei, prominent nucleoli, and lightly basophilic cytoplasm. A lobular pattern of tumor is most common in the eyelid, though full-thickness involvement and Pagetoid spread of tumor cells in the conjunctiva or epidermis are also encountered. The tumor cells around the periphery of the lobules often have less cytoplasm and are more basophilic than those toward the center of the lobule. Oil red O stains for lipid within the tumor cells is rarely needed for diagnosis.

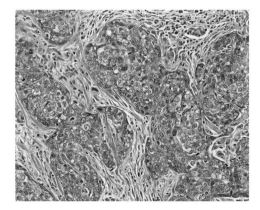 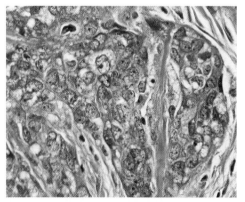

Sebaceous Cell Carcinoma (Contd.)

DIFFERENTIAL DIAGNOSIS   The differential diagnosis includes basal cell carcinoma, squamous cell carcinoma, papilloma, blepharitis, chalazion, ocular cicatricial pemphigoid, cutaneous horns, discoid lupus, pyogenic granulomas, lacrimal sac tumors, and superior limbic keratoconjunctivitis.

TREATMENT   Any suspicious eyelid lesion or one that does not respond to medical therapy or recurs in the same location deserves a biopsy. Because eyelid margin sebaceous carcinomas often originate in the deep tarsus, superficial shave biopsies may reveal chronic inflammation but miss the underlying tumor. A full-thickness eyelid biopsy with permanent sections may be required to determine the correct diagnosis. Alternately, a punch biopsy of full-thickness tarsal plate may be diagnostic. Wide surgical excision with microscopic monitoring of the margins is the treatment of choice. Mohs' micrographic surgical excision may be used, but it may not be as successful as in basal cell carcinoma or squamous cell carcinoma due to the possibility of multicentric skip lesions and pagetoid spread. If the tumor is very large or recurrent with spread to the bulbar conjunctiva or to orbital tissues, a subtotal or complete exenteration may be necessary. If evidence of spread to regional lymph nodes is present, the patient will require lymph node or radical neck dissection. Radiation therapy can be considered as an adjunct to local surgery. However, primary treatment with irradiation alone is inadequate, and recurrence usually occurs within three years.

REFERENCES

Boniuk M, Zimmerman LE. Sebaceous carcinoma of the eyelid, eyebrow, caruncle, and orbit. Trans Am Acad Ophthalmol Otolaryngol 1968; 72:619–641.

DePotter P, Shields CL, Shields CL. Sebaceous gland carcinoma of the eyelids. Int Ophthalmol Clin 1993; 33:5–9.

Dixon RS, Mikhail GR, Slater HC. Sebaceous carcinoma of the eyelid. J Am Acad Dermatol 1980; 3:241–243.

Doxanas MT, Green WR. Sebaceous gland carcinoma. Arch Ophthalmol 1984; 102:245–249.

Dzubow LM. Sebaceous carcinoma of the eyelid: treatment with Mohs surgery. Dermatol Surg Oncol 1985; 11:40–44.

Folberg R, Whitaker DC, Tse DT, Nerad JA. Recurrent and residual sebaceous carcinoma after Mohs' excision of the primary lesion. Am J Opthalmol 1987; 103:817–823.

Font RL. Eyelids and lacrimal drainage system. In: Spencer WH, ed. Ophthalmic Pathology: An Atlas and Textbook, 4th ed. Philadelphia: WB Saunders 1996:2218–2433.

Harvey JT, Anderson RL. The management of meibomian gland carcinoma. Ophthalmic Surg 1982; 13:56–61 .

Kass LG, Hornblass A. Sebaceous carcinoma of the ocular adnexa. Surv Ophthlamol 1989; 33:477–490.

Khan JA, Grove AS, Joseph MP, Goodman M. Sebaceous gland carcinoma: diuretic use, lacrimal system spread, and surgical margins. Ophthalmic Plast Reconstr Surgery 1989; 5:227–234.

Kostick DA, Linberg JV, McCormick SA. Sebaceous gland carcinoma. In: Mannis MJ, Macsai MS, Huntley AC, eds. Eye and Skin Disease. Philadelphia: Lippincott-Raven Publishers 1996:413–417.

Lisman RD, Jakobiec FA, Small P. Sebaceous carcinoma of the eyelids. The role of adjunctive cryotherapy in the management of conjunctival pagetoid spread. Ophthalmology 1989; 96:1021–1026.

Ni C. Sebaceous cell carcinoma of the ocular adnexa. In: Ni C, Albert DM, eds. Tumors of the Eyelid. Vol. 22. Boston: Little Brown, 1982:23–61.

Nunery WR, Welsh MG, McCord CD Jr. Recurrence of sebaceous carcinoma of the eyelid after radiation therapy. Am J Ophthalmol 1983; 96:10–15.

Rao NA, Hidayat AA, McLean IW, Zimmerman LE. Sebaceous carcinoma of the ocular adnexa: a clinicopathological study of 104 cases. Hum Pathol 1982; 13:113–122.

Russell WG, Page DL, Hough AJ, Rogers LW. Sebaceous carcinoma of meibomian gland origin. The diagnostic importance of pagetoid spread of neoplastic cells. Am J Clin Pathol 1980; 73:504–511.

Seborrheic Keratosis

INTRODUCTION   Seborrheic keratosis is the most common eyelid tumor and the incidence increases with age. They are more common in light-skinned individuals. Also known as a *senile verruca* and *seborrheic wart*, this is a benign epithelial neoplasm that can occur on any part of the body. The reticulated type is usually found on the sun-exposed areas of the face and eyelids, and may develop from solar lentigines. These lesions usually affect middle-aged and older adults.

CLINICAL PRESENTATION   Seborrheic keratoses initially present as painless, movable, sharply defined slightly elevated macules with a variable degree of pigmentation that varies from tan to brown. They sometimes appear in large numbers. As they grow they typically develop a greasy papillomatous or verrucous, stuck-on appearance. They are usually sessile, but can sometimes be pedunculated. Older lesions tend to be more verrucous and folded, with multiple keratin plugs creating a pitted surface. Irritation can cause inflammation, swelling, and sometimes bleeding, and crusting. In the variant called *dermatosis papulosa nigra* a large number of darkly pigmented lesions occurs on the cheeks of black patients. A rapid increase in size and number may represent the *sign of Leser-Trélat* (multiple eruptive seborrheic keratosis), which may occur in patients with an occult malignancy.

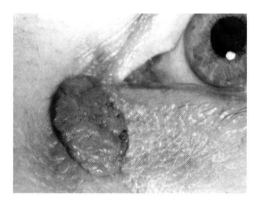 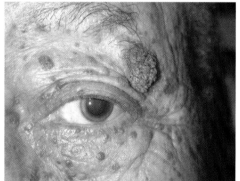

HISTOPATHOLOGY   Seborrheic keratoses are sharply defined tumors that have multiple histological types that overlap frequently [acanthotic, papillomatous (hyperkeratotic), adenoid [reticulated], irritated, and clonal]. Acanthotic seborrheic keratoses (shown below) are encountered most frequently and are composed of broad columns of basaloid cells that interdigitate. Varying amounts of

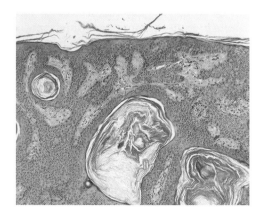 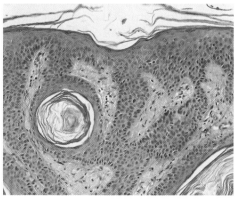

squamoid cells are admixed with the basaloid cells. Invaginations of keratin and horn cysts are typical features of acanthotic seborrheic keratosis.

DIFFERENTIAL DIAGNOSIS   Seborrheic keratosis can be confused with melanocytic nevus, verruca vulgaris, actinic keratosis, pigmented basal cell carcinoma, and malignant melanoma.

TREATMENT   These lesions are primarily of cosmetic concern only, although they can be an annoyance when they rub or catch on clothing. They may be removed for biopsy or cosmesis, or to prevent irritation. Therapy includes light cryotherapy followed by curettage, laser ablation, and surgical excision. They usually do not recur after treatment. Malignant melanoma has been reported within a seborrheic keratosis. In up to 10% of lesions they may not be able to be distinguished from melanoma so that biopsy is appropriate if there is any doubt about the diagnosis.

REFERENCES

Cribier B. Seborrheic keratosis. Ann Dermatol Venereol 2005; 132:292–295.

Ellis DL, Yates RA. Sign of Leser-Trelat. Clin Dermatol 1993; 11:141–148.

Harrison MA Jr, Reed RN, Derbes VJ. Dermatosis papulosa nigra. Arch Dermatol 1964; 89:655.

Herron MD, Bowen AR, Krueger GG. Seborrheic keratosis: a study comparing the standard cryosurgery with topical calcipotriene, topical tazarotene, and topical imiquimod. Int J Dermatol 2004; 43:300–302.

Kobalter AS, Roth A. Benign epithelial neoplasms. In: Mannis MJ, Macsai MS, Huntley AC, eds. Eye and Skin Disease. Philadelphia: Lippincott-Raven Publishers, 1996:345–355.

Sanderson KV. The structure of seborrheic keratosis. Br J Dermatol 1963; 80:588–593.

Scully J. Treatment of seborrheic keratosis. JAMA 1970; 213:1498.

Thomas I, Kihiczak NI, Rothenberg J, Ahmed S, Schwartz RA. Melanoma within the seborrheic keratosis. Dermatol Surg 2004; 30:559–561.

Squamous Cell Carcinoma

INTRODUCTION   Squamous cell carcinoma is a malignant tumor that most commonly affects elderly, fair-skinned individuals. It arises from keratinocytes of the epidermis. Unlike the more common basal cell carcinoma, squamous cell carcinoma tends to arise in precancerous areas of skin alteration or in areas of skin damaged by chronic sun exposure, ionizing radiation, carcinogens (e.g., arsenic), psoralen plus ultraviolet A (PUVA) therapy for psoriasis, and the human papilloma virus. Intrinsic factors that may contribute to its development include xeroderma pigmentosum, oculocutaneous albinism, and immunodeficiency. Chronic skin dermatoses, inflammation, ulceration, and contracted scars also are associated with the development of this tumor. In fact, scarring of the skin is the most common intrinsic factor leading to this tumor in black patients. Lymphatic spread and perineural invasion are possible.

CLINICAL PRESENTATION   The most common site of eyelid involvement is the lower lid. Initial changes can look like a chronic eczema-like lesion. The tumor often originates in an actinic keratosis, but tends to be thicker, larger and have a more heaped-up keratinization. These lesions have a tendency to ulcerate, and growth may be endophytic or more exophytic with raised papillary verrucous borders. Occasionally it can take on the appearance of a cutaneous horn. Long-standing lesions become friable and bleed easily. Necrosis may follow with superimposed bacterial infection. Orbital extension has been reported in up to 16% of cases. Palpable regional lymph nodes indicate metastatic spread.

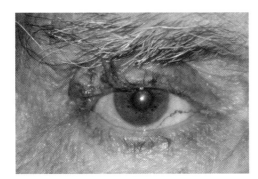
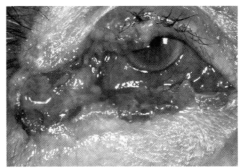

(Courtesy of Richard L. Anderson, M.D.)

HISTOPATHOLOGY   The typical squamous cell carcinoma has nests and tongues of squamous epithelial cells that arise from the epidermis and extend into the dermis. Squamous cells are recognizable by their eosinophilic cytoplasm and large nuclei. Keratinization and horn pearl formation are present in tumors that are better differentiated. A mild to moderate infiltrate of lymphocytes around the periphery of the tumor is common.

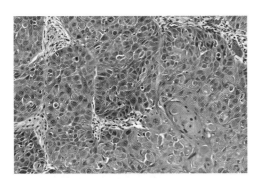
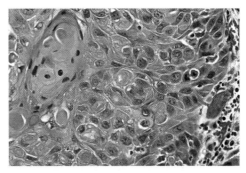

DIFFERENTIAL DIAGNOSIS   The differential diagnosis includes basal cell carcinoma, sebaceous cell carcinoma, Bowen's disease, actinic keratosis, keratoacanthoma, inverted follicular keratosis, papilloma, pseudoepitheliomatous hyperplasia, seborrheic keratosis, trichilemomma, fungal infection, and verruca vulgaris.

TREATMENT   Diagnosis requires a biopsy for histologic confirmation. Once the diagnosis is established the goal of therapy is complete removal of tumor cells with preservation of unaffected eyelid and periorbital tissues needed for reconstruction. Mohs' micrographic surgery provides the highest cure rate with the most effective preservation of normal tissue. Excisional biopsy with frozen section control is an acceptable alternative technique. Radiation therapy is generally not recommended as the initial treatment, but it may be useful in the treatment of advanced or deeply invasive recurrent lesions. Doses are in the range of 4000 to 7000 cGy. A recurrence rate of 12% with radiation has been reported. Cryotherapy is often used to treat nonperiorbital lesions, but when applied to the eyelids complications such as marginal notching, ectropion, sympblepharon formation, fornix foreshortening, and depigmentation of eyelid skin have all been reported. Cryotherapy is also associated with a higher recurrence rate. Advanced cases may be associated with metastasis to the pre-auricular and submandibular lymph nodes, which heralds a more guarded prognosis. Invasion into deep orbital tissues can be seen, often requiring orbital exenteration for definitive management.

REFERENCES

Bowyer JD, Sullivan TJ, Whitehead KJ, Kelly LE, Allison RW. The management of perineural spread of squamous cell carcinoma to the ocular adnexae. Ophthal Plast Reconstr Surg 2003; 19:275–281.

Dailey JR, Kennedy RH, Flaharty PM, Eagle RC Jr, Flanagan JC. Squamous cell carcinoma of the eyelid. Ophthalmol Plast Reconstr Surg 1994; 10:153–159.

Donaldson MJ, Sullivan TJ, Whitehead KJ, Williamson RM. Squamous cell carcinoma of the eyelids. Br J Ophthalmol 2002; 86:1161–1165.

Doxanas MT, Iliff NT, Green WR. Squamous cell carcinoma of the eyelids. Ophthalmology 1987; 94:538–541.

Epstein E, Epstein NN, Bragg K, Linden G. Metastases from squamous cell carcinoma of the skin. Arch Dermatol 1968; 97:245–251.

Font RL. Eyelids and lacrimal drainage system. In: Spencer WH, ed. Ophthalmic Pathology: An Atlas and Textbook. 4th ed. Vol. 4. Philadelphia: WB Saunders, 1996:2218–2433.

Hass AF, Tucker SM. Squamous cell carcinoma. In: Mannis MJ, Macsai, Huntley AC, eds. Eye and Skin Disease. Philadelphia: Lippincott-Raven Publishers, 1996:405–411.

Kwitko ML, Boniuk M, Zimmerman LE. Eyelid tumors with reference to lesions confused with squamous cell carcinoma. I. Incidence and errors in diagnosis. Arch Ophthalmol 1963; 69:693–697.

Lederman M. Discussion of carcinomas of conjunctiva and eyelid. In: Boniuk M, ed. Ocular and Adnexal Tumors. St Louis: CV Mosby, 1964:104–109.

Lund HZ. How often does squamous cell carcinoma of the skin metastasize? Arch Dermatol 1965; 92:635–637.

Mencia-Gutierrez E, Fernandez Gonzalez MC, Gutierrez Diaz E, et al. Squamous cell carcinomas of the eyelids: 18 cases. Arch Soc Esp Oftalmol 2000; 75:665–669.

Mora RG, Perniliaro C. Cancer of the skin in blacks. I. A review of 163 black patients with cutaneous squamous cell carcinoma. J Am Acad Dermatol 1981; 5:405–411.

Reifler DM, Hornblass A. Squamous cell carcinoma of the eyelid. Surv Ophthalmol 1986; 30:349–365.

Syringoma

INTRODUCTION   Syringoma is a common adnexal tumor formed by well-differentiated ductal elements. Immunohistochemistry shows the presence of eccrine enzymes and the pattern of cytokine expression suggests differentiation toward the uppermost part of the dermal duct. It is unclear if these lesions represent true adnexal neoplasms or a hyperplastic response to an inflammatory reaction. These lesions are mostly benign, asymptomatic and occur primarily in young females. A very rare malignant syringoma has been described on the eyelids, characterized by larger size, isolated nature, and subcutaneous and perineural invasion.

CLINICAL PRESENTATION   The lesions typically occur at the time of puberty and present as multiple small (1–3 mm), skin-colored to yellowish papules with a rounded or flat surface. They can sometimes appear translucent or cystic. Lesions are usually multiple and distributed symmetrically on the upper cheek and lower eyelids.

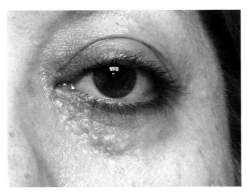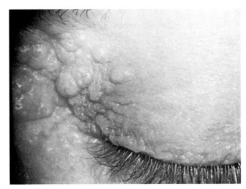

(Courtesy of Robert A. Goldberg, M.D.)

HISTOPATHOLOGY   Syringomas are dermal tumors composed of small ductules usually lined by two layers of flattened cuboidal cells. An epithelial strand at the end of a ductule may create a tadpole or comma-like appearance. Solid nests and strands of epithelial cells are also present commonly. The lack of deep extension and perineural invasion differentiates syringoma from microcystic adnexal carcinoma.

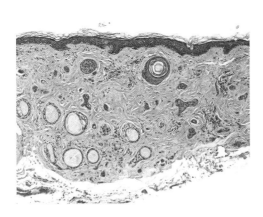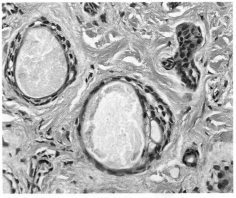

DIFFERENTIAL DIAGNOSIS   The differential diagnosis includes flat warts, milia, sarcoid nodules, trichoepithelioma, and basal cell carcinoma.

TREATMENT   Syringomas are of cosmetic concern only. The most common forms of treatment include surgical excision, electrodessication, CO2 laser ablation, tricholoracetic acid, and cryotherapy. All forms of treatment carry a risk of scarring and the cosmetic result following removal may be less acceptable than the original condition.

REFERENCES

Glatt HJ, Proia AD, Tsoy EA, et al. Malignant syringoma of the eyelid. Ophthalmology 1984; 91:987–990.

Hashimoto K, Gross BG, Lever WF. Syringoma: histochemical and electron microscopic studies. J Invest Dermatol 1966; 46:150–166.

Lee JH, Chang JY, Lee KH. Syringoma: a clinicopathologic and immunohistochemical study and results of treatment. Yonsei Med J 2007; 48:35–40.

Lipper S, Peiper SC. Sweat gland carcinoma with syringomatous features: a light microscopic and ultrastructural study. Cancer 1979; 44:157–163.

Nerad JA, Anderson RL. CO2 laser treatment of eyelid syringomas. Ophthalmic Plast Reconstr Surg 1988; 4:91–94.

Ni C, Dryja TP, Albert DM. Sweat gland tumors in the eyelids: a clinicopathological analysis of 55 cases. Int Ophthalmol Clin 1982; 22:1–22.

Sugano DM, Lucci LM, Avila MP et al. Eyelid trichoepithelioma-report of 2 cases. Arq Bras Ofta;mol 2005; 68:136–139.

Winklemann RK, Gottlieb BF. Syringoma: an enzymatic study. Cancer 1963; 16:665–669.

Trichilemmal (Sebaceous) Cyst

INTRODUCTION   The trichilemmal cyst is also referred to as a sebaceous or pilar cyst. It is derived from the outer root sheath of the deeper parts of a hair follicle and consists of a well-keratinized epidermal wall surrounding semi-solid hair keratin and cholesterol-rich debris, rather than just sebaceous material. Trichilemmal cysts are more common in females and most cases occur in the sixth and seventh decades of life. They differ from epidermoid cysts in that they lack a granular layer in the lining epithelium. Foci of proliferating cells and mitoses can occasionally be seen producing the proliferating trichilemmal cyst or pilar tumor. Some authors regard these as malignant tumors.

CLINICAL PRESENTATION   Clinically the trichilemmal cyst is indistinguishable from the epidermoid cyst. Unlike the epidermoid cyst no central punctum is seen. They occur on hair-bearing skin including the scalp and face as single or multiple round smooth, mobile cysts within the dermis that may rupture and discharge a thick stringy, cheesy white material. Occasionally they may form a cutaneous horn. The wall can rupture the contents into the dermis resulting in an inflammatory reaction or infection, becoming red and tender with the formation of granulation tissue which at times can resemble a well-differentiated squamous cell carcinoma.

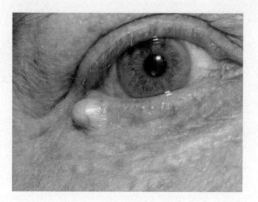

HISTOPATHOLOGY   Trichilemmal cysts have a fibrous capsule on which rests a layer of darkly staining basal cells. The basal cells merge with stratified squamous epithelium whose cells increase in size and vertical diameter as they mature and abruptly change into the eosinophilic-staining keratin within the lumen. The epithelial lining lacks a granular cell layer. The keratinous material in the lumen commonly has cholesterol clefts.

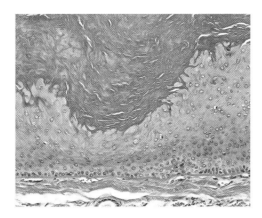 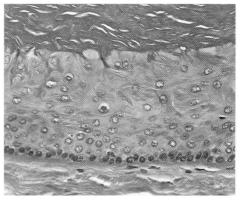

DIFFERENTIAL DIAGNOSIS   The differential diagnosis includes dermoid cyst, epidermoid cyst, pilomatrixoma, acne comedones, dermatofibroma, lipoma, milia, and cystic squamous cell and basal cell carcinoma.

TREATMENT   Treatment of trichilemmal cysts is not necessary. When of cosmetic concern they are removed surgically with excision of the intact cyst wall. The rare proliferating trichilemmal cyst can be locally aggressive and rare cases of malignant transformation have bee reported. It is important to distinguish them from squamous cell carcinoma. They should be completely excised with clear margins.

REFERENCES

Brownstein MH, Arluk DJ. Proliferating tricholemmal cyst: a stimulant of squamous cell carcinoma. Cancer 1981; 48:1207–1214.

Brownstein MH. Trichilemmal horn: cutaneous horn showing tricholemmal keratinization. Br J Dermatol 1979; 100:303–309.

Folpe AL, Reisenauer AK, Mentzel T, Rutten A, Solomon AR. Proliferating tricholemmal tumors: clinicopathologic evaluation is a guide to biologic behavior. J Cutan Pathol 2003; 30:492–498.

Haas N, Audring H, Sterry W. Carcinoma arising in a proliferating tricholemmal cyst expressing fetal and tricholemmal hair phenotype. Am J Dermatopathol 2002; 24:340–344.

Headington JT. Tumors of the hair follicle: a review. Am J Pathol 1976; 85:480–505.

Janitz J, Wiedersberg H. Trichilemmal pilar tumors. Cancer 1980; 45:1594–1597.

Leopard BJ, Sanderson KV. The natural history of trichilemmal cysts. Br J Dermatol 1976; 94:379–390.

McGavran MH, Binnington B. Keratinous cysts of the skin. Identification and differentiation of pilar cysts from epidermal cysts. Arch Dermatol 1966; 94:499–508.

Pinkus H. Sebaceous cysts are tricholemmal cysts. Arch Dermatol 1969; 99:544–555.

Sethi S, Singh UR. Proliferating tricholemmal cyst: report of two cases, one benign and the other malignant. J Dermatol 2002; 29:214–220.

Shet T, Rege J, Naik L. Cytodiagnosis of simple and proliferating tricholemmal cysts. Acta Cytol 2001; 45:582–588.

Weiss J, Heine M, Grimmel M, Jung EG. Malignant proliferating tricholemmal cyst. J Am Acad Dermatol 1995; 32:870–873.

Trichoepithelioma

INTRODUCTION   Trichoepithelioma is a benign adnexal tumor of hair follicle origin that may occur as a solitary lesion or as an inherited form with multiple lesions, each with a predilection for the face. They can occur at any age, but the mean age is 45 years. Solitary lesions tend to present in older patients. These lesions are nonaggressive and assymptomatic, but may cause significant cosmetic disfigurement. Multiple lesions may occur in an inherited, autosomal dominant pattern called *epithelioma adenoids cysticum of Brooke*. This syndrome begins in the second decade of life with the appearance of multiple lesions that tend to involve the face, particularly in the region of the nasolabial folds, lips, nose, and eyelids. The scalp, neck, and trunk may also be involved.

CLINICAL PRESENTATION   The solitary lesion presents as an asymptomatic, flesh-colored to yellowish, firm dome-shaped papule, 2 to 8 m in diameter. Telangiectatic vessels may be seen. In overall configuration it may mimic the appearance of a basal cell carcinoma. With time, these lesions may increase in size and number. Only rarely will they ulcerate.

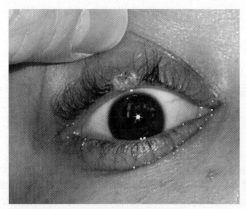
(Courtesy of Morris Hartstein, M.D.)

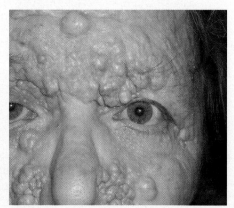
(Courtesy of Robert Dryden, M.D. and Brett Koltus, M.D.)

HISTOPATHOLOGY   Trichoepitheliomas are dermal tumors composed of islands of basaloid cells that may exhibit peripheral palisading. Trichoepitheliomas often have small keratinous cysts lined by stratified squamous epithelium. Epithelial structures resembling hair papillae or abortive hair follicles usually allow the trichoepithelioma to be differentiated from a basal cell carcinoma.

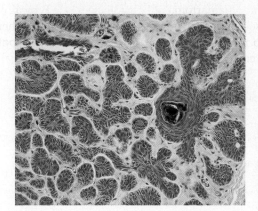

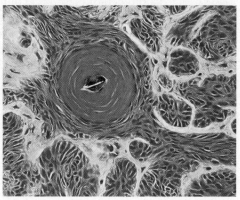

In some cases, immunostaining with antibodies to bcl-2 may be needed to distinguish a trichoepithelioma from a basal cell carcinoma: bcl-2 is predominantly peripheral in trichoepithelioma, while it is expressed diffusely in basal cell carcinoma.

DIFFERENTIAL DIAGNOSIS   Differential diagnosis includes basal cell carcinoma, syringoma, cylindroma, mila, trichilemmoma, and trichofolliculoma.

TREATMENT   Treatment includes surgical excision of solitary lesions, and dermabrasion, cryosurgery, or laser ablation for multiple lesions.

REFERENCES

Anderson DE, Howell JB. Epithelioma adenoids cysticum: genetic update. Br J Dermatol 1976; 95:225–232.

Aygum C, Blum JE. Trichoepithelioma 100 years later: a case report supporting the use of radiotherapy. Dermatology 1993; 187:209–212.

Gray HR, Helwig EB. Epithelioma adenoids cysticum and solitary trichoepithelioma. Arch Dermatol 1963; 87:102–114.

Hidayat AA, Font RL. Tricholemmoma of the eyelid and eyebrow. A clinicopathologic study of 31 cases. Arch Ophthalmol 1980; 98:844–847.

Jelinek JE. Aspects of heredity syndromic associations and course of conditions in which cutaneous lesions occur solitarily or multiplicity. J Am Acad Dermatol 1982; 7:526–540.

Simpson W, Garner A, Collin JR. Benign hair-follicle derived tumours in the differential diagnosis of basal-cell carcinoma of the eyelids: a clinicopathological comparison. Br J Ophthalmol 1989; 73:347–353.

Sternberg I, Buckman G, Levine MR, Sterin W. Trichoepithelioma. Ophthalmology 1986; 93:531–533.

Sugano DM, Lucci LM, Avila MP, et al. Eyelid trichoepithelioma—report of 2 cases. Arq Bras Oftalmol 2005; 68:136–139.

Wheelnad RG, Bailin PL, Kroanberg E. Carbon dioxide (CO2) laser vaporization for the treatment of multiple trichoepithelioma. J Dermatol Surg Oncol 1984; 10:470–475.

Trichofolliculoma

INTRODUCTION   Trichofolliculoma is an uncommon hamartoma of hair follicle tissue typically occurring on the face of adults. They are not associated with systemic disease or with other skin disorders. Trichofolliculomas are believed to represent abortive differentiation of pluripotent skin cells on their way to develop into hair follicles. They are associated with minimal clinical morbidity. There is no sexual or racial predilection.

CLINICAL PRESENTATION   Trichofolliculoma presents as a solitary, small, dome-shaped, flesh-colored papule or nodule with a diagnostic central keratin filled pore. Telangiectatic vessels may be apparent on the surface. If the lesion is actively trichogenic, tiny tufts or wisps of white cottony hairs may protrude from the central core. In the absence of such hairs, these lesions appear more like a nodular basal cell carcinoma or nevus.`

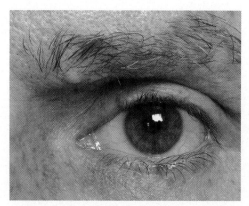

(Courtesy of Robert A. Goldberg, M.D.)

HISTOPATHOLOGY   Trichofolliculomas have a dilated hair follicle, containing keratinous debris and hair shaft fragments, from which radiate numerous small follicles that exhibit variable degrees of maturation (shown below). The follicles that radiate from the central follicle may branch further to give rise to secondary or tertiary follicles. The radiating follicles may contain hair shafts, rudimentary pilar structures, or there may be only cords of epithelial cells.

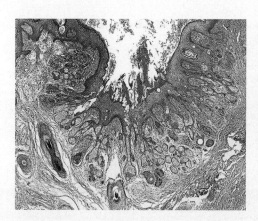
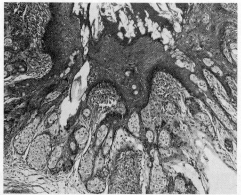

DIFFERENTIAL DIAGNOSIS   The differential diagnosis includes basal cell carcinoma, pilar cyst, epidermal inclusion cyst, nevus, and trichopithelioma.

TREATMENT   The lesion has no malignant potential and is cured by simple surgical excision. Recurrence is rare.

REFERENCES

Carreras B Jr, Lopez-Marin I Jr, Mellado VG, Gutierrez MT. Trichofolliculoma of the eyelid. Br J Ophthalmol 1981; 65:214–215.

Gray HR, Helwig EB. Trichofolliculoma. Arch Dermatol 1962; 86:619–625.

Morton AD, Nelson CC, Headington JT, Elner VM. Recurrent Trichofolliculoma of the upper eyelid margin. Ophthal Plast Reconstr Surg 1997; 13:287–288.

Pinkus H, Sutton R. Trichofolliculoma. Arch Dermatol 1965; 91:46–49.

Simpson W, Garner A, Collin JRO. Benign hair-follicle derived tumours in the differential diagnosis of basal cell carcinoma of the eyelids: a clinicopathologic comparison. Br J Ophthalmol 1989; 37:347–353.

Steffen C, Leaming DV. Trichofolliculoma of the upper eyelid. Cutis 1982; 30:343–345.

Taniguchi S, Hamada T. Trichofolliculoma of the eyelid. Eye 1996; 10:751–752.

INTRODUCTION   Varices of the eyelids are usually associated with orbital varices with an extension forward into the lid. A varix is an abnormal dilatation of one or more normal veins. They probably relate to an acquired or congenital weakness of the involved vein, or to an obstruction of the venous circulation, or both. Varices can result from compression by a tumor or an arterial aneurysm over an adjacent vein, an arteriovenous malformation, or any trauma or infection that involves the wall or lumen of the vein. Varices that result from infection or trauma may become thrombosed.

CLINICAL PRESENTATION   A palpebral varix is a well-circumscribed soft dark blue to brown lesion with no associated audible bruit or thrill. The lesion often enlarges with any activity that increases venous pressure such as bending over or a Valsalva maneuver (right photo). In some cases it can be associated with an organizing thrombus with hemosiderin and dystrophic calcification. When thrombus is present the lesion is firm and less compressible. Varices can rupture with minor trauma or vomiting resulting in hemorrhage and ecchymosis. If orbital extension is present, acute pain, proptosis and motility restriction may be associated with deep hemorrhage.

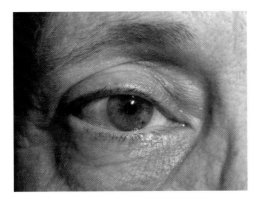 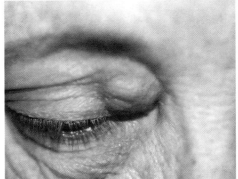

HISTOPATHOLOGY   An ectatic vein typifies a varix. The vessel wall may be fibrotic, and the lumen may be thrombosed or contain phleboliths resulting from calcification of old thrombus.

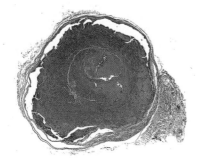 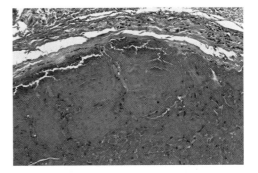

DIFFERENTIAL DIAGNOSIS   The differential diagnosis includes both capillary and cavernous hemangioma, dacryocele, arteriovenous malformation, and lymphangioma.

TREATMENT   In most cases the varix can safely be observed. Because most eyelid varices can have an orbital component, a CT scan is indicated especially if there are any orbital signs. When it is desired to treat it because of eyelid dysfunction or cosmesis surgical excision has been the best approach. Sclerotherapy performed with a 0.75% solution of sodium tetradecyl sulfate has also been successful in promoting resolution of ectatic periocular veins.

REFERENCES

Fante RG, Goldman MP. Removal of periocular veins by sclerotherapy. Ophthalmology 2001; 108:433–434.

Green D. Removal of periocular veins by sclerotherapy. Ophthalmology 2001; 108:442–448.

Morikawa M, Rothman MI, Numaguchi Y. Varix of the eyelid: a unique CT finding. AJR Am J Roentgenol 1994; 162:1505–1506.

Mudgil AV, Meyer DR, Dipillo MA. Varix of the angular vein manifesting as a medial canthal mass. Am J Ophthalmol 1993; 116:245–246.

Reifler DM, Leder D, Rexford T. Orbital hemorrhage and eyelid ecchymosis in acute orbital myositis. Am J Ophthalmol 1989; 107:111–113.

Rochels R. Varicosis of the angular vein—a rare differential diagnosis. Klin Monatsbl Augenheilkd 1984; 184:558–559.

Wright JE, Sullivan TJ, Garner A, Wulc AE, Moseley I. Orbital venous anomalies. Ophthalmology 1997; 104:905–913.

Xiao LH, Wang Y, Yang XJ, Zhu H, Quan Y. Bilateral orbital varicose vein complicated with right eyelid hemorrhage. A case report. Zhonghua Yan Ke Za Zhi 2004; 40:494.

Verruca Vulgaris

INTRODUCTION   Also known as a *viral wart*, or a *viral papilloma*, this lesion is a papilloma caused by an epidermal infection with the human papillomavirus, which is spread by direct contact and fomites. Immunocompromised patients are more susceptible to infection. Verruca vulgaris is more common in children and young adults between the ages of 5 and 20 years. They may occur anywhere on the skin, including the eyelids. Two common variants exist: *Verruca filiformis* or filiform warts (which include the subgroup known as digitate warts) and *verruca plana*, or flat warts.

CLINICAL PRESENTATION   These lesions begin as small tan or gray papules that slowly enlarge to become elevated papules with an irregular hyperkeratotic, papillomatous surface. The filiform variety is the most common variety on the face and eyelid, and is distinguished by columnar, hyperkeratotic projections. The digitate variety has several such spikes joined at the base. Lesions along the eyelid margin may induce a mild papillary conjunctivitis due to shedding of virus particles into the tear film. Patients also may develop a superficial punctate keratitis, and may have pannus formation. Primary conjunctival lesions may also occur.

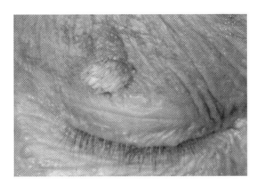

HISTOPATHOLOGY   Verruca vulgaris is characterized by marked hyperkeratosis and acanthosis. Papillomatosis is prominent in the filiform variant of verruca vulgaris. Parakeratosis, often arranged as vertical tiers, overlies the papillomatous projections. The granular cell layer is usually prominent, and the cells contain coarse clumps of basophilic keratohyaline granules. Dilated capillary loops may be conspicuous in the core of the papillary projections.

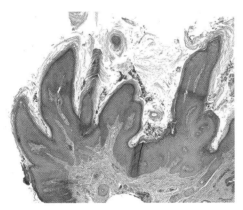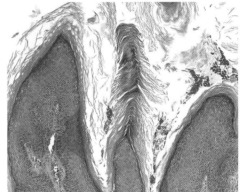

DIFFERENTIAL DIAGNOSIS   The differential diagnosis includes squamous papilloma, nevi, inverted follicular keratosis, cutaneous horns, and seborrheic keratoses.

TREATMENT   Observation is recommended if no ocular complications occur, as these are benign lesions. Treatment, if necessary, includes the use of cryotherapy, keratolytic agents, chemical cautery, electrodessication, local antimetabolite therapy, or complete surgical excision, as incomplete excision may cause multiple recurrences. Caution is advised to prevent spread of the virus that can occur when cutting across the stalk of pedunculated lesions, or leaving residual tumor behind.

Verruca Vulgaris (Contd.)

REFERENCES

Bock RH. Treatment of palpebral warts with cantharon. Am J Ophthalmol 1965; 60:529–530.

Friedman-Kien A. In: Demis D, ed. Clinical Dermatology, Vol. 3. Philadelphia: Harper & Row, 1984, Unit 14–14.

Gross G, Pfister H, Hagedorn M, Gissmann L. Correlation between human papilloma virus (HPV) type and histology of warts. J Invest Dermatol 1982; 78:160–164.

Lee S, Kim JG, Chun SI. Treatment of verruca plana with 5% 5-fluorouracil ointment. Dermatologica 1980; 160:383–389.

Noojin RO. Multiple ophthalmic verrucae. Arch Dermatol 1968; 97:176.

Tagami H, Takigawa M, Ogino A, Imamura S, Ofugi S. Spontaneous regression of plane warts after inflammation: clinical and histologic studies in 25 cases. Arch Dermatol 1977; 113:1209–1213.

Xanthelasma

INTRODUCTION   Xanthelasmas are common, plaque-like yellow lipid deposits occurring in middle-aged and older adults, particularly in women. The peak age of occurrence is in the fourth and fifth decades. Eyelid xanthelasmas are the most common cutaneous xanthomas. They occur more commonly near the inner canthus, and involve the upper lid more frequently than the lower lid. Although xanthelasmas often occur in patients with normal serum cholesterol levels, up to 50% of cases are associated with elevated plasma lipid levels or with congenital disorders of lipid metabolism.

CLINICAL PRESENTATION   Xanthelasmas appear as soft yellowish plaques that occur typically on the medial half of the upper and lower eyelids. Frequently all four lids will be involved. Although they usually do not affect eyelid function, large lesions can cause a mechanical ptosis. Infrequently, these lesions may be surmounted by small milia or epidermal inclusion cysts. Lesions tend to enlarge slowly and coalesce. They may extend into deeper tissues to involve the orbicularis muscle.

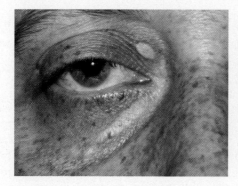 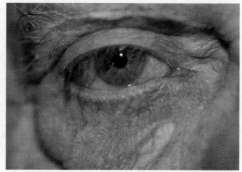

HISTOPATHOLOGY   Xanthelasmas have small aggregates of lipid-laden foam cells (macrophages) within the superficial dermis. Fibrosis is absent or only minimal. Other inflammatory cells are absent.

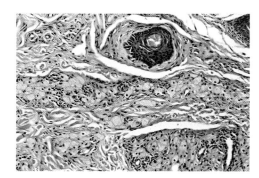 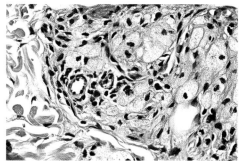

DIFFERENTIAL DIAGNOSIS   Differential diagnosis includes necrobiotic xanthogranuloma, juvenile xanthogranuloma, Erdheim-Chester disease, primary amyloidosis, sarcoidosis, lipoid proteinosis, and atypical lymphoid infiltrate.

TREATMENT   The presence of xanthelasma, particularly in young patients, justifies evaluation for serum lipid abnormalities and diabetes which can cause secondary hyperlipidemia. Treatment is indicated mainly for cosmetic concerns. Surgical excision is appropriate for most lesions and the incisions can usually be placed in crease lines appropriate for cosmetic blepharoplasty. For large lesions or in younger patients where there is not enough skin laxity to excise the lesion completely, CO_2 or argon laser ablation can be used. However, laser treatment can cause scarring and skin contraction resulting in ectropion. Chemical cauterization using 100% trichloracetic acid (TCA) will precipitate and coagulate proteins and dissolve lipids, and can be effective at treating larger lesions with minimal scarring. Cryotherapy can also be effective but may require repeat treatment and can cause scarring and hypopigmentation. Recurrences are common regardless of the method of treatment.

REFERENCES

Basar E, Oguz H, Ozdemir H, Ozkan S, Uslu H. Treatment of xanthelasma palbebrarum with argon laser photocoagulation. Argon laser and xanthelasma palpebrarum. Int Ophthalmol 2004; 25:9–11.

Bergman R. The pathogenesis and clinical significance of xanthelasma palpebrarum. J Am Acad Dermatol 1994; 30:236–242.

Haygood LJ, Bennett JD, Brodell RT. Treatment of xanthelasma palpebrarum with bichloroacetic acid. Dermatol Surg 1998; 24:1027–1031.

Pedace F, Winkelmann R. Xanthelasma palpebrum. JAMA 1965; 193:893–894.

Ribera M, Pinto X, Argimon JM, et al. Lipid metabolism and apolipoprtein E phenotypes in patients with xanthelasma. Am J Med 1995; 99:484–490.

Rohrich RJ, Janis JE, Pownell PH. Xanthelasma palpebrarum: a review and current management principles. Plast Reconstr Surg 2002; 110:1310–1314.

Tosti A, Varotti C, Tosti G, Giovannini A. Bilateral extensive xanthelasma palpebrarum. Cutis 1988; 41:113–114.

Ustunsoy E, Demir Z, Coskunfirat K, et al. Extensive bilateral eyelid ptosis caused by xanthelasma palpebrarum. Ann Plast Surg 1997; 38:177–178.

Vinger P, Sach B. Ocular manifestations of hyperlipidemia. Am J Ophthalmol 1970; 70:563–573.

Youn SJ, Park HS, Kim WS, Lee ES, Yang JM. Bilateral xanthelasma palpebrarum on both eyelids in a 9-year old boy. Pediatr Dermatol 2006; 23:95–97.

Xanthogranuloma

INTRODUCTION   Xanthogranulomas are lesions of lipid accumulation with foamy histiocytes. Different forms of xanthogranuloma are based on specific histologic findings and on clinical associations such as ocular lesions (juvenile xanthogranuloma), paraproteinemia and necrobiosis (necrobiotic xanthogranuloma), adult lesions with or without new onset asthma (adult onset xanthogranuloma), and visceral deposits with bone lesions (Erdheim-Chester Disease). They occur most commonly on the face, scalp, and upper trunk, and whites are affected more than blacks. These lesions can be associated with elevated serum lipid levels but usually lipids are normal.

CLINICAL PRESENTATION   Cutaneous lesions may be single or multiple, well-demarcated to diffuse, elevated, painless plaques that can occur unilaterally or bilaterally. They are yellowish in color with an orange peel-like surface. Lesions can be soft or more indurated and rubbery in consistency. Multiple lesions are more likely to have eye findings associated with juvenile xanthogranuloma. The eyelid lesions may extend into the anterior orbit by infiltration of muscles, lacrimal gland, and retrobulbar fat. With orbital involvement the patient may present with lid retraction, ptosis, chemosis, motility disturbance, proptosis, or an afferent papillary defect from extension along the optic nerve.

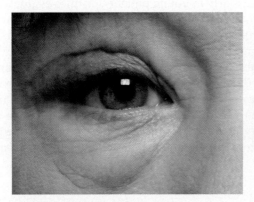
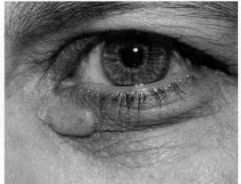

(Courtesy of Robert A. Goldberg, M.D.)

HISTOPATHOLOGY   Xanthogranulomas in adults may resemble juvenile xanthogranulomas histologically with lipid-laden macrophages (foam cells) and Touton giant cells along with interspersed lymphocytes and plasma cells.

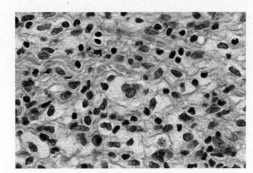
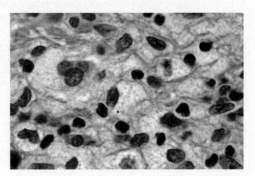

DIFFERENTIAL DIAGNOSIS   The differential diagnosis includes juvenile xanthogranuloma, low grade necrobiotic xanthogranuloma, Erdheim-Chester disease, xanthelasma, dermatofibroma, lipoid proteinosis, tuberous xanthoma, lipoma, fibrous histiocytoma, lymphoma, neurofibroma, and amyloidosis.

TREATMENT   While xanthogranulomas are benign they can be associated with significant morbidity and mortality when there is systemic involvement. Therefore all patients should have systemic evaluation to rule out Erdheim-Chester disease and necrobiotic xanthogranuloma. Surgical excision of the lesion will provide cosmetic improvement. Corticosteroid injections with triamcinolone acetonide have been effective and avoid the systemic complications of cytotoxic agents. Low dose periorbital radiotherapy is also an option. For resistant lesions cytotoxic agents may be required.

REFERENCES

DeStafano JJ, Carlson JA, Meyer DR. Solitary spindle-cell xanthogranuloma of the eyelid. Ophthalmology 2002; 109:258–261.

Elner VM, Mintz R, Demirci H, Hassan AS. Local corticosteroid treatment of eyelid and orbital xanthogranuloma. Ophthal Plast Reconstr Surg 2006; 22:36–40.

Hammond MD, Niemi EW, Ward TP, Eiseman AS. Adult orbital xanthogranuloma with associated adult-onset asthma. Ophthal Plast Reconstr Surg 2004; 20:329–332.

Jakobiec FA, Mills MD, Hidayat AA, et al. Periocular xanthogranulomas associated with severe adult-onset asthma. Trans Am Ophtalmol Soc 1993; 91:99–125.

Karcioglu ZA, Sharara N, Boles TL, Nasr AM. Orbital xanthogranuloma: clinical and morphological features in eight patients. Ophthal Plast Reconstr Surg 2003; 19:372–381.

Miszkiel KA, Sohaib SAA, Rose GE, Cree IA, Moseley IF. Radiological and clinical features of orbital xanthogranuloma. Br J Ophthalmol 2000; 84:251–258.

Pfenningsdorf S, Lieb WE. Papular xanthomas of the eyelids. Klin Monatsbl Augenheilkd 1997; 210:113–115.

Rose GE, Patel BC, Garner A, Wright JE. Orbital xanthogranuloma in adults. Br J Ophthalmol 1991; 75:680–684.

Shields JA, Karcioglu ZA, Shields CJ, Eagle RC Jr, Wong S. Orbital and eyelid involvement with Erdheim-Chester Disease. Arch Ophthalmol 1991; 109:850–854.

Index

Bold numbers refer to pages of primary discussion (i.e., where the subject appears under its own heading).

Impetigo, 165, **168–196,** 210
Incisional biopsy, **49**
Infundibular cyst, 152
Insect bite, 157–158, 162, **169–171**
Intradermal nevus, 32, 196–197, 206, 219, 226
Intravascular papillary endothelial hyperplasia, **171–172,** 173
Intravascular pyogenic granuloma, **173–174**
Inverted follicular keratosis, 28, 106, 140, **174–175,** 198, 208, 249, 259

Junctional nevus, 185, 196
Juvenile xanthogranuloma, **175–177,** 215, 261–263

Kaposi's sarcoma, 112, 125, 173, **177–179,** 195, 233, 238
Kearns-Sayre syndrome, 64
Keloid, 144, **179–180**
Keratinous cyst, 152, 203, 254
Keratoacanthoma, 28, 32, 121, 144, 175, **181–182,** 200, 206, 226, 236, 243, 249
Keratohyalin, **42**
Keratosis
    actinic, **105–107,** 121, 139–140, 184, 226, 228, 248–149
    inverted follicular, 106, 140, **174–175,** 198, 208, 249, 259
    seborrheic, 106, 139–140, 150, 174–175, 182, 184, 195, 197–198, 226, 144, **247–249**
    senile, 175
    solar, 140
Knobloch syndrome, 97
Koilocyte, **43**

Lagophthalmos, 14
Lamellar ichthyosis, 166–167
Langerhans' giant cell, **43**
Laxity of eyelid, 14
Lentigo, 32, 106
    maligna, 28, **183–185,** 194, 198
    malignant melanoma, 184
    senilis, 28, 183, **184–186**
Leser-Trélat sign, 247
Leukemia cutis, 32, **186–187**
Levator muscle function, 15
Lichen-type scale, **22**
Lichenification, **24**
Lichenoid inflammation, **43**
Lipoid proteinosis, 68, 108, 242, 261, 263
Lupus erythematosus, 126, **188–190,** 240, 242
Lymphangioma, 32, 117, 127, 129, 171, **190–191,** 235, 258
Lymphoma, 28, 178, **192–194,** 200, 209, 211–212, 233, 263

Macule, **20**
Madarosis, **86–87,** 245
Malignant melanoma, 28, 32, 103–104, 106, 121, 125, 131, 144, 183–184, **194–196,** 198, 200–201, 224, 238, 248
MALT lymphoma, 192
Marcus Gunn Jaw winking syndrome, 60, **87–88**

Meibomian glands, 34, 122–124, 133–135, 239, 244–246
Meige's syndrome, 78
Melanocytic nevus, 28, 131, 144, **196–198,** 248
Melanoma
    acral lentiginous, 194
    lentigo malignant, **183–185,** 194, 198
    malignant, 103–104, 106, 121, 125, 131, 144, 183–184, **194–196,** 198, 200–201, 224, 238, 248
    nodular, 194–195
    superficial spreading, 194
Melanoma-in-situ, 103
Melanophage, **44**
Melanosis, 32, 103–105, 183–184, 223
    oculi, 225
    precancerous, 85
    primary acquired (PAM), 105–106, 185
Merkel cell tumor, 32, **199–100**
Metastatic tumors, 28, 140, 142, 158, 178, **200–202,** 208
Microblepharon, **89**
Microcystic adnexal carcinoma, **202–204,** 151
Milia, 32, 148, 153, **204–205,** 213, 251, 253, 260
Mitomycin C, 105
Mixed tumor of skin, 135
Modifications of eyelid lesions, **22–24**
Mohs microsurgery, **50,** 121–122, 182, 184, 195, 200, 203–204, 208–209, 236, 246, 249
Moll's glands, 32, 113–114, 133
Molluscum contagiosum, 32, 176, 182, **205–207,** 242
Morphology of eyelid lesions, **24–27**
Mucoepidermoid carcinoma, **207–209**
Mucormycosis, 133, 154, **209–211,** 217
Muir-Torre syndrome, 181–182, 243–244
Multiple myeloma, 107, 214, 232–233
Myasthenia gravis, 60
Mycosis fungoides, **211–212,** 215
Myxoma, 32, **213–214**

Necrobiosis, **44**
Necrobiotic xanthogranuloma, **214–216,** 262–263
Necrotizing fasciitis, 153–154, 169, 172, **216–218**
Nerves of the eyelids, **108**
Neurofibroma, 28, 33, 117, 136, 142, 145, 153, 191, 198, 214, **218–220,** 223, 263
    plexiform, 117, 191, **234–235**
Neurofibromatosis, 142, 218–219, 234
Nevocellular nevus, 195–196
Nevoid basal cell carcinoma syndrome, 120, 142
Nevus flammeus, 127, **220–221**
Nevus fuscocaeruleus ophthamomaxillaris, 223
Nevus of ota, 104, 221, 223; *See also* Oculodermal melanocytosis
Nevus
    blue, **124–126,** 144, 224
    cellular blue, 124, 125, **130–131**
    compound, 196–198
    intradermal, 32, 196–197, 206, 219, 226
    junctional, 185, 196
    melanocytic, 131, 144, **196–198,** 248
    nevocellular, 195–196
    strawberry, 126
Nodular fasciitis, **222–223**
Nodular hidradenoma, 114, **149–150**
Nodular melanoma, 194–195